New Techniques, Materials and Technologies in Dentistry: Second Edition

New Techniques, Materials and Technologies in Dentistry: Second Edition

Guest Editors

José João Mendes
Ricardo Castro Alves
Ana Cristina Mano Azul

MDPI

Basel • Beijing • Wuhan • Barcelona • Belgrade • Novi Sad • Cluj • Manchester

Guest Editors
José João Mendes
Clinical Research Unit (CRU),
CiiEM
Egas Moniz School of Health
and Science
Almada
Portugal

Ricardo Castro Alves
Clinical Research Unit (CRU),
CiiEM
Egas Moniz School of Health
and Science
Almada
Portugal

Ana Cristina Mano Azul
Clinical Research Unit (CRU),
CiiEM
Egas Moniz School of Health
and Science
Almada
Portugal

Editorial Office
MDPI AG
Grosspeteranlage 5
4052 Basel, Switzerland

This is a reprint of the Special Issue, published open access by the journal *Applied Sciences* (ISSN 2076-3417), freely accessible at: https://www.mdpi.com/journal/applsci/special_issues/X7PBB4N309.

For citation purposes, cite each article independently as indicated on the article page online and as indicated below:

Lastname, A.A.; Lastname, B.B. Article Title. *Journal Name* **Year**, *Volume Number*, Page Range.

ISBN 978-3-7258-7436-1 (Hbk)
ISBN 978-3-7258-7437-8 (PDF)
https://doi.org/10.3390/books978-3-7258-7437-8

Contents

About the Editors vii

Ricardo Alves, Ana Azul and José João Mendes
Special Issue on New Techniques, Materials and Technologies in Dentistry—Second Edition
Reprinted from: *Appl. Sci.* **2026**, *16*, 2308, https://doi.org/10.3390/app16052308 1

Rita Noites, Inês Tavares, Miguel Cardoso, Isabel M. Carreira, Maria Bartolomeu, Ana S. Duarte and Ilda P. Ribeiro
Human Gingival Fibroblasts Response to Different Endodontic Sealers: An In Vitro Study
Reprinted from: *Appl. Sci.* **2023**, *13*, 10976, https://doi.org/10.3390/app131910976 5

Zoran Urošević, Violeta Petrović, Ivana Milanović, Vojislav Komlenić, Tatjana Savić-Stanković and Jugoslav Ilić
Push-Out Bond Strength of Three Bioceramic Sealers to Root Canal Dentin After Different Irrigation Protocols
Reprinted from: *Appl. Sci.* **2025**, *15*, 9259, https://doi.org/10.3390/app15179359 16

Diana Marian, Ramona Amina Popovici, Iustin Olariu, Dana Emanuela Pitic (Cot), Maria-Monica Marta and Ioana Veja (Ilyes)
Patterns and Practices in the Use of Endodontic Materials: Insights from Romanian Dental Practices
Reprinted from: *Appl. Sci.* **2025**, *15*, 1272, https://doi.org/10.3390/app15031272 29

Ana Bettencourt, Catarina Jorge, Vitor Anes and Cristina Bettencourt Neves
Effect of the Incorporation of Compounds into Digitally Manufactured Dental Materials—A Systematic Review
Reprinted from: *Appl. Sci.* **2024**, *14*, 2931, https://doi.org/10.3390/app14072931 45

Angel Lobito, Catarina Colaço, Joana Costa, Jorge Caldeira, Luís Proença and José João Mendes
In Vitro Evaluation of Surface Roughness and Color Variation after Two Brushing Protocols with Toothpastes Containing Different Whitening Technologies
Reprinted from: *Appl. Sci.* **2024**, *14*, 4053, https://doi.org/10.3390/app14104053 64

Cigdem Cebi Tuysuz, Necla Demir and Emir Yuzbasioglu
Does Repolishing Affect the Gloss and Roughness of Lithium Disilicate and Monolithic Zirconia Ceramics?
Reprinted from: *Appl. Sci.* **2025**, *15*, 4622, https://doi.org/10.3390/app15094622 75

Isadora Martini Garcia, Andressa Simionato, Virgínia Serra Souza, Jackson Damiani Scholten, Mary Anne Sampaio Melo and Fabrício Mezzomo Collares
Tuning BMI.NTf$_2$ Ionic Liquid Concentration in Dental Adhesives Towards a Rational Design of Antibacterial Materials
Reprinted from: *Appl. Sci.* **2025**, *15*, 3810, https://doi.org/10.3390/app15073810 97

Celso Massahiro Ogawa, Everton Flaiban, Ana Lúcia Franco Ricardo, Diana Lorena Garcia Lopes, Lays Assolini Pinheiro de Oliveira, Bruna Maciel de Almeida, et al.
Comparative Evaluation of Temporomandibular Condylar Changes Using Texture Analysis of CT and MRI Images
Reprinted from: *Appl. Sci.* **2024**, *14*, 7020, https://doi.org/10.3390/app14167020 106

Hela Allani, Ana Teresa Santos and Honorato Ribeiro-Vidal
Multidisciplinary Applications of AI in Dentistry: Bibliometric Review
Reprinted from: *Appl. Sci.* **2024**, *14*, 7624, https://doi.org/10.3390/app14177624 . . . . **117**

Cesar Augusto Signori Arruda, Filipa Passos Sousa and Ricardo Castro Alves
Modified Lip Repositioning Surgery in the Treatment of Gummy Smile
Reprinted from: *Appl. Sci.* **2024**, *14*, 5580, https://doi.org/10.3390/app14135580 . . . . **130**

Tomomi Yamada, Kazunori Nozaki, Makoto Tsubokura, Mikako Hayashi and Chung-Gang Li
Toward Quieter Dental Devices: Transient CFD Simulation of Airflow and Noise in Air Turbine Handpieces
Reprinted from: *Appl. Sci.* **2025**, *15*, 8187, https://doi.org/10.3390/app15158187 . . . . **145**

About the Editors

José João Mendes

José João Mendes (Prof. Dr.) has served as President of the Egas Moniz School of Health and Science since 2017, and is the elected President of the Egas Moniz Center for Interdisciplinary Research. He completed a DDS at the Egas Moniz School of Health and Science in Portugal in 1995, completed his postgraduate studies in Implantology at the Universitat Bern (Switzerland,1997), obtained an MBA in Health Unit Management from Universidade Católica Portuguesa (2002) and received his PhD in Biomedical Sciences from the ICBAS School of Medicine and Biomedical Sciences (2010). He is Section Editor of the *European Journal of Dentistry* and Associate Editor of *Frontiers in Oral Medicine*. Furthermore, he served as Assistant Professor of Conservative Dentistry (MSc in Dentistry of the ISCSEM/IUEM) in 1996, Assistant Professor of Physiology in 1999 (MSc in Dentistry of the ISCSEM/IUEM)—and has been Head of the same Curricular Unit since 2020—Head of the Integrated Dental Clinic Curricular Unit (MSc in Dentistry of the ISCSEM/IUEM) in 2008 and Head of the Curricular Unit on Management and Entrepreneurship in Dental Medicine in 2020. Since 2010, he has held the position of Clinical Director at the Egas Moniz Dental Clinic.

Ricardo Castro Alves

Ricardo Castro Alves graduated from the Egas Moniz School of Health and Science (Portugal) in 2003, obtained his MSc in Dentistry from Egas Moniz in 2010 and completed his PhD at Granada University (Spain) in 2016. He is a Specialist in Periodontology of the Portuguese Dental Association (OMD) and current vice-president and former secretary of the general assembly of the Portuguese Society of Periodontology.

Between 2007 and 2016, he was an Assistant Professor of Periodontology. Since 2018, he has been Head of the Periodontology Department at Egas Moniz. He is the coordinator of the postgraduate program in Periodontology at Egas Moniz, Head of the Clinical Research Unit of Centro de Investigação Interdisciplinar Egas Moniz and former Secretary and member of the Egas Moniz Ethics Committee. He is also a member of the continuing education center of the Portuguese Dental Association.

Ana Cristina Mano Azul

Ana Cristina Mano Azul completed her international education at Lycée Français Charles Lepierre (Lisbon). She graduated from the Faculty of Dental Medicine (Lisbon) and obtained a European PhD degree from the Universitat de València (Spain). Ana is an Associate Professor at the Egas Moniz School of Health and Science. Over the last 38 years, she has focused on teaching dental material and conservative dentistry as Head of the School's Conservative Dentistry units. She also serves as Coordinator of the Integrated MSc in Dentistry and the PG Diploma in International Clinical Endodontics. Ana is an integrated member of the Egas Moniz Center for Interdisciplinary Research, and her research focuses on materials science and aesthetic dentistry. She has served as President of the Fiscal Council of the Portuguese Dental Association and as a member of its General Council. She formerly served as President of the General Assembly of the Portuguese Society of Stomatology and Dental Medicine and is currently Vice-President of its Fiscal Council.

applied sciences

MDPI

Editorial

Special Issue on New Techniques, Materials and Technologies in Dentistry—Second Edition

Ricardo Alves *, Ana Azul and José João Mendes

Clinical Research Unit (CRU), CiiEM, Egas Moniz Cooperativa de Ensino Superior, 2829-511 Caparica, Portugal; aazul@egasmoniz.edu.pt (A.A.); jmendes@egasmoniz.edu.pt (J.J.M.)
* Correspondence: ralves@egasmoniz.edu.pt

1. Introduction

The continuous evolution of dentistry is closely linked to advances in materials science, digital technologies, and innovative clinical techniques [1,2]. Contemporary dental practice increasingly relies on interdisciplinary research that bridges engineering, biology, and clinical sciences, enabling more predictable, efficient, and patient-centered treatments. In parallel, the growing demand for minimally invasive procedures, enhanced esthetics, and long-term functional outcomes has accelerated the translation of laboratory-based innovations into daily clinical practice [3].

In recent decades, dentistry has undergone a profound transformation driven by the integration of digital workflows, advanced manufacturing processes, and data-driven technologies. Computer-aided design and manufacturing (CAD/CAM), additive manufacturing, and high-resolution imaging have redefined diagnostic accuracy, treatment planning, and restorative precision [1,2]. Simultaneously, the development of novel biomaterials—ranging from bioactive ceramics to multifunctional polymer-based systems—has expanded the therapeutic possibilities available to clinicians, fostering a shift from passive restorative approaches toward biologically interactive and preventive strategies [3].

Another defining feature of contemporary dental research is the increasing convergence between clinical dentistry and emerging technological fields such as artificial intelligence, computational modeling, and image analysis. These tools not only enhance diagnostic capabilities and treatment predictability, but also generate large volumes of data that require rigorous validation, ethical oversight, and clinical interpretation [4]. As a result, modern dentistry faces the dual challenge of embracing innovation while ensuring that new techniques and technologies are supported by robust scientific evidence and aligned with patient safety and clinical relevance.

In this context, the Second Edition of the Special Issue "New Techniques, Materials and Technologies in Dentistry" in *Applied Sciences* aims to further explore and consolidate recent scientific progress shaping modern oral healthcare. This Second Edition goes beyond a descriptive overview of technological advances, highlighting how recent innovations are reshaping clinical decision-making, material selection, interdisciplinary research paradigms, and educational models in contemporary dentistry. By bringing together fundamental research, applied clinical studies, and emerging digital methodologies, this Special Issue seeks to provide a comprehensive snapshot of current trends while identifying future directions for research and clinical practice.

2. New Techniques, Materials and Technologies in Dentistry

This Special Issue gathers original research articles and reviews addressing key challenges and opportunities across multiple dental disciplines. A strong emphasis is placed on dental materials and their biological, mechanical, and clinical performance. Several contributions focus on endodontic materials, evaluating both their biological response and clinical behavior. In vitro investigations into the cytocompatibility of endodontic sealers with human gingival fibroblasts highlight the importance of biocompatibility in material selection (Contribution 1), while studies on push-out bond strength and irrigation protocols provide clinically relevant insights into adhesion and sealing performance (Contribution 2). In parallel, surveys of clinical practice patterns offer valuable perspectives on the real-world use of endodontic materials (Contribution 3). Collectively, these contributions also expose persistent challenges, including the translational gap between in vitro findings and long-term clinical outcomes, as well as the need for standardized protocols and the robust clinical validation of emerging materials and technologies.

Another prominent theme of this Special Issue is the development and optimization of restorative and digital dental materials. Systematic analyses of digitally manufactured materials enriched with functional compounds underline current trends toward enhanced performance and bioactivity (Contribution 4). Experimental studies addressing the surface roughness, gloss, and color stability of ceramics and resin-based materials after brushing, repolishing, or whitening procedures contribute to a deeper understanding of material longevity and esthetics (Contributions 5, 6). Additionally, innovative approaches to the design of antibacterial dental adhesives, including the incorporation of ionic liquids, illustrate the growing focus on preventive and bioactive restorative solutions (Contribution 7).

The issue also reflects the expanding role of advanced technologies and digital methodologies in dentistry. Image-based diagnostic tools, including texture analysis applied to CT and MRI data, demonstrate the potential of quantitative imaging for the assessment of temporomandibular joint changes (Contribution 8). Furthermore, the integration of artificial intelligence into dental research and practice is addressed through bibliometric and multidisciplinary analyses, emphasizing AI's increasing impact on diagnostics, treatment planning, and decision support systems (Contribution 9). At the same time, these developments underline the importance of ethical frameworks, data quality, and clinical validation to ensure that artificial intelligence acts as a decision support tool rather than a substitute for clinical judgment.

Clinical innovation is further represented by contributions exploring novel therapeutic and surgical approaches, such as modified lip repositioning techniques for the management of gummy smile, reinforcing the importance of minimally invasive and esthetic-driven treatments (Contribution 10). From an engineering perspective, computational fluid dynamics simulations applied to dental handpieces highlight efforts to improve device performance and patient comfort by reducing operational noise (Contribution 11).

Collectively, the articles included in this Special Issue illustrate the dynamic and multifaceted nature of contemporary dental research. By combining fundamental material studies, applied clinical research, and emerging digital technologies, this collection aims to support evidence-based practice and stimulate further interdisciplinary collaboration. We hope that this Second Edition will serve as a valuable reference for researchers, clinicians, and industry professionals, and will inspire continued innovation in dentistry.

Beyond their clinical and technological relevance, the studies included in this Special Issue also have important implications for dental education. The growing complexity of materials, digital workflows, and data-driven tools reinforces the need for updated training models that integrate evidence-based practice, digital literacy, and critical appraisal skills in undergraduate and postgraduate curricula.

https://doi.org/10.3390/app16052308

3. Future Perspectives

Several important topics could not be addressed in this Special Issue, and others will require further research. Technical and technological developments in dentistry continue to progress at an extraordinary pace.

Although this Special Issue has now concluded, its success has encouraged us to launch a third edition of "New Techniques, Materials and Technologies in Dentistry." Submissions are currently open, and we warmly invite researchers to contribute and share their work.

Acknowledgments: This Special Issue was made possible through the collaboration of many talented authors. We would like to express our sincere appreciation to all reviewers for their valuable contributions in enhancing the quality of the submitted manuscripts. Lastly, we extend our thanks to the editorial team of *Applied Sciences*, with special appreciation to the Section Managing Editor of the MDPI Beijing Office.

Conflicts of Interest: The authors declare no conflicts of interest.

List of Contributions:

1. Noites, R.; Tavares, I.; Cardoso, M.; Carreira, I.; Bartolomeu, M.; Duarte, A.; Ribeiro, I. Human Gingival Fibroblasts Response to Different Endodontic Sealers: An In Vitro Study. *Appl. Sci.* **2023**, *13*, 10976. https://doi.org/10.3390/app131910976.
2. Urošević, Z.; Petrović, V.; Milanović, I.; Komlenić, V.; Savić-Stanković, T.; Ilić, J. Push-Out Bond Strength of Three Bioceramic Sealers to Root Canal Dentin After Different Irrigation Protocols. *Appl. Sci.* **2025**, *15*, 9359. https://doi.org/10.3390/app15179359.
3. Marian, D.; Popovici, R.; Olariu, I.; Pitic (Cot), D.; Marta, M.; Veja (Ilyes), I. Patterns and Practices in the Use of Endodontic Materials: Insights from Romanian Dental Practices. *Appl. Sci.* **2025**, *15*, 1272. https://doi.org/10.3390/app15031272.
4. Bettencourt, A.; Jorge, C.; Anes, V.; Neves, C. Effect of the Incorporation of Compounds into Digitally Manufactured Dental Materials—A Systematic Review. *Appl. Sci.* **2024**, *14*, 2931. https://doi.org/10.3390/app14072931.
5. Lobito, A.; Colaço, C.; Costa, J.; Caldeira, J.; Proença, L.; Mendes, J. In Vitro Evaluation of Surface Roughness and Color Variation after Two Brushing Protocols with Toothpastes Containing Different Whitening Technologies. *Appl. Sci.* **2024**, *14*, 4053. https://doi.org/10.3390/app14104053.
6. Cebi Tuysuz, C.; Demir, N.; Yuzbasioglu, E. Does Repolishing Affect the Gloss and Roughness of Lithium Disilicate and Monolithic Zirconia Ceramics? *Appl. Sci.* **2025**, *15*, 4622. https://doi.org/10.3390/app15094622.
7. Garcia, I.; Simionato, A.; Souza, V.; Scholten, J.; Melo, M.; Collares, F. Tuning BMI.NTf$_2$ Ionic Liquid Concentration in Dental Adhesives Towards a Rational Design of Antibacterial Materials. *Appl. Sci.* **2025**, *15*, 3810. https://doi.org/10.3390/app15073810.
8. Ogawa, C.; Flaiban, E.; Ricardo, A.; Lopes, D.; de Oliveira, L.; de Almeida, B.; de Oliveira Lira, A.; Orhan, K.; de Castro Lopes, S.; Costa, A. Comparative Evaluation of Temporomandibular Condylar Changes Using Texture Analysis of CT and MRI Images. *Appl. Sci.* **2024**, *14*, 7020. https://doi.org/10.3390/app14167020.
9. Allani, H.; Santos, A.; Ribeiro-Vidal, H. Multidisciplinary Applications of AI in Dentistry: Bibliometric Review. *Appl. Sci.* **2024**, *14*, 7624. https://doi.org/10.3390/app14177624.
10. Arruda, C.; Sousa, F.; Alves, R. Modified Lip Repositioning Surgery in the Treatment of Gummy Smile. *Appl. Sci.* **2024**, *14*, 5580. https://doi.org/10.3390/app14135580.
11. Yamada, T.; Nozaki, K.; Tsubokura, M.; Hayashi, M.; Li, C. Toward Quieter Dental Devices: Transient CFD Simulation of Airflow and Noise in Air Turbine Handpieces. *Appl. Sci.* **2025**, *15*, 8187. https://doi.org/10.3390/app15158187.

https://doi.org/10.3390/app16052308

References

1. Miyazaki, T.; Hotta, Y.; Kunii, J.; Kuriyama, S.; Tamaki, Y. A review of dental CAD/CAM: Current status and future perspectives. *Dent. Mater. J.* **2009**, *28*, 44–56. [CrossRef] [PubMed]
2. Van Noort, R. The future of dental devices is digital. *Dent. Mater.* **2012**, *28*, 3–12. [CrossRef] [PubMed]
3. Jandt, K.D.; Watts, D.C. Nanotechnology in dentistry: Present and future perspectives on dental nanomaterials. *Dent. Mater.* **2020**, *36*, 1365–1378. [CrossRef] [PubMed]
4. Schwendicke, F.; Samek, W.; Krois, J. Artificial intelligence in dentistry: Chances and challenges. *J. Dent. Res.* **2020**, *99*, 769–774. [CrossRef] [PubMed]

https://doi.org/10.3390/app16052308

applied sciences

MDPI

Article

Human Gingival Fibroblasts Response to Different Endodontic Sealers: An In Vitro Study

Rita Noites [1,*], Inês Tavares [2], Miguel Cardoso [1], Isabel M. Carreira [2,3,4,5], Maria Bartolomeu [1], Ana S. Duarte [1] and Ilda P. Ribeiro [2,3,4,5]

1 Center for Interdisciplinary Research in Health (CIIS), Faculty of Dental Medicine (FMD), Universidade Católica Portuguesa, 3504-505 Viseu, Portugal; mabcardoso@ucp.pt (M.C.); mbartolomeu@ucp.pt (M.B.); asduarte@ucp.pt (A.S.D.)
2 Cytogenetics and Genomics Laboratory, Institute of Cellular and Molecular Biology, Faculty of Medicine, University of Coimbra, 3000-548 Coimbra, Portugal; inesmouratavares@hotmail.com (I.T.); icarreira@fmed.uc.pt (I.M.C.); ptiribeiro@uc.pt (I.P.R.)
3 Faculty of Medicine, Coimbra Institute for Clinical and Biomedical Research (iCBR), Center of Investigation on Environment Genetics and Oncobiology (CIMAGO), University of Coimbra, 3000-548 Coimbra, Portugal
4 Center for Innovative Biomedicine and Biotechnology (CIBB), University of Coimbra, 3000-548 Coimbra, Portugal
5 Clinical Academic Center of Coimbra (CACC), 3004-531 Coimbra, Portugal
* Correspondence: rita.noites@ucp.pt

Abstract: Endodontic treatment aims to eliminate infection of the root canals and fill the dental pulp space. The biocompatibility studies of the sealers used in root canals obturation are crucial since they are applied in direct contact with periradicular tissues. **Objective:** The aim of this study was to evaluate the cytotoxicity of three root canal sealers—AH Plus, Bio MTA+, and Bio C sealer—on immortalized human gingival fibroblasts. **Methods:** AH Plus, Bio MTA+, and Bio C sealers were evaluated through incubation in real-time and material-conditioned media. Cells were incubated for 24 h and 72 h, at three different concentrations (1, 10, and 100 mg/mL) of each sealer. The cytotoxic activity of the sealers was assessed by Methyl tetrazolium (MTT) and Sulforhodamine B (SRB) assays. Cell morphology and cytogenetic alterations were studied microscopically. **Results:** MTT and SRB assays revealed similar results within both approaches. Cell culture exposed to sealers through incubation in real-time revealed a cytotoxic effect of AH Plus at 100 mg/mL. Material-conditioned media study revealed a cytotoxic effect of Bio MTA+ and Bio C, increasing with higher compound concentration and reaching 50% with 100 mg/mL. Regarding the cell's morphology, Bio C sealer revealed a decrease in cell confluence and several morphological changes. AH Plus and Bio MTA+ did not seem to affect the cell confluence however morphology alterations were observed. In the cytogenetic study, a severe decrease of the mitotic index and a large number of chromosomal aberrations were observed. The present study represents an advance in the understanding of the biocompatibility of AH Plus, Bio MTA+, and Bio C sealers. These sealers demonstrated some cytotoxicity, depending on the concentration used. Although more validation studies are still needed, this study brings very relevant results in terms of cytotoxicity, cell morphology, and cytogenetic alterations. **Conclusions:** These results could help in the selection of the most appropriate compounds to be used in clinical practice as well as to determine the maximum recommended amounts of each sealer. **Clinical Relevance:** This study highlights the potential cytotoxic effects of three commonly used root canal sealers on human gingival fibroblasts, with varying degrees of impact depending on the concentration used. The results emphasize the importance of careful consideration when selecting and applying these materials in clinical practice.

Keywords: endodontic sealers; AH Plus; Bio MTA+; Bio C sealer; cytotoxicity; cell morphology; cytogenetic alterations; biocompatibility; human gingival fibroblasts; HGF-1 cell line

1. Introduction

Endodontic treatment aims to prevent apical and coronal infiltration and microorganisms' proliferation by eliminating root canal infection and filling the dental pulp space [1–4]. Thus, the obturation of root canal systems is one of the most important steps of endodontic treatment [1]. Since endodontic sealers used to fill the root canals are applied in direct contact with the periapical tissues, such as the periodontal ligament, it is very important to evaluate the cellular effects of these materials [5,6]. In this context, minimal invasive endodontics enters as an approach to root canal treatment that emphasizes preserving the natural tooth structure as much as possible while effectively treating the infection or inflammation within the tooth. Thus, the removal of healthy tooth structure is minimized and consequently the long-term success of the treatment is enhanced while the patient discomfort is reduced [7]. The bioactivity, alongside with other properties of the sealers used in the endodontic treatment will imply the long-term success of the treatment.

There are several types of sealers, with different physical, chemical, and biological characteristics, which translate into different sealing abilities, adhesive properties, antimicrobial efficacy, radiodensity, and biocompatibility [8]. Sealers are categorized according to their main chemical constituents: zinc oxide eugenol, calcium hydroxide, glass ionomer, silicone, resin, and bioceramic-based sealers [9,10]. AH Plus (Dentsply DeTrey GmbH, Konstanz, Germany), an epoxy-resin-based sealer, is considered a gold standard due to its high bond strength to the dentin and physical properties, being one of the most used in clinical practice [6,11]. However, this endodontic sealer does not present bioactive properties [6]. Bio MTA+ (PPH CERKAMED Wojciech Pawłowski, Stalowa Wola, Poland), one of the most recent sealers, is a silico-calcium-based material that contributes to tissue regeneration after perforation of the canal wall. In vitro studies have shown that mineral trioxide aggregate (MTA), in general, has good biocompatibility, nonmutagenic sealing ability, and bioinductive properties [12]. Bio MTA+, a similar material to the conventional MTA, with decreased-sized grains and the insertion of nanoceramic particles and hydroxyapatite, provides higher penetration of calcium ions to the demineralized tissue, and increased sealing process [12,13].

Bio C sealer (Angelus Indústria de Produtos Odontológicos S/A, Londrina, PR, Brazil) is a novel bioceramic, nonresin sealer, composed of calcium silicates, calcium aluminate, calcium oxide, zirconium oxide, iron oxide and silicon oxide and its bioactivity is also related to the release of calcium ions that stimulates periapical healing [8,11]. This endodontic sealer has presented adequate flow and radiopacity, low volumetric change, and good biocompatibility, resulting in the allowance of the rapid regression of inflammatory reaction [6,14].

Our study aimed to compare the biocompatibility of Bio MTA+ and Bio C sealer with the most used sealer in clinical practice, AH Plus. Thus, a comprehensive evaluation of the biocompatibility of these three root canal sealers, AH Plus, Bio MTA+, and Bio C sealer, from cytotoxicity to genotoxicity, was performed on immortalized human gingival fibroblasts, at different concentrations and over 24 and 72 h, using two different methodologies. Cell viability and proliferation, as well as the cytotoxicity of compounds, may be assessed by the 3-(4,5-dimethylthiazol-2-yl) bromide-2,5-diphenyltetrazolium (MTT) assay [15], which measures the mitochondrial activity of cells, and the Sulforhodamine B (SRB) assay [16] that allows cell density determination, based on the quantification of cellular protein content. In this study, both methodologies were used as complementary methods.

2. Materials and Methods

2.1. Endodontic Sealers

Three endodontic sealers were used in this study, AH Plus (Dentsply DeTrey GmbH, Konstanz, Germany), Bio MTA+ (PPH CERKAMED Wojciech Pawłowski, Stalowa Wola, Poland), and Bio C sealer (Angelus Indústria de Produtos Odontológicos S/A, Londrina, PR, Brazil). The sealers were prepared according to the manufacturer's instructions and shaped with 1.5-mm-thick polyvinyl chloride molds with a diameter of 3 mm. To allow complete setting, the sealers were stored at 37 °C. After setting, the disks were removed from the molds, weighed, and sterilized (on both surfaces) by ultraviolet irradiation for 20 min.

2.2. Cell Culture

Immortalized human gingival fibroblast-1, HGF-1 (ATCC CRL-2014) obtained from the American Type Culture Collection (ATCC®, Manassas, VA, USA) were cultured in Ham's F-10 Nutrient Mix cell culture medium (Gibco, Life Technologies Corporation, New York, NY, USA) supplemented with 15% fetal bovine serum (FBS; Gibco, Life Technologies Corporation, New York, NY, USA), 1% L-Glutamine and 1% Penicillin-streptomycin (Gibco, Life Technologies Corporation, New York, NY, USA). Cells were incubated in a humidified atmosphere with 5% CO_2, at 37 °C.

2.3. Cells Exposure to Endodontic Sealers

HGF-1 cells were seeded in 24-well plates at 7.5×10^4 cells/well containing 1 mL of culture medium and allowed to attach overnight in a humidified atmosphere with 5% CO_2, at 37 °C. After attachment, the cells were exposed to 0, 1, 10, or 100 mg/mL of each sealer for 24 h and 72 h in a humidified atmosphere with 5% CO_2, at 37 °C. The sealers were placed over permeable cell culture inserts (VWR International), as previously described [17,18]. After 24 h or 72 h, the inserts were removed and transferred to a new plate and the experiment was carried out a second time with the same sealers. This experiment was repeated twice to guarantee four experiments for each assay.

2.4. Cell Exposure to Medium Conditioned with the Endodontic Sealers

Material-conditioned medium were prepared at 100 mg/mL of each sealer, as recommended by the American Society for Testing Material (ASTM, 1992). Cell culture medium was incubated with the sealers in a ratio of 100 mg of the material per mL of culture medium for 24 h at 4 °C. The sealers were removed before using the conditioned medium. The pH of the conditioned medium was evaluated before dilution. These conditioned medium was diluted in fresh culture medium, to obtain three final concentrations of the sealers extracts used to perform the cytotoxicity tests: undiluted, conditioned by 100 mg/mL; 1:10, corresponding to 10 mg/mL; 1:100, corresponding to 1 mg/mL.

2.5. Cytotoxic Effects of the Endodontic Sealers

Cytotoxicity of the three sealers was determined by MTT and SRB assays, according to ISO 10993-5 recommendations. For the MTT assay, the culture medium was removed, and cells were washed with Phosphate buffered saline (PBS). Afterwards, 200 µL of MTT solution was added to each well and the cells were incubated overnight at 37 °C. After incubation, 200 µL of isopropanol was added to each well to solubilize the formazan crystals resulting from the cleavage of MTT salt ring by viable cells. Aliquots (200 µL) of each well were transferred to a 96-well plate and the optical density of formazan dye was read at 570 nm and 620 nm using a multi-well plate reader (Synergy HT spectrophotometer; BioTek Instruments, Winooski, VT, USA). For the SRB assay, the culture medium was removed, cells were washed with PBS, and then allowed to dry. The cells were then fixed with 1% acetic acid in methanol for 1 h, at 4 °C. The fixation solution was removed, and the wells were allowed to dry. Two hundred µL of SRB was added and the plate was incubated for 1 h, at room temperature, protected from light. Then, the wells were washed with distilled water, several times, until the unbound dye was completely eliminated. Bounded SRB was solubilized with 200 µL of Tris base buffer and the spectrophotometric absorbance was read at 540 nm and 690 nm, using a multiwell plate reader (Synergy HT spectrophotometer; BioTek Instruments, Winooski, VT, USA).

2.6. Cell Morphology Evaluation

Cell morphology was analyzed before and after exposition to the three different sealers. Cells were cultured in 24-well plates with silicon wafers at 7.5×10^4 cell/well containing 1 mL of culture medium and allowed to attach overnight in a humidified atmosphere with 5% CO_2, at 37 °C. After attachment, cells were exposed to material-conditioned media at 100 mg/mL of each sealer for 24 h in a humidified atmosphere with 5% CO_2, at 37 °C. Cells incubated in normal culture medium were also analyzed as the control group. After 24 h of incubation, the silicon wafers were removed and washed with distilled water to remove medium residues and were placed on stubs with a carbon sticker. Observations were carried out using a variable-pressure Scanning Electron Microscope (FlexSEM 1000; Hitachi High-Tech Corporation, Hitachinaka, Japan).

2.7. Cytogenetic Studies

Cytogenetic analysis was performed using material-conditioned medium with AH Plus, as one of the most used sealers in the clinical practice. Cells were incubated for 24 h in material-conditioned medium with 10 mg/mL and 100 mg/mL of AH Plus. Cells incubated in normal culture medium were also studied as the control group. Metaphase chromosomes were prepared and analyzed by GTG-banding using standard protocols [19]. Metaphases were digitally imaged and karyotyped resorting to a microscope (Eclipse E400; Nikon, Tokyo, Japan) and CytoVision™ software version 3.93.2 (Applied Imaging System, San Jose, CA, USA).

2.8. Statistical Analysis

Statistical analysis was performed using the software GraphPad Prism software (GraphPad Software, San Diego, CA, USA). Normal distribution of quantitative variables was assessed using the Shapiro-Wilk test. Since not all the groups passed the normality test, data were analyzed using the Kruskal-Wallis test and Dunn's multiple comparisons test was used to compare the mean of each group with the mean of the control group. An alpha value of 0.05 was considered as the threshold for statistical significance.

3. Results

3.1. Cytotoxicity Evaluation of the Endodontic Sealers

3.1.1. Endodontic Sealers Exposure through Incubation in Real-Time

MTT assay revealed a cytotoxic effect of AH Plus, which determined a significant decrease in the metabolic activity to 29.85% and 8.39% after 24 h ($p < 0.001$; Figure 1A) and 72 h ($p < 0.0001$; Figure 1B), respectively, after exposure to 100 mg/mL. No cytotoxic effect was detected after exposure to Bio MTA+ and Bio C sealer for 24 h (Figure 1A) at the same final concentration of 100 mg/mL, while minor cytotoxicity was observed after exposure for 72 h, maintaining a metabolic activity of 76.35% and 83.09% (Figure 1B). The study of cell viability, by SRB assay, revealed similar results. Thus, a decrease in cell viability to 26.77% ($p < 0.001$; Figure 1C) and to 18.72% ($p < 0.0001$; Figure 1D) occurred when the cells were exposed to 100 mg/mL of AH Plus during 24 h and 72 h, respectively.

3.1.2. Endodontic Sealers Exposure through Conditioned Media

MTT assay, performed after exposure to material-conditioned media for 24 h, revealed a cytotoxic effect of Bio MTA+ and Bio C sealer with a growing decrease of metabolic activity with increasing compound concentration. After exposure to Bio MTA+ a decrease of metabolic activity to 50.79% after 24 h with 100 mg/mL ($p < 0.0001$; Figure 2) was observed. With Bio C sealer we verified a decrease in metabolic activity to 50.26% ($p < 0.0001$; Figure 2) after exposure to 100 mg/mL for 24 h. Interestingly, AH Plus did not seem to affect metabolic activity when exposure was through the material-conditioned medium. The pH of the Bio C sealer conditioned medium was significantly higher, pH 10, while AH Plus and the Bio MTA+ conditioned media did not vary significantly (pH 7.5).

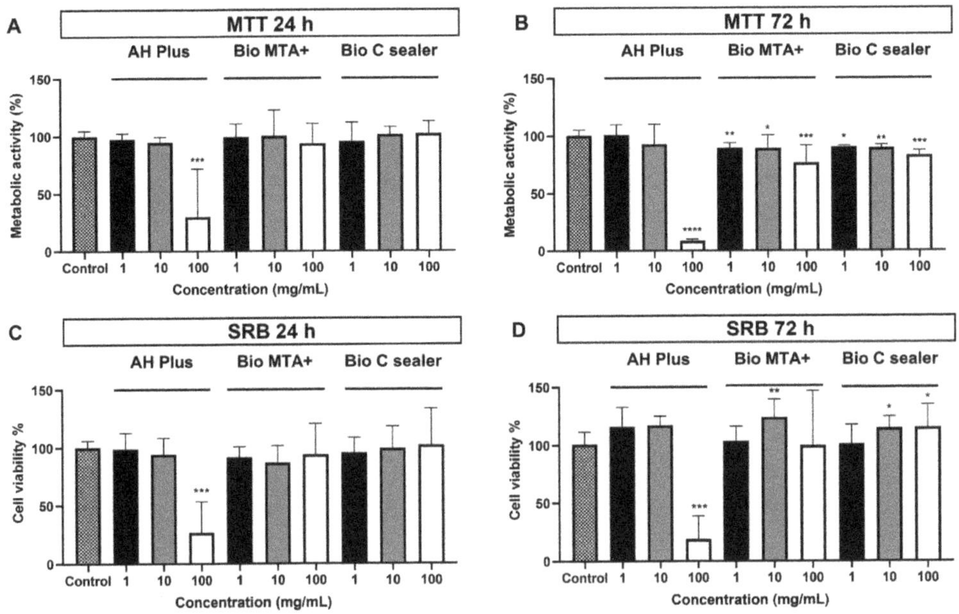

Figure 1. Cytotoxicity of AH Plus, Bio MTA+ and Bio C endodontic sealers to immortalized human gingival fibroblasts. Cells were exposed through incubation in real-time with three different concentrations (1 mg/mL, 10 mg/mL, and 100 mg/mL) using cell culture inserts. The results are presented as the average and standard error of four experiments. The asterisk indicates the cases where significant differences to the control group were observed: * $p < 0.05$; ** $p < 0.01$; *** $p < 0.001$; **** $p < 0.0001$. Legend: (**A**) Metabolic activity of the HGF-1 cells after 24 h of incubation with the sealers; (**B**) Metabolic activity of the HGF-1 cells after 72 h of incubation with the sealers; (**C**) Viability of the HGF-1 cells after 24 h of incubation with the sealers; (**D**) Viability of the HGF-1 cells after 72 h of incubation with the sealers.

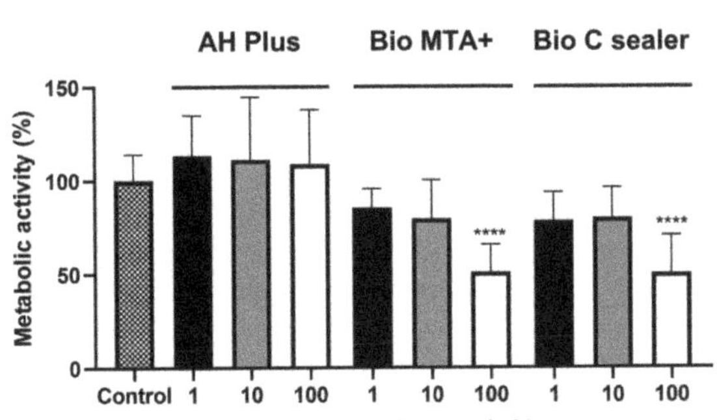

Figure 2. Cytotoxicity of AH Plus, Bio MTA+ and Bio C endodontic sealers to immortalized human gingival fibroblasts. Cells were exposed through material-conditioned media (1 mg/mL, 10 mg/mL, and 100 mg/mL). The results are presented as the average and standard error of three experiments. The asterisk indicates the cases where significant differences to the control group were observed: **** $p < 0.0001$.

3.2. Cell Morphology Evaluation

SEM evaluation revealed a normal morphology of control group cells, with a good confluence (Figure 3A), normal extensions, and an intact membrane (Figure 4A). With AH Plus, cell confluence was similar to the control group (Figure 3B), but the cells showed a more irregular morphology, with compromised membranes and loss of cell content (Figure 4B). Regarding the treatment with Bio MTA+, the silicon wafer was covered with fibroblasts, close to the control group (Figure 3C), but the morphology of the cells presented some alterations, namely rounded cells and compromised cell membrane with loss of cell content (Figure 4C). The Bio C sealer was the compound that showed a more drastic effect on cell morphology, with a decrease in cell confluence and several morphological changes, including rounded cell shape, loss of membrane integrity, and leakage of cellular content (Figures 3D and 4D).

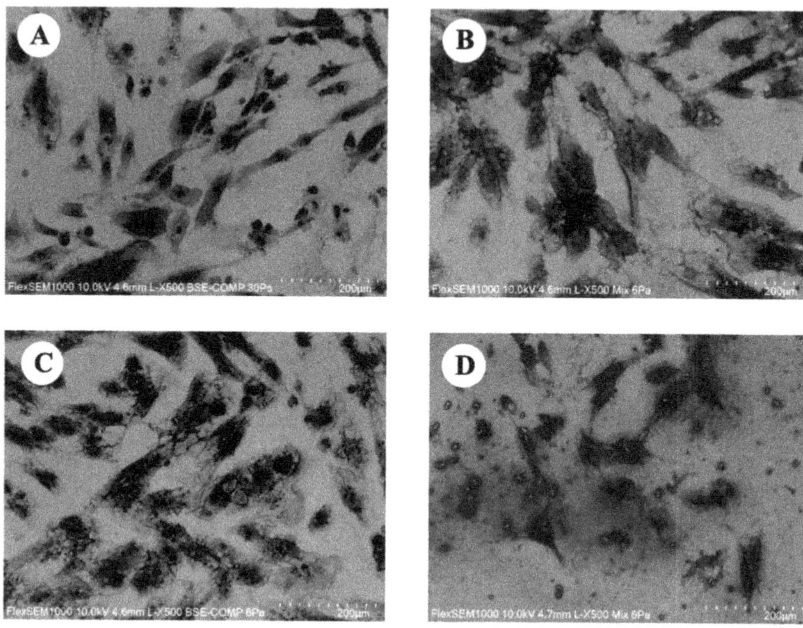

Figure 3. Morphology study after 24 h of HGF-1 fibroblasts incubation with material-conditioned media with 100 mg/mL of each sealer (500×). (**A**) Control group: cells organized in large number on the surface; (**B**) AH Plus group: the cells were distributed homogeneously on the glass substrate; (**C**) Bio MTA+ group: normal cell confluence was also observed; (**D**) Bio C group: presence of cell-free areas with a decrease in cell confluence.

3.3. Cytogenetic Studies

As a preliminary approach for the cytogenetic studies, we studied the effects of the most common sealer (AH Plus) used in routine dental consultations. The cytogenetic study was performed on the HGF-1 cells exposed to material-conditioned medium with AH Plus sealer and to a normal culture medium as the control group. Forty GTG metaphases of cells exposed to a normal culture medium and a total of 90 GTG metaphases, with both 10 mg/mL and 100 mg/mL of AH Plus concentration, were analyzed. Cells exposed exclusively to normal culture medium exhibited certain chromosomal abnormalities, with the majority of the cells remaining normal. However, after the incubation with AH Plus we observed a severe decrease in mitotic index and a five-fold increase in chromosomal aberrations, most structural associated with breakage, involving chromosomes 3, 4, 5, 6, 7, 8, 9, 11, 13, 14, 15, 16, 17, 19 and 22. Are examples of these chromosomal alterations several unbalanced translocations, marker chromosomes, and other complex rearrangements.

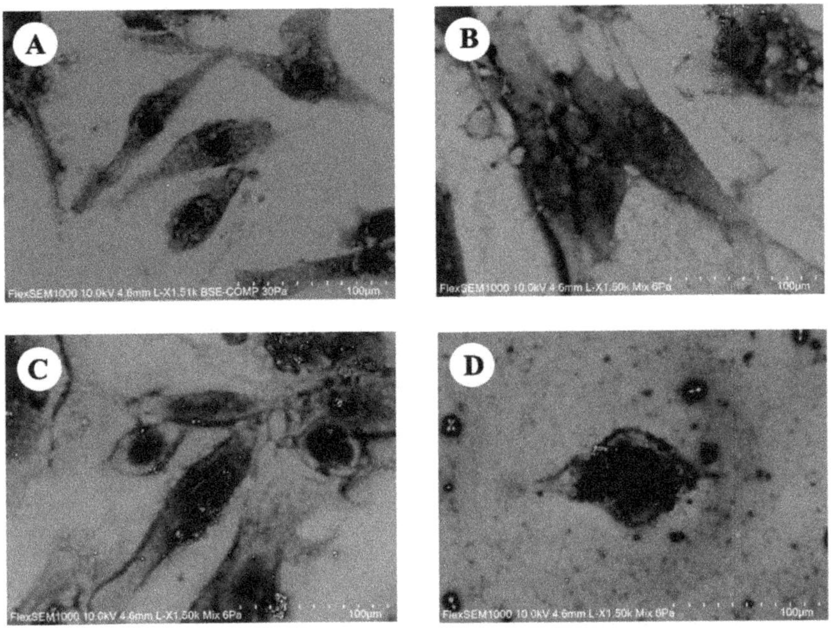

Figure 4. Morphology study after 24 h of HGF-1 fibroblasts incubation with each sealer with material-conditioned media with 100 mg/mL (500×). (**A**) Control group: cells with normal extensions and intact membranes; (**B**) AH Plus group: cells with irregular morphology, with compromised membranes and loss of cell content; (**C**) Bio MTA+ group: cells with some morphological alterations namely rounded cells and compromised cell membranes with loss of cell content; (**D**) Bio C group: several morphological changes including rounded cell shape, loss of membrane integrity and leakage of cellular content.

4. Discussion

Although endodontic sealers have a significant impact on endodontic treatment resolution, no extensive comparative studies have been made regarding the cytotoxicity and biocompatibility of the newly developed sealers [20]. The study of cytotoxicity and biocompatibility of the root canal sealers is crucial considering that they are applied in direct contact with periapical tissue [5,21]. Therefore, the selection of the best sealer to be used in clinical practice—particularly in a minimal invasive endodontic approach since the goal is to preserve more of the natural tooth structure—must be taken into account. The chemical and physical properties, as well as the sealing ability of endodontic sealers, should ensure the effective sealing of the remaining root canal space to prevent reinfections or further damages. Also, their biocompatibility determines the interaction with the surrounding tissues, by releasing antimicrobial substances and tissue regeneration molecules that promote the healing process [5,7,8,21].

In this context, a cell line of immortalized human gingival fibroblast (HGF-1) was considered as a cellular model since fibroblasts are predominant cells in connective tissue, being highly predominant in pediodontal and periimplant connective tissues, responsible for the maintenance and production of the extracellular matrix [22].

Several methods have been used to evaluate the toxicity of root canal sealers in vitro [3,4]. Two different methods were applied: incubation in real-time (using a cell culture system with inserts) and material-conditioned media. Thereby, we were able to evaluate both the effect of the sealers through incubation in real-time with the cells and the effect of the root canal sealers diffusing substances on the culture medium. Regarding the incubation in real-time exposure, both MTT and SRB assays revealed a cytotoxic effect of AH Plus at 100 mg/mL after 24 h (p-value < 0.001), making this effect even more pronounced after 72 h of incubation. No cytotoxic effects were detected by using Bio MTA+ and Bio C sealer for 24 h, while slight cytotoxicity was observed by testing these compounds for 72 h. Previous studies revealed similar results regarding AH Plus toxicity [3,11,23,24]. This cytotoxicity has been attributed to the release of formaldehyde from amines added to accelerate the polymerization of epoxy resin, as well as to the presence of bisphenol-A (BPA) in its composition that had been identified as a mutagenic component [11,25,26]. BPA, commercially used in the manufacture of epoxy resins, was identified as one of the first produced synthetic estrogens, and has endorsed the recent discussion about endocrine-disrupting chemicals regarding their presence and potential leakage from the products whose composition they integrate, as dental sealants. Although the data concerning the effective leakage of BPA from resin-based dental sealants has shown to be contradictory, this possibility must remain a concern [27].

Moreover, other studies also demonstrated that Bio C sealer, along with another bioceramic premixed root canal sealer, showed higher cell viability and biocompatibility than AH Plus [11,14], also attributed to the calcium ions, present in their composition, elution into the medium [11]. Also, it was previously suggested that calcium silicate-based sealers, such as Bio C sealer, have more pronounced biological properties than resin-based sealers, such as AH Plus [28]. Although some primary studies have been made to investigate the effect of the mineral trioxide aggregate (MTA) based bioceramic material revealing an expected high bioactivity and biocompatibility [29,30], as far as we know, no cytotoxicity studies have been performed until now using Bio MTA+.

On the other hand, AH Plus did not seem to cause any cytotoxic effect on cells when applied in the material-conditioned medium, while Bio MTA+ and Bio C sealers revealed growing cytotoxicity with increasing compound concentration, reaching a decrease in the metabolic activity of HGF-1 cells of 50% with 100 mg/mL. The material-conditioned medium with Bio C sealer revealed a significantly higher pH than the control medium. This indicates that Bio C sealer has a strong capacity to release hydroxyl ions and the alkaline pH is a possible cause of high cytotoxicity, which could explain the results shown by this material [31]. In addition, previous studies have shown that AH Plus has low solubility while Bio C sealer has high solubility [32]. This high solubility of Bio C sealer may suggest an increased solute degradation in the culture medium, possibly responsible for the cytotoxic effects demonstrated by Bio C sealer conditioned-medium tests. Despite the fact that, as mentioned above, some studies have revealed a cytotoxic effect of AH Plus, some other studies reported similar results to those that we obtained in the material-conditioned medium, where no cytotoxic effect of AH Plus was detected [1,5,33,34]. These discrepant results may be due to the lack of standardized methodologies. Thus, further studies are needed to clarify this effect of AH Plus.

In general, it has been reported that there is a possible association between the antimicrobial properties of the endodontic sealers and their cytotoxic effects, regarded as the lack of selective toxicity towards the microorganisms [35,36].

The antimicrobial properties of the endodontic sealers are an important aspect of the success of the endodontic treatment since an efficient antimicrobial behaviour from the sealers will reduce the residual amount of microorganisms left by the root canal's cleaning procedures. Regarding the sealers' antimicrobial behaviour, an increase in the pH of the environment may be translated into higher antimicrobial efficiency, namely against *Enterococcus faecalis*, the most prevalent bacteria in (re)infected root canals. [37]. The pH increase of the medium during the Bio C sealer incubation will most likely result in an efficient antimicrobial behaviour by this sealer. Previous studies have demonstrated good antimicrobial activity (against both Gram-positive and Gram-negative bacteria) by calcium silicate-based sealers also containing oxide compounds [38]. Additionally, Shin et al. have also demonstrated that the antimicrobial activity of the endodontic sealers is higher for the freshly mixed sealers, and tends to decrease after sealers setting [38].

Related to AH Plus, its antimicrobial activity was previously demonstrated [39], and more recently Mak et al. have shown that although this sealer has a strong antimicrobial activity when freshly prepared (from the formaldehyde released during the polymerization process), it decreases after time [40], which could be related with the low solubility of this sealer.

Although no antimicrobial studies have been made specifically using Bio MTA+ sealer, studies have been made using other Mineral Trioxide Aggregate (MTA) based sealers, demonstrating that the high amounts of oxide compounds, such as iron oxide, aluminum oxide, sodium oxide, and magnesium oxide, are capable of cell wall's damaging [38].

Beyond the study of cytotoxicity, we also performed the analysis of the cell morphology after incubation with the material-conditioned media. SEM analysis was in line with the results of the cytotoxicity study by material-conditioned media. With AH Plus a cellular confluence similar to the control group was observed, despite some minor changes in morphology. Similar results with the use of AH Plus have already been observed in a previous study [5]. Bio C sealer was the sealer that showed a more drastic effect on cells morphology with a decrease in cell confluence and several morphological changes. Unlike Bio C sealer, Bio MTA+ did not display a sudden decline in cell confluence, but many changes in cell morphology were observed.

The cytogenetic study was performed using the most common sealer used in dental treatments, AH Plus. The analysis of 40 GTG metaphases revealed that, although the majority of the cells were normal, some chromosomal aberrations were identified. The occurrence of these rearrangements could be due to the cultivation of these cells over different passages, which might induce some chromosomal changes. On the other hand, after the addition of AH Plus, several cytogenetic harvesting procedures were needed, and a larger number of metaphases had to be observed because of the severe decrease in mitotic index, and the high number of chromosomal aberrations. Most of the cytogenetic alterations were structural but some numerical changes were also observed. The study of a total of 90 GTG metaphases, with both the 10 mg/mL and the 100 mg/mL of AH Plus concentration, revealed several unbalanced translocations, aneuploidies, marker chromosomes, and other complex rearrangements. These results could be due to a directly induced chromosomal instability by the sealer but also due to the selection in the culture of cells with previous specific aberrations- However, some previous studies suggested that the epoxy resin in the AH Plus sealer has mutagenic behaviour, which can be translated in breaks in cellular DNA [41]. One of the most frequently observed chromosomal changes was the duplication of almost the whole long arm of chromosome 11 and the loss of the Y chromosome, which were always observed simultaneously, in a total of 31 metaphases (20 metaphases of 100 mg/mL and 11 metaphases of 10 mg/mL). This chromosomal alteration was also observed in metaphase cells exposed to the normal culture medium. Therefore, the high number of metaphases with this alteration after incubation with the compound is suggestive of a selection of the cells showing this specific alteration.

5. Conclusions

In conclusion, this study allowed us to verify that these root canal sealers exhibit some cytotoxicity, regarding cell viability, morphology of cells, and chromosomal stability, depending on the concentration used, and also contributes to the importance' confirmation of the endodontic sealers composition in the assurance of their biocompatibility towards the periapical cells/tissue. Although more studies are still needed, this work evaluates and compares these three sealers reaching important results that could help in the selection of the most appropriate compounds to be used in clinical practice and to determine the maximum recommended amounts of each sealer, as well as the importance of the sealers composition, and their antimicrobial behaviour. Our research into the biocompatibility of endodontic sealers, specifically Bio C sealer and Bio MTA+, has enhanced our comprehension of their impact on cells and provided valuable insights to guide and support future research. Ultimately, this knowledge aims to ensure the safe and effective application of these sealers in clinical practice.

Author Contributions: R.N., I.T., M.C., I.M.C., A.S.D. and I.P.R. participated in the conception and design of the study. All the authors participated in the acquisition, analysis, or interpretation of the data. All the authors participated in the writing of the manuscript. All authors have read and agreed to the published version of the manuscript.

Funding: The Center for Innovative Biomedicine and Biotechnology (CIBB) was funded by the Foundation for Science and Technology, I.P, (FCT, Portugal) through the Strategic Project UIDB/04539/2020 and UIDP/04539/2020. The Center for Interdisciplinary Research in Health (CIIS) was funded by FCT through the Strategic Project UIDB/04279/2020 and UIDP/04279/2020.

Institutional Review Board Statement: Not applicable.

Informed Consent Statement: Not applicable.

Data Availability Statement: The authors confirm that the data supporting the findings of this study are available within the article.

Acknowledgments: The authors thank to Foundation for Science and Technology (FCT, Portugal) for funding Center for Innovative Biomedicine and Biotechnology (CIBB) through the Strategic Project UIDB/04539/2020 and UIDP/04539/2020; and also for the financial support of Center for Interdisciplinary Research in Health (CIIS) under the project UIDB/04279/2020 and UIDP/04279/2020. Thanks are also due to FCT and UCP for the CEEC institutional financing of Ana Sofia Duarte (CEECINST/00137/2018/CP1520/CT0013). Maria Bartolomeu and thanks to the UCP for the Junior Researcher position project InDig (POCH-02-53I2-FSE-000025) supported by National Funds through Programa Operacional Capital Humano e Fundo Social Europeu (FSE).

Conflicts of Interest: The authors declare no conflict of interest.

References

1. Poggio, C.; Riva, P.; Chiesa, M.; Colombo, M.; Pietrocola, G. Comparative Cytotoxicity Evaluation of Eight Root Canal Sealers. *J. Clin. Exp. Dent.* **2017**, *9*, e574–e578. [CrossRef] [PubMed]
2. Badole, G.P.; Warhadpande, M.M.; Meshram, G.K.; Bahadure, R.N.; Tawani, S.G.; Tawani, G.; Badole, S.G. A Comparative Evaluation of Cytotoxicity of Root Canal Sealers: An in Vitro Study. *Restor. Dent. Endod.* **2013**, *38*, 204. [CrossRef] [PubMed]
3. Jung, S.; Libricht, V.; Sielker, S.; Hanisch, M.R.; Schäfer, E.; Dammaschke, T. Evaluation of the Biocompatibility of Root Canal Sealers on Human Periodontal Ligament Cells Ex Vivo. *Odontology* **2019**, *107*, 54–63. [CrossRef] [PubMed]
4. Jung, S.; Sielker, S.; Hanisch, M.R.; Libricht, V.; Schäfer, E.; Dammaschke, T. Cytotoxic Effects of Four Different Root Canal Sealers on Human Osteoblasts. *PLoS ONE* **2018**, *13*, e0194467. [CrossRef] [PubMed]
5. Teixeira, L.; Basso, F.G.; Hebling, J.; Costa, C.A.d.S.; Mori, G.G.; Silva-Sousa, Y.T.C.; Oliveira, C.F.d. Cytotoxicity Evaluation of Root Canal Sealers Using an In Vitro Experimental Model with Roots. *Braz. Dent. J.* **2017**, *28*, 165–171. [CrossRef]
6. Tolosa-Monfà, A.; Veroni, A.; Blasi-Cabús, J.; Ballester-Palacios, M.-L.; Berástegui-Jimeno, E. Cytotoxicity Comparison of Bio C Sealer against Multiple Root Canal Sealers. *J. Clin. Exp. Dent.* **2023**, *15*, e110.
7. Marvaniya, J.; Agarwal, K.; Mehta, D.N.; Parmar, N.; Shyamal, R.; Patel, J. Minimal Invasive Endodontics: A Comprehensive Narrative Review. *Cureus* **2022**, *14*, e25984. [CrossRef]
8. Kulkarni, D.; Bansal, A.; Mishra, N.; Chhabra, S.; Trivedi, S.; Kukreja, N.; Trivedi, A.; Gill, P. Evaluation of Sealing Ability of Three Root Canal Sealers: An In Vitro Study. *J. Contemp. Dent. Pract.* **2020**, *21*, 291–295. [CrossRef]
9. AL-Haddad, A.; Che Ab Aziz, Z.A. Bioceramic-Based Root Canal Sealers: A Review. *Int. J. Biomater.* **2016**, *2016*, 9753210. [CrossRef]
10. Lee, J.K.; Kwak, S.W.; Ha, J.-H.; Lee, W.; Kim, H.-C. Physicochemical Properties of Epoxy Resin-Based and Bioceramic-Based Root Canal Sealers. *Bioinorg. Chem. Appl.* **2017**, *2017*, 2582849. [CrossRef]
11. López-García, S.; Pecci-Lloret, M.R.; Guerrero-Gironés, J.; Pecci-Lloret, M.P.; Lozano, A.; Llena, C.; Rodríguez-Lozano, F.J.; Forner, L. Comparative Cytocompatibility and Mineralization Potential of Bio-C Sealer and TotalFill BC Sealer. *Materials* **2019**, *12*, 3087. [CrossRef] [PubMed]
12. Peskersoy, C.; Lukarcanin, J.; Turkun, M. Efficacy of Different Calcium Silicate Materials as Pulp-Capping Agents: Randomized Clinical Trial. *J. Dent. Sci.* **2021**, *16*, 723–731. [CrossRef] [PubMed]
13. Chalas, R.; Mielko, E.; Zubrzycka-Wrobel, J.; Nowak, J. A Chemical Activity Evaluation of Two Dental Calcium Silicate-Based Materials. *Curr. Issues Pharm. Med. Sci.* **2015**, *28*, 89–91. [CrossRef]
14. Alves Silva, E.C.; Tanomaru-Filho, M.; da Silva, G.F.; Delfino, M.M.; Cerri, P.S.; Guerreiro-Tanomaru, J.M. Biocompatibility and Bioactive Potential of New Calcium Silicate–Based Endodontic Sealers: Bio-C Sealer and Sealer Plus BC. *J. Endod.* **2020**, *46*, 1470–1477. [CrossRef] [PubMed]
15. Ghasemi, M.; Turnbull, T.; Sebastian, S.; Kempson, I. The MTT Assay: Utility, Limitations, Pitfalls, and Interpretation in Bulk and Single-Cell Analysis. *Int. J. Mol. Sci.* **2021**, *22*, 12827. [CrossRef]
16. Vichai, V.; Kirtikara, K. Sulforhodamine B Colorimetric Assay for Cytotoxicity Screening. *Nat. Protoc.* **2006**, *1*, 1112–1116. [CrossRef]

17. Moghaddame-Jafari, S.; Mantellini, M.; Botero, T.; McDonald, N.; Nor, J. Effect of ProRoot MTA on Pulp Cell Apoptosis and Proliferation In Vitro. *J. Endod.* **2005**, *31*, 387–391. [CrossRef] [PubMed]
18. Mantellini, M.G.; Botero, T.M.; Yaman, P.; Dennison, J.B.; Hanks, C.T.; Nör, J.E. Adhesive Resin Induces Apoptosis and Cell-Cycle Arrest of Pulp Cells. *J. Dent. Res.* **2003**, *82*, 592–596. [CrossRef]
19. Ribeiro, I.P.; Rodrigues, J.M.; Mascarenhas, A.; Marques, V.; Caramelo, F.; Julião, M.J.; Liehr, T.; Melo, J.B.; Carreira, I.M. (Cyto)Genomic and Epigenetic Characterization of BICR 10 Cell Line and Three New Established Primary Human Head and Neck Squamous Cell Carcinoma Cultures. *Genes. Genom.* **2019**, *41*, 1207–1221. [CrossRef]
20. Özdemir, O.; Kopac, T. Cytotoxicity and Biocompatibility of Root Canal Sealers: A Review on Recent Studies. *J. Appl. Biomater. Funct. Mater.* **2022**, *20*, 228080002210763. [CrossRef]
21. Geurtsen, W. Biocompatibility Of Root Canal Filling Materials. *Aust. Endod. J.* **2001**, *27*, 12–21. [CrossRef] [PubMed]
22. Coura, G.S.; Zortéa Jr, A.J.; Savi, L.A.; Simões, C.M.O.; Magini, R.S. Preliminar Protocol Of Human Gingival Fibroblast Culture. *RBP Rev. Bras. Implantol. Prótese Sobre Implant.* **2005**, *12*, 190–196.
23. Lee, B.-N.; Hong, J.-U.; Kim, S.-M.; Jang, J.-H.; Chang, H.-S.; Hwang, Y.-C.; Hwang, I.-N.; Oh, W.-M. Anti-Inflammatory and Osteogenic Effects of Calcium Silicate–Based Root Canal Sealers. *J. Endod.* **2019**, *45*, 73–78. [CrossRef]
24. Giacomino, C.M.; Wealleans, J.A.; Kuhn, N.; Diogenes, A. Comparative Biocompatibility and Osteogenic Potential of Two Bioceramic Sealers. *J. Endod.* **2019**, *45*, 51–56. [CrossRef] [PubMed]
25. Zhou, H.; Du, T.; Shen, Y.; Wang, Z.; Zheng, Y.; Haapasalo, M. In Vitro Cytotoxicity of Calcium Silicate–Containing Endodontic Sealers. *J. Endod.* **2015**, *41*, 56–61. [CrossRef] [PubMed]
26. Shah, N.; Logani, A.; Mishra, N.; Kaur, A. Biotoxicity of Commonly Used Root Canal Sealers: A Meta-Analysis. *J. Conserv. Dent.* **2015**, *18*, 83. [CrossRef] [PubMed]
27. Löfroth, M.; Ghasemimehr, M.; Falk, A.; Vult von Steyern, P. Bisphenol A in Dental Materials—Existence, Leakage and Biological Effects. *Heliyon* **2019**, *5*, e01711. [CrossRef]
28. Seo, D.-G.; Lee, D.; Kim, Y.-M.; Song, D.; Kim, S.-Y. Biocompatibility and Mineralization Activity of Three Calcium Silicate-Based Root Canal Sealers Compared to Conventional Resin-Based Sealer in Human Dental Pulp Stem Cells. *Materials* **2019**, *12*, 2482. [CrossRef]
29. Pelliccioni, G.; Vellani, C.; Gatto, M.; Gandolfi, M.; Marchetti, C.; Prati, C. Proroot Mineral Trioxide Aggregate Cement Used as a Retrograde Filling without Addition of Water: An In Vitro Evaluation of Its Microleakage. *J. Endod.* **2007**, *33*, 1082–1085. [CrossRef]
30. Benetti, F.; de Azevedo Queiroz, Í.O.; Oliveira, P.H.C.d.; Conti, L.C.; Azuma, M.M.; Oliveira, S.H.P.d.; Cintra, L.T.A. Cytotoxicity and Biocompatibility of a New Bioceramic Endodontic Sealer Containing Calcium Hydroxide. *Braz. Oral. Res.* **2019**, *33*, e042. [CrossRef]
31. Silva, E.J.N.L.; Rosa, T.P.; Herrera, D.R.; Jacinto, R.C.; Gomes, B.P.F.A.; Zaia, A.A. Evaluation of Cytotoxicity and Physicochemical Properties of Calcium Silicate-Based Endodontic Sealer MTA Fillapex. *J. Endod.* **2013**, *39*, 274–277. [CrossRef] [PubMed]
32. Zordan-Bronzel, C.L.; Esteves Torres, F.F.; Tanomaru-Filho, M.; Chávez-Andrade, G.M.; Bosso-Martelo, R.; Guerreiro-Tanomaru, J.M. Evaluation of Physicochemical Properties of a New Calcium Silicate–Based Sealer, Bio-C Sealer. *J. Endod.* **2019**, *45*, 1248–1252. [CrossRef] [PubMed]
33. Al-Hiyasat, A.S.; Tayyar, M.; Darmani, H. Cytotoxicity Evaluation of Various Resin Based Root Canal Sealers. *Int. Endod. J.* **2010**, *43*, 148–153. [CrossRef] [PubMed]
34. Karapınar-Kazandağ, M.; Bayrak, Ö.F.; Yalvaç, M.E.; Ersev, H.; Tanalp, J.; Şahin, F.; Bayırlı, G. Cytotoxicity of 5 Endodontic Sealers on L929 Cell Line and Human Dental Pulp Cells. *Int. Endod. J.* **2011**, *44*, 626–634. [CrossRef]
35. Zhang, H.; Shen, Y.; Ruse, N.D.; Haapasalo, M. Antibacterial Activity of Endodontic Sealers by Modified Direct Contact Test Against Enterococcus Faecalis. *J. Endod.* **2009**, *35*, 1051–1055. [CrossRef]
36. Siqueira, J.F., Jr.; Favieri, A.; Gahyva, S.M.; Moraes, S.R.; Lima, K.C.; Lopes, H.P. Antimicrobial Activity and Flow Rate of Newer and Established Root Canal Sealers. *J. Endod.* **2000**, *26*, 274–277. [CrossRef]
37. Alghamdi, F.; Shakir, M. The Influence of Enterococcus Faecalis as a Dental Root Canal Pathogen on Endodontic Treatment: A Systematic Review. *Cureus* **2020**, *12*, e7257. [CrossRef]
38. Shin, J.H.; Lee, D.Y.; Lee, S.H. Comparison of Antimicrobial Activity of Traditional and New Developed Root Sealers against Pathogens Related Root Canal. *J. Dent. Sci.* **2018**, *13*, 54–59. [CrossRef]
39. Huang, Y.; Li, X.; Mandal, P.; Wu, Y.; Liu, L.; Gui, H.; Liu, J. The in Vitro Antimicrobial Activities of Four Endodontic Sealers. *BMC Oral. Health* **2019**, *19*, 118. [CrossRef]
40. Mak, S.T.; Leong, X.F.; Tew, I.M.; Kumolosasi, E.; Wong, L. In Vitro Evaluation of the Antibacterial Activity of EndoSeal MTA, IRoot SP, and AH Plus against Planktonic Bacteria. *Materials* **2022**, *15*, 2012. [CrossRef]
41. Schweikl, H.; Schmalz, G.; Federlin, M. Mutagenicity of the Root Canal Sealer AHPlus in the Ames Test. *Clin. Oral. Investig.* **1998**, *2*, 125–129. [CrossRef] [PubMed]

applied sciences

MDPI

Article

Push-Out Bond Strength of Three Bioceramic Sealers to Root Canal Dentin After Different Irrigation Protocols

Zoran Urošević [1], Violeta Petrović [2], Ivana Milanović [2], Vojislav Komlenić [2], Tatjana Savić-Stanković [2] and Jugoslav Ilić [2,*]

[1] Clinic for Dental Medicine, Military Medical Academy, 11000 Belgrade, Serbia; urosevic82@gmail.com
[2] Department of Restorative Odontology and Endodontics, School of Dental Medicine University of Belgrade, 11000 Belgrade, Serbia; violeta.petrovic@stomf.bg.ac.rs (V.P.); ivana.milanovic@stomf.bg.ac.rs (I.M.); vojislav.komlenic@stomf.bg.ac.rs (V.K.); tanja.savic@stomf.bg.ac.rs (T.S.-S.)
* Correspondence: jugoslav.ilic@stomf.bg.ac.rs; Tel.: +381-112685288

Abstract

The adhesion of endodontic sealers to dentin may be influenced both by the chemical composition of the sealer and the final irrigation protocol. The aim of this study was to examine the push-out bond strength of three differently formulated bioceramic sealers to root canal dentin, after different irrigation protocols. Four cavities were prepared in dentine discs obtained from middle thirds of third molars with fused roots. Discs were randomly divided into three groups ($n = 8$). Group 1: specimens were immersed in 2.5% NaOCl; group 2: in 2.5% NaOCl followed by 17% EDTA; and group 3: in a solution of 2.5% NaOCl with 9% etidronic acid (HEDP). The cavities on each disk were filled with four tested sealers: AH Plus Bioceramic, Bio C Angelus, BioRoot RCS, and AH Plus ($n = 8$ per sealer). The push-out bond strength test was performed after 7 days. The data were statistically analyzed using two-way analysis of variance with the Bonferroni post hoc test ($\alpha = 0.05$). Irrigation with NaOCl resulted in significantly lower bond strength values of the sealers in comparison to NaOCl/EDTA and NaOCl/HEDP groups. In the NaOCl and NaOCl/HEDP groups, BioRoot RCS showed similar push-out bond strength compared to AH Plus and significantly higher compared to Bio-C and AH Plus Bioceramic. In the NaOCl/EDTA group, bioceramic sealers achieved a significantly weaker bond strength compared to AH Plus. The bond strength of BioRoot RCS was significantly higher compared to Bio-C and AH Plus Bioceramic. The irrigation protocols and the chemical composition of the sealers significantly influenced their bond strength to dentin. Epoxy resin-based sealer achieved the strongest bond strength, while within bioceramic sealers, the highest values were obtained for BioRoot RCS and the lowest for AH Plus Bioceramic.

Keywords: bioceramic sealers; irrigation protocols; push-out bond strength

1. Introduction

Three-dimensional hermetic root canal obturation is achieved using gutta-percha and root canal sealers [1]. Considering that gutta-percha lacks adhesive properties, sealers play a crucial role in creating a reliable bond between the root canal filling, dentin, and gutta-percha. This bonding helps prevent microleakage and bacterial infiltration while also stabilizing the filling during tooth function and operative procedures [2]. Due to its adhesiveness [3], dimensional stability, and insolubility in tissue fluids [4], AH Plus, an epoxy resin-based sealer, is considered the gold standard among endodontic sealers.

However, shortcomings such as cytotoxicity during setting [5], and a lack of bioactivity [6], have been reported.

Recently, scientific and professional attention has been focused on bioceramic, i.e., calcium silicate-based sealers, created by modifying bioactive calcium silicate cements such as MTA and similar materials. Unlike resin-based sealers, bioceramic sealers are hydraulic in nature and set in a moist environment through the hydration of hydrophilic tricalcium and dicalcium silicate particles [7]. During hydration, calcium hydroxide is released, responsible for the alkaline pH [8], antimicrobial properties [9], and bioactivity of the sealers, i.e., the formation of hydroxyapatite crystals, at the sealer-dentin interface, through the reaction of calcium from the released calcium hydroxide and phosphates from tissue fluids [10,11]. The adhesiveness of these sealers and the bond strength to the dentin of the root canal have been investigated but with inconsistent results, which are most likely associated with different methodological approaches [12,13]. Furthermore, in line with continuous improvements of these sealers, a number of new, predominantly single-syringe (one-component) formulations are currently available. Although introduced as bioceramic sealers, these new products may differ in composition, regarding the amount of calcium silicate particles, as well as the type of vehicles and additives used [14]. In relation to the aforementioned context, Bio-C Sealer (Angelus, Londrina, PR, Brazil) is a recently developed, single-syringe, pre-mixed endodontic sealer. In addition to calcium silicates, its formulation includes tricalcium aluminate and employs propylene glycol as a vehicle [14]. Previous research suggests the biocompatibility [5,15], bioactivity [16], and mineralization potential [15] of this sealer.

AH Plus Bioceramic (Dentsply Sirona, Ballaigues, Switzerland) is one of the latest premixed, single-component bioceramic sealers, predominantly consisting of a radiopacifier and vehicle (dimethyl sulfoxide). This sealer contains only 5–15% tricalcium silicates particles, which is significantly less compared to the first premixed formulations of bioceramic sealers [14]. However, recent studies have reported on the cytocompatibility [6,17,18] and bioactivity [6,17,19] of this sealer.

The data are scarce regarding how differences in the amount of calcium silicate particles, as well as different vehicles and additives in the sealer's composition, affect the push-out bond strength of the new commercially available products.

On the other hand, the specific hydraulic nature and chemical composition of the bioceramic sealers have raised the question about appropriate final irrigation prior to obturation. Namely, it was reported that EDTA, traditionally used to remove the smear layer, negatively affected the push-out bond strength of the BioRoot RCS [20]. Therefore, alternative chelating agents and irrigation protocols have been proposed. It has been suggested that etidronic acid (1 hydroxyethylidene-1, 1-bisphosphonate) used in a protocol of a continuous chelation (mixed with NaOCl) is effective at smear layer removal [21,22]. Also, previous studies reported the positive effect of continuous chelation on the push-out bond strength of some commercially available bioceramic sealers [23]. However, the push-out bond strength of the newly-synthesized bioceramic sealers after different irrigation protocols has not been thoroughly investigated yet.

In line with what was mentioned above, the objective of this study was to examine the push-out bond strength of three bioceramic sealers of different compositions and formulations, to root canal dentin following different irrigation protocols, and compare the obtained values with the bond strength of the control epoxy resin-based sealer.

Null hypotheses were (i) the different irrigation protocols do not affect the bond strength of sealers; and (ii) there is no difference in the bond strength to dentinal walls among the tested sealers.

2. Materials and Methods

2.1. Materials

The study was approved by the Ethics Committee of the School of Dental Medicine University of Belgrade (36/3, 2025). Four sealers were selected for examination in this study. Sealers composition, formulations, and manufacturers are listed in Table 1.

Table 1. Manufacturers, formulation, and composition of the sealers used in the study.

Sealer Brand Name and Manufacturer	Formulation	Composition
AH Plus Bioceramic Dentsply Sirona, Ballaigues, Switzerland	Premixed One-component	Tricalcium silicate (5–15%), zirconium dioxide (50–70%), dimethyl sulfoxide (10–30%), lithium carbonate (<0.5%), and thickening agents (<6%)
Bio C Angelus, Londrina, PR Brazil	Premixed One-component	Calcium silicates, tricalcium aluminate, calcium oxide, zirconium oxide, iron oxide, silicon dioxide, and dispersing agents (propylene glycol)
BioRoot RCS Septodont, Saint-Maur-des-Fossés, France	Powder/liquid Two-component	Powder: tricalcium silicate, zirconium oxide (20–50%), calcium carbonate 25–50%, and povidone Liquid: aqueous solution of calcium chloride with polycarboxylate
AH Plus Dentsply De Trey GmbH, Konstanz, Germany	Paste–paste Two-component	Paste A: bisphenol-A epoxy resin, bisphenol-F epoxy resin, calcium tungstate, zirconium oxide, silica, and iron oxide pigments Paste B: dibenzyl-diamine, aminoadamantane, tricyclodecane-diamine, calcium tungstate, zirconium oxide, silica, and silicone oil

2.2. Preparation of Specimens

Intact third molars with fused roots, extracted for orthodontic reasons, were used in the study. After cleaning and disinfection, the teeth were molded in self-bonding acrylate (Duracryl plus, Spofa dental, KavoKerr corporation, Brea, CA, USA). Subsequently, teeth were cut perpendicular to the longitudinal axis of the tooth in the area of the middle third of the root, using a 0.7 mm diameter diamond saw, under water cooling (Isomet Saw; Buehler, Lake Bluff, IL, USA). In this way, two transverse discs with a thickness of 1 ± 0.1 mm were obtained from each tooth (Figure 1), making 24 discs in total. On each disc, four cavities (diameter of 1.2 mm) were prepared using a fissured cylindrical carbide bur (Densply Maillefer, Ballaigues, Switzerland) mounted in a specially designed table drill. The cavities were prepared in the paracanal dentin so that they were at least 1 mm away from the root canal, root cementum, and adjacent cavity [24].

Dentin discs were then randomly divided into three groups ($n = 8$) based on the irrigation protocol: Group 1: 2.5% NaOCl (i-dental, Lithuania), Group 2: sequential chelation with 2.5% NaOCl and 17% EDTA (MD-Cleanser, Meta Biomed Europe GmbH, Germany), and Group 3: continuous chelation with a mixture of 2.5% NaOCl and 9% etidronic acid (Dual Rinse HEDP; Medcem GmbH, Vienna, Austria). The irrigation protocols involved successive immersion of the discs in the respective irrigants [23], as illustrated in Figure 2.

The discs were then slightly dried with paper towels, coated with paraffin foil to prevent leaking out of the sealers, and attached to glass slides with self-adhesive tape.

Each of the four cavities prepared on every disc was filled with one of the four tested sealers, with eight samples allocated to each sealer group ($n = 8$). Two-component BioRoot RCS was prepared according to the manufacturer's instructions, while one-component, premixed bioceramic sealers (Bio-C and AH Plus Bioceramic) were used directly from the syringe. Control, epoxy resin-based sealer (AH Plus) was prepared according to the manufacturer's instructions. The sealers were delivered into the cavities with a probe, with constant vibration, after which the excess sealer was removed with a plastic instrument. Glass slides with samples were wrapped in gauze soaked in artificial tissue fluid (Hank's balanced saline solution, Sigma Aldrich, Darmstadt, Germany) and incubated in sealed plastic containers at 37 °C and 100% humidity for 7 days [24].

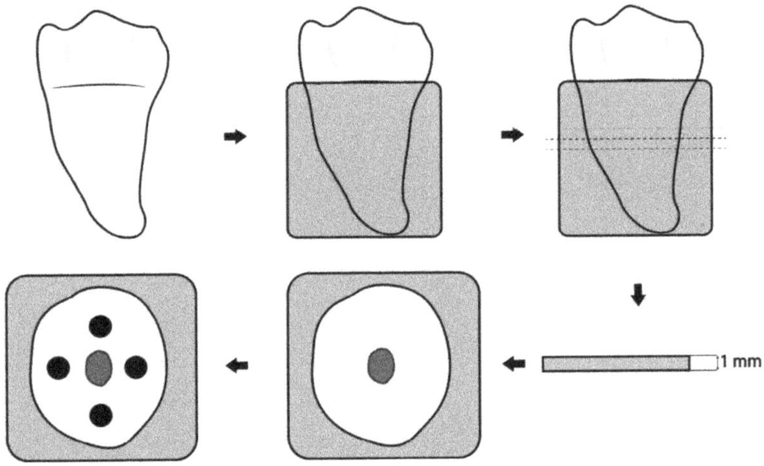

Figure 1. Preparation of the specimens. The intact third molars with fused roots were molded in self-bonding acrylate. Teeth were cut perpendicular to the longitudinal axis of the tooth in the area of the middle third of the root obtaining two transverse discs per tooth (thickness = 1 ± 0.1mm). Four cavities (d = 1.2 mm) were prepared in the paracanal dentin so that they were at least 1 mm away from the root canal, root cementum, and adjacent cavity. Each cavity was filled with one of the tested fillers.

2.3. *Push-Out Bond Strength Test*

The measurement of the bond strength of the sealers to the dentin was carried out by push-out test on a universal testing machine (PCE-FM 200, PCE group, Germany) with the use of an indenter with a diameter of 1 mm and at a speed of 1 mm/min. The samples were placed on two glass plates with a spacing sufficient to allow for the unimpeded dislocation of the sealer. Force values at the moment of dislocation of the sealer were recorded in the belonging Lutron program. The procedure was carried out for each of the four sealers applied on one disc. The bond strength of the sealers to the root canal dentin, expressed in MPa, was calculated according to the following formula: bond strength (σ) = $F/\pi \times d \times h$, where F is the maximum measured force value (N), π constant (3.14), d—cavity diameter (1.2 mm), and h—disk thickness (1 mm) [23,24].

2.4. *Statistical Analysis*

The obtained results were statistically analyzed using two-way analysis of variance (ANOVA) with the Bonferroni post hoc *t*-test for multiple comparisons since data were normally distributed (Shapiro-Wilk test, $p = 0.6$). The significance level was set at $\alpha = 0.05$. The power of the test was 1.0 for the factor "type of the sealer" and 0.813 for the factor "irrigation protocol". Statistical analyses were performed using the SigmaPlot 14.0 software (Palo Alto, CA, USA).

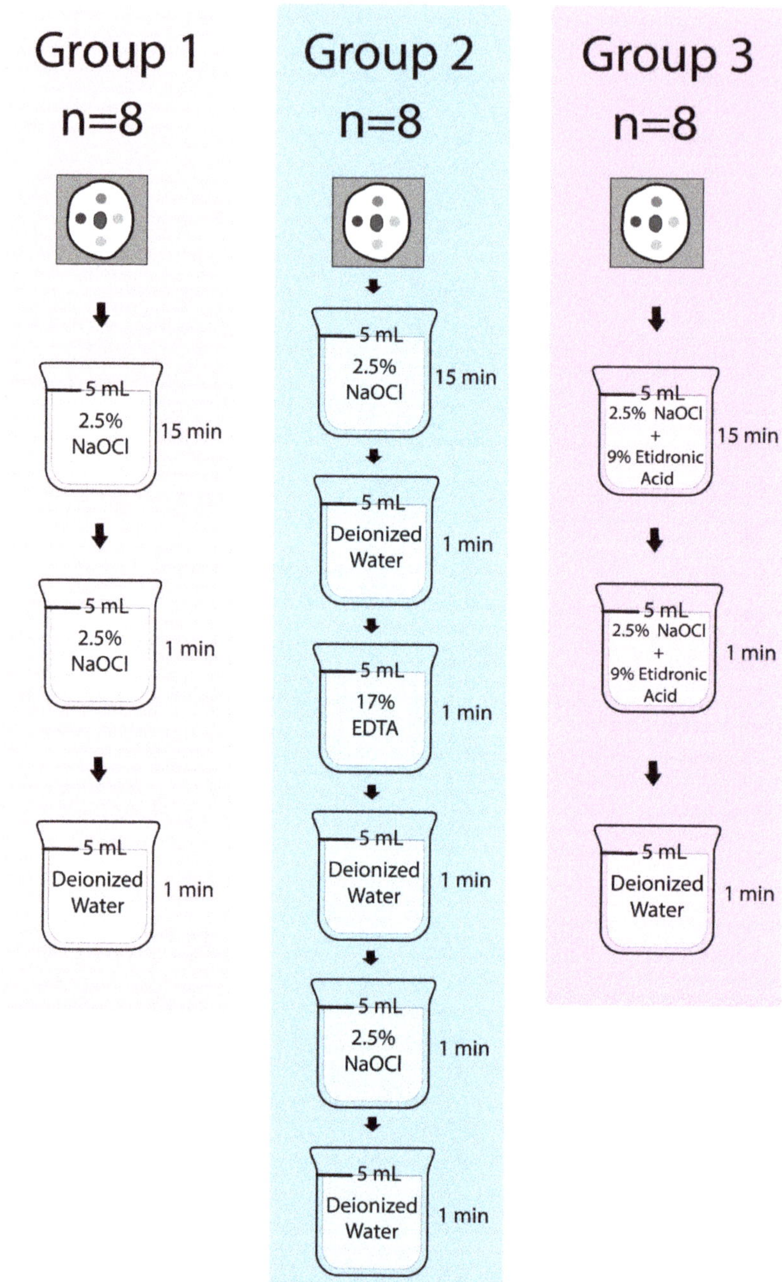

Figure 2. Irrigation protocols in experimental groups. Group 1: 5 mL of 2.5% NaOCl for 15 min followed by 5 mL of fresh 2.5% NaOCl for 1 min; Group 2: 5 mL 2.5% NaOCl for 15 min followed by 5 mL of 17% EDTA for 1 min followed by 5 mL of 2.5% NaOCl for 1 min; and Group 3: 5 mL of a mixture of 2.5% NaOCl and 9% etidronic acid for 15 min followed by 5 mL of a fresh mixture for 1 min. In all groups, between the irrigants, discs were immersed in 5 mL of deionized water for 1 min. After each irrigation protocol, discs were additionally immersed in 5 mL of deionized water for 1 min.

3. Results

The type of endodontic sealer and the irrigation protocol utilized both had a statistically significant effect on the push-out bond strength of the evaluated sealers ($p < 0.001$ and $p = 0.003$, respectively). Their effect was mutually independent since significant interaction between these two examined factors was not identified ($p = 0.359$).

In the NaOCl group, although all tested bioceramic sealers demonstrated weaker bond strength compared to epoxy resin-based AH Plus sealer, these differences were significant for Bio-C and AH Plus Bioceramic. Notably, BioRoot RCS showed significantly higher push-out bond strength compared to AHBC (Figure 3). In the NaOCl/EDTA group, the bond strength of BioRoot RCS and Bio-C sealer was similar and significantly stronger compared to AH Plus Bioceramic. The bond strength of all tested bioceramic sealers was weaker compared to AH Plus (Figure 4). In the NaOCl/HEDP group, the values measured for AH Plus and BioRoot RCS sealers were mutually close and significantly higher compared to Bio-C and AH Plus Bioceramic (Figure 5).

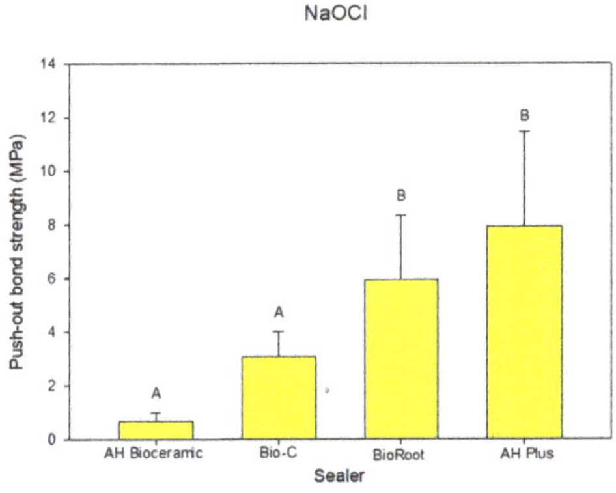

Figure 3. Push-out bond strength in experimental group with NaOCl irrigation protocol. The group consisted of dentin discs ($n = 8$) with four prepared cavities on each disc, filled with each of tested sealers. Values are presented as mean (vertical bars) and standard deviations (lines) of bond strength of tested sealers to root canal dentin. Columns sharing the same uppercase letter are not significantly different ($p > 0.05$).

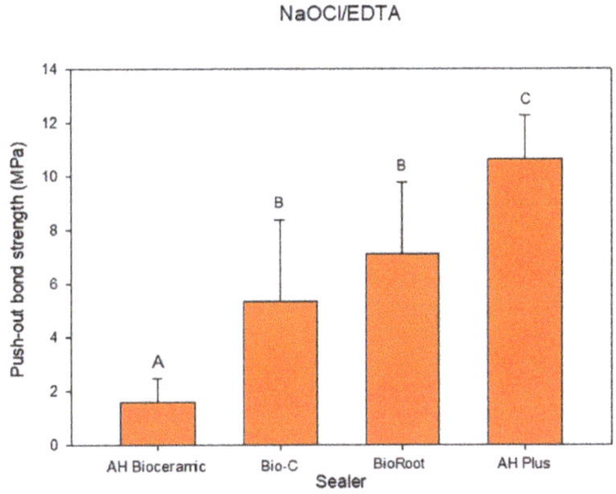

Figure 4. Push-out bond strength in experimental group with NaOCl/EDTA irrigation protocol. The group consisted of dentin discs ($n = 8$) with four prepared cavities on each disc, filled with each of tested sealers. Values are presented as mean (vertical bars) and standard deviations (lines) of bond strength of tested sealers to root canal dentin. Columns sharing the same uppercase letter are not significantly different ($p > 0.05$).

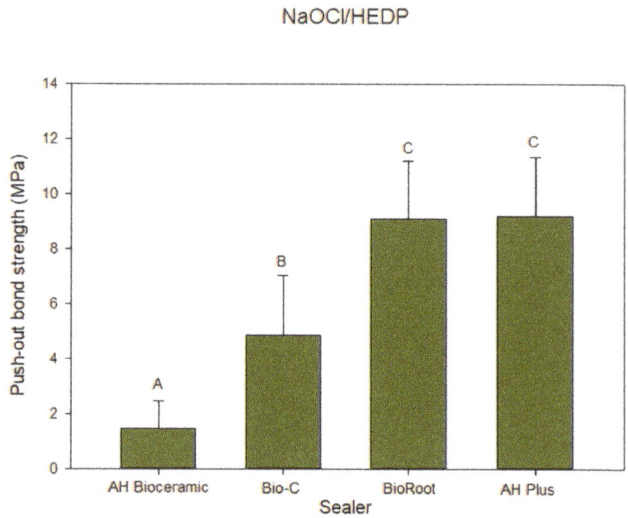

Figure 5. Push-out bond strength in experimental group with NaOCl/HEDP irrigation protocol. The group consisted of dentin discs ($n = 8$) with four prepared cavities on each disc, filled with each of tested sealers. Values are presented as mean (vertical bars) and standard deviations (lines) of bond strength of tested sealers to root canal dentin. Columns sharing the same uppercase letter are not significantly different ($p > 0.05$).

Irrigation with solely NaOCl resulted in significantly lower bond strength values in comparison to two other investigated protocols (Figure 6). However, in all experimental irrigation protocols the strongest bond with dentine was measured for AH Plus and the weakest bond for AH Plus Bioceramic sealer. BioRoot RCS showed significantly higher bond strength with dentin in NaOCl\HEDP protocol compared to the use of NaOCl (Table 2).

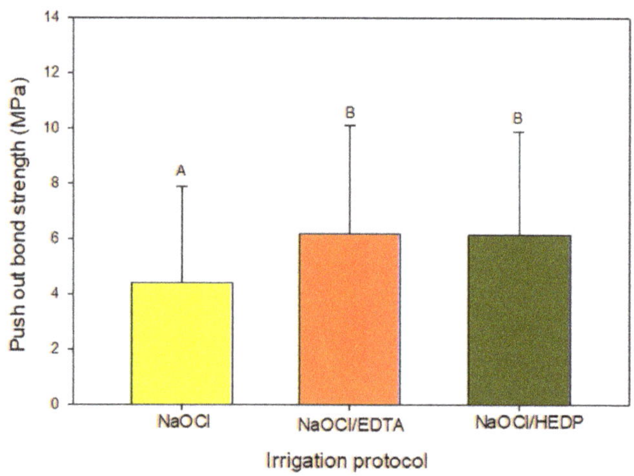

Figure 6. Mean values (vertical bars) and standard deviations (lines) of push-out bond strength values obtained with tested irrigation protocols. Irrigation protocol with NaOCl resulted in significantly lower bond strength values in comparison to two other investigated protocols. Columns sharing the same uppercase letter are not significantly different ($p > 0.05$).

Table 2. Values (mean ± SD) of push-out bond strength for tested sealers after application of different irrigation protocols. In all experimental irrigation protocols, the strongest bond with dentine was measured for AH Plus and the weakest bond for AH Plus Bioceramic sealer. Letter A in superscript indicates significantly higher bond strength value for BioRoot RCS in NaOCl\HEDP group compared to NaOCl group (p = 0.02).

	Irrigating Protocol		
Sealer	**NaOCl**	**NaOCl\EDTA**	**NaOCl\HEDP**
AHBC	0.657 ± 0.352	1.601 ± 0.888	1.450 ± 1.023
Bio-C	3.057 ± 0.949	5.350 ± 3.017	4.854 ± 2.167
BioRoot	5.908 ± 2.437	7.117 ± 2.660	9.091 ± 2.115 ^{A}
AH Plus	7.943 ± 3.496	10.639 ± 1.628	9.196 ± 2.150

4. Discussion

The present study evaluated the push-out bond strength of three bioceramic sealers, which are mutually different regarding chemical composition and formulation, and the epoxy resin-based sealer used as control sealer, after three different irrigation protocols. Since different irrigation protocols significantly affected the bond strength of investigated bioceramic sealers to root canal dentin, the first hypothesis was rejected. Additionally, we found that the bond strength of sealers to root canal dentin was also significantly influenced by the type of sealers, i.e., their chemical composition. Therefore, the second hypothesis was rejected, too.

The bond strength was evaluated with a push-out test, commonly used for assessing the adhesiveness of materials [12,13], in accordance to methodology described by Scelza, et al. [24]. This methodology enables better standardization of the prepared cavities and a smaller number of samples and teeth required for research compared to methodologies where only one material per disc is evaluated. Since all the sealers were evaluated on the same dentin disc samples, the influence of age, degree of mineralization, and strength of dentin on the obtained results was equally distributed, thus reducing the incorporated selection bias. Notably, the number of included teeth was comparable between our study and the abovementioned study.

Regarding irrigations protocols, the samples of the first group were treated only with NaOCl. In the second and third groups, chelating agents were used in order to improve the cleaning of the dentine walls through the removal of inorganic debris and the smear layer, created by the use of burs during the preparation of artificial cavities. In the second group, 17% EDTA solution, the most used chelating agent during root canal irrigation, was applied, followed by NaOCl (sequential chelation protocol). The third group of samples was treated with a mixture of sodium hypochlorite solution and HEDP (continuous chelation protocol). This protocol was introduced with the aim of simplifying the irrigation protocol during root canal preparation [25]. HEDP is a mild chelating agent, effective in removing the smear layer but with slower action than EDTA [26]. Unlike EDTA, which reduces the antibacterial and organolytic capacity of NaOCl, the mixture of NaOCl and etidronic acid retains the good properties of both agents, therefore reducing the formation of a smear layer and the accumulation of inorganic debris during instrumentation [27]. Also, it dissolves the remains of pulp tissue [28] and effectively eliminates bacterial biofilms from paracanal dentin and dentinal tubules [29].

The results of this study demonstrate a significant increase in bond strength values in the groups where chelating agents were used, compared to NaOCl group where the smear layer was not removed. This confirms the statement that the application of chelating agents ensures cleaner walls of the root canal, enabling the penetration of obturation sealers into dentinal tubules and achieving a more efficient bond between the sealer and the dentin of the root canal [30]. Our results are in a line with Emekli et al., who also observed higher values of push-out bond strength of bioceramic sealers after applying chelating agents [31]. On the contrary, Donnermeyer, et al. reported lower push-out bond strength values of BioRoot after the application of EDTA and higher after NaOCl, using them as final irrigants [20]. In addition to other methodological differences, in the mentioned study, the contact time of EDTA with root canal dentin was much longer compared to our study, and EDTA was not flushed from the canals either with NaOCl or using distillated water. Prolonged exposure time and, possibly, remaining EDTA could lead to the reduction in calcium ions at the sealer-dentin interface, resulting in lower push-out bond strength. In our study, in Group 2 (sequential chelation), after the smear layer was removed with EDTA, NaOCl was used as a final irrigant. According to Fernandes Zancan et al., irrigation with NaOCl after chelating agents provides the most favorable dentin surface for bonding with bioceramic sealers [32].

The application of two different smear layer removal protocols, sequential and continuous chelation, resulted in similar bond strength values of the tested sealers. The obtained results are in accordance with recently published data [31] and suggest that continuous chelation could be an effective alternative to the traditional sequential irrigation protocol, before obturation with bioceramic sealers, but with a need for further investigations.

The different chemical composition of the sealers tested in this study resulted in differences in push-out bond strength. Superior bond strength values of epoxy resin- based AH Plus sealer compared to bioceramic sealers obtained in this study are in line with previous studies [3,20,24,33–35]. The adhesiveness of AH Plus sealer is attributed to the formation of covalent bonds between the epoxy rings of the sealer and the amino groups of dentin collagen, low values of polymerization contraction, and distinct cohesion of molecules within the sealer [36]. Noteworthily, in the NaOCl group, the bond strength of AH Plus was slightly weaker compared to the other two protocols where chelating agents were used. It is possible that using NaOCl only resulted in less available collagen for bonding with AH Plus [31].

The bonding mechanism of Bioceramic sealers with dentin is different compared to that of epoxy resin-based sealers. Those sealers, due to their chemical composition, achieve a micromechanical bond with the dentin of the root canal. During setting in a wet environment, the reaction of calcium from the sealers with phosphates from tissue fluids leads to the formation of apatite crystals that are first deposited on the contact surface of the material and dentin, filling the existing micro spaces [37]. Over time, as the number of crystals increases, they are deposited in the form of finger-like extensions in the dentin tubules (Mineral infiltration zone) [32,38,39]. Since the mineralization is a time-dependent phenomenon, prolonged contact with tissue fluids can contribute to the push-out bond strength of the bioceramic sealers [10,23,40].

BioRoot, Bio-C, and AH Plus Bioceramic sealers evaluated in this study, although classified in the same group as the bioceramic sealers, have demonstrated different push-out bond strengths. Two-component BioRoot RCS exhibited superior bond strength compared to one-component, pre-mixed sealers Bio-C and AH Plus Bioceramic. Lopes, et al. also reported higher values of BioRoot RCS bond strength compared to Bio-C sealer [34]. AH Bioceramic exhibited the lowest values of push-out bond strength, significantly lower even compared to Bio-C sealer. The weak bond strength of the AH Plus Bioceramic sealer obtained in the present study is in line with the recently published data [41,42].

The superior bonding of BioRoot RCS can be attributed to the greater release of calcium ions compared to one-component sealers. According to the manufacturer, AH Plus Bioceramic sealer contains only 5–15% of tricalcium silicate particles. Recently, Chen et al. detected near three times less calcium in the AH Plus Bioceramic leachates compared to leachates of BioRoot RCS after 28 days and almost five times less after 90 days [43]. It has been proven that a lower content of calcium silicate in the material results in the weaker formation of calcium hydroxide and lower release of calcium ions, which can consequently result in a smaller number of formed apatite crystals responsible for the micromechanical bonding of sealers with dentin [10].

The obtained results could be also attributed to the different formulations of evaluated bioceramic sealers and consequential different degrees of hydration, i.e., setting after storage. The setting of the two-component BioRoot RCS starts via the mixing powder and liquid component and continues with further hydration in the root canal. In one-component bioceramic sealers such as Bio-C and AH Bioceramic, calcium silicate particles are dispersed in non-aqueous carriers and exclusively use the moisture of the dentinal tubules for setting [14]. During this research, after the application of the sealers, the samples were wrapped in gauze soaked in artificial tissue fluid and left to set for 7 days, like in methodologically similar research [24,33]. It is possible that this period of time was not enough for the adequate hydration of these one-component formulations and achieving adequate micromechanical bonding.

The distinct mechanisms through which sealer type and irrigation protocol influence push-out bond strength have been shown—via statistical analysis—to function independently, indicating that their effects are not interdependent. Nevertheless, their combined application may produce additive benefits that enhance the overall clinical performance of root canal obturation.

The main limitation of this in vitro study is the impossibility of direct interpolation of results to the clinical situation. Namely, the complex influences and relationships that affect the strength of the sealer's bond to the dentinal wall in the root canal are very difficult to fully reproduce in experimental conditions. Nevertheless, careful interpretation of these findings in the context of clinical application suggests that utilizing chelation protocols in conjunction with a two-component bioceramic sealer may offer advantages in achieving a reliable and effective endodontic seal. Regarding sample size, the achieved strengths of the test in the analysis indicate meaningful findings. Nevertheless, a larger sample size would give additional strength to the findings, primarily regarding the mutual interaction of examined factors. Additionally, the visualization and examination of the dentin-sealer interface as well as the inclusion of more factors such as the influence of temperature changes and prolonged observation could provide valuable information on the long-term projection of bond stability and should be considered the next step in the analysis of this research problem. Our results certainly suggest that differently formulated bioceramic sealers available on the market would consequently have different properties.

5. Conclusions

Under the conditions of this in vitro study, the irrigation protocols and the chemical composition of the sealers significantly influenced their bond strength to dentin. Irrigation protocols that included chelating agents positively influenced the bond strength of the tested sealers. In all the irrigation protocols, epoxy resin-based sealer achieved the strongest bond to dentin, while within bioceramic sealers the highest values were obtained for BioRoot® RCS and the lowest for the AH Plus® Bioceramic.

Author Contributions: Conceptualization, J.I. and V.P.; methodology, J.I., V.P. and I.M.; software, J.I. and T.S.-S. validation, V.P. and Z.U.; formal analysis, V.P. and J.I.; investigation, I.M.; resources, T.S.-S.; data curation, V.K.; writing—original draft preparation, Z.U. and V.P.; writing—review and editing, V.P. and J.I. visualization, T.S.-S.; and supervision, V.P. All authors have read and agreed to the published version of the manuscript.

Funding: This research received no external funding.

Institutional Review Board Statement: The study was conducted in accordance with the Declaration of Helsinki and approved by the Ethics Committee of University of Belgrade, School of Dental Medicine (36/3 2025).

Informed Consent Statement: Not applicable.

Data Availability Statement: The original contributions presented in the study are included in the article; further inquiries can be directed to the corresponding author.

Acknowledgments: This study was supported by funds of University of Belgrade, School of Dental Medicine.

Conflicts of Interest: The authors declare no conflicts of interest.

References

1. Schäfer, E.; Olthoff, G. Effect of Three Different Sealers on the Sealing Ability of Both Thermafil Obturators and Cold Laterally Compacted Gutta-Percha. *J. Endod.* **2002**, *28*, 638–642. [CrossRef]
2. Schwartz, R.S. Adhesive Dentistry and Endodontics. Part 2: Bonding in the Root Canal System- The Promise and the Problems: A Review. *J. Endod.* **2006**, *32*, 1125–1134. [CrossRef]
3. Oliveira, D.; Cardoso, M.; Queiroz, T.; Silva, E.; Souza, E.; De-Deus, G. Suboptimal push-out bond strength of calcium silicate-based sealers. *Int. Endod. J.* **2016**, *49*, 796–801. [CrossRef]
4. Tanomaru-Filho, M.; Torres, F.F.E.; Chávez-Andrande, G.M.; Almeida, M.d.; Navarro, L.G.; Steier, L.; Guerreiro-Tanomaru, J.M. Physicochemical Properties and Volumetric Change of Silicone/Bioactive Glass and Calcium Silicate-based Endodotic Sealers. *J. Endod.* **2017**, *43*, 2097–2101. [CrossRef]
5. Kwak, S.W.; Koo, J.; Song, M.; Jang, I.H.; Gambarini, G.; Kim, H.C. Physicochemical Properties and Biocompatibility of Various Bioceramic Root Canal Sealers: In Vitro study. *J. Endod.* **2023**, *49*, 871–879. [CrossRef]
6. Souza, L.C.d.; Neves, G.S.T.; Kirkpatrick, T.; Letra, A.; Silva, R. Physicochemical and Biological Properties of AH Plus Bioceramic. *J. Endod.* **2023**, *49*, 69–76. [CrossRef]
7. Sfeir, G.; Zogheib, C.; Patel, S.; Giraud, T.; Nagendrababu, V.; Bukiet, F. Calcium Silicate-Based Root Canal Sealers: A Narrative Review and Clinical Perspectives. *Materials* **2021**, *14*, 3965. [CrossRef]
8. Donnermeyer, D.; Bürklein, S.; Dammaschke, T.; Schäfer, E. Endodontic sealers based on calcium silicates: A systematic review. *Odontology* **2019**, *107*, 421–436. [CrossRef]
9. Bukhari, S.; Karabucak, B. The Antimicrobial Effect of Bioceramic Sealer on an 8-week Maturated Enterococcus faecalis Biofilm Attached to Root Canal Dentinal Surface. *J. Endod.* **2019**, *45*, 1047–1052. [CrossRef]
10. Han, L.; Okiji, T. Bioactivity evaluation of three calcium silicate-based endodontic materials. *Int. Endod. J.* **2013**, *46*, 808–814. [CrossRef]
11. Moraes, T.G.d.; Menezes, A.S.d.; Grazziotin-Soares, R.; Moraes, R.U.M.e.; Ferreira, P.V.C.; Carvalho, C.N.; Bauer, J.; Carvalho, E.M. Impact of Immersion Media on Physical Properties and Bioactivity of Epoxy Resin-Based and Bioceramic Endodontic Sealers. *Polymers* **2022**, *14*, 729. [CrossRef]
12. Neelakantan, P.; Ahmed, H.M.A.; Wong, M.C.M.; Matinlinna, J.P.; Cheung, G.S.P. Effect of root canal irrigation protocols on the dislocation resistance of mineral trioxide aggregate-based materials: A systematic review of laboratory studies. *Int. Endod. J.* **2018**, *51*, 847–861. [CrossRef]
13. Bricko, J.; Burrow, M.F.; Parashos, P. Design variability of the Push-out Bond Test in Endodontic Research: A Systematic Review. *J. Endod.* **2018**, *44*, 1237–1245. [CrossRef]
14. Cardinali, F.; Camilleri, J. A critical review of the material properties guiding the clinician's choice of root canal sealers. *Clin. Oral Investig.* **2023**, *27*, 4147–4155. [CrossRef]
15. López-García, S.; Pecci-Lloret, M.R.; Guerrero-Gironés, J.; Pecci-Lloret, M.P.; Lozano, A.; Llena, C.; Rodríguez-Lozano, F.J.; Forner, L. Comparative Cytocompatibility and Mineralization Potential of Bio-C Sealer and TotalFill BC Sealer. *Materials* **2019**, *12*, 3087. [CrossRef]
16. Silva, E.C.A.; Tanomaru-Filho, M.; Silva, G.F.d.; Delfino, M.M.; Cerri, P.S.; Guerreiro-Tanomaru, M. Biocompatibility and Bioactive Potential of New Calcium Silicate -based Endodontic Sealers: Bio-C sealer and Sealer Plus BC. *J. Endod.* **2020**, *46*, 1470. [CrossRef]
17. Sanz, J.L.; López-García, S.; Rodríguez-Lozano, F.J.; Melo, M.; Lozano, A.; Llena, C.; Forner, L. Cytocompatibility and bioactive potential of AH Plus Bioceramic sealer: An in vitro study. *Int. Endod. J.* **2022**, *55*, 1066–1080. [CrossRef]

18. Sanz, J.L.; López-García, S.; Garcia-Bernal, D.; Rodriguez-Lozano, F.J.; Forner, L.; Lozano, A.; Murcia, L. Comparative bioactivity and immunomodulatory potential of the new BioRoot Flow and AH Plus Bioceramic sealer: An in vitro study on hPDLSCs. *Clin. Oral Investig.* **2024**, *28*, 195. [CrossRef]
19. Zamparini, F.; Prati, C.; Taddei, P.; Spinelli, A.; Foggia, M.d.; Gandolfi, M.G. Chemical-Physical Properties and Bioactivity of New Premixed Calcium Silicate-Bioceramic Root Canal Sealers. *Int. J. Mol. Sci.* **2022**, *23*, 13914. [CrossRef]
20. Donnermeyer, D.; Vahdat-Pajouh, N.; Schäfer, E.; Dammaschke, T. Influence of the final irrigation solution on the push-out bond strength of calcium silicate-based, epoxy resin-based and silicone-based endodontic sealers. *Odontology* **2019**, *107*, 231–236. [CrossRef] [PubMed]
21. Hazar, E.; Hazar, A. Effect of phytic acid and etidronic acid using continuous and sequential chelation on the removal of smear layer, dentin microhardness, and push-out bond strength of calcium silicate-based cement. *BMC Oral Health* **2025**, *25*, 633. [CrossRef]
22. Razumova, S.; Brago, A.; Kryuchkova, A.; Troitskiy, V.; Bragunova, R.; Barakat, H. Evaluation of the efficiency of smear layer removal during endodontic treatment using scanning electron microscopy: An in vitro study. *BMC Oral Health* **2025**, *25*, 151. [CrossRef]
23. Neelakantan, P.; Nandagopal, M.; Shemesh, H.; Wesselink, P. The effect of root dentin conditioning protocols on the push-out bond strength of three calcium silicate sealers. *Int. J. Adhes. Adhes.* **2015**, *60*, 104–108. [CrossRef]
24. Scelza, M.Z.; Silva, D.; Scelza, P.; Noronha, F.d.; Barbosa, I.B.; Souza, E.; De Deus, G. Influence of a new push-out test method on the bond strength of three resin-based sealers. *Int. Endod. J.* **2015**, *48*, 801–806. [CrossRef]
25. Zehnder, M.; Schmidlin, P.; Sener, B.; Waltimo, T. Chelation in Root Canal Therapy Reconsidered. *J. Endod.* **2005**, *31*, 817–820. [CrossRef]
26. De Deus, G.; Zehnder, M.; Reis, C.; Fidel, S.; Fidel, R.A. Longitudinal Co-site Optical Microscopy Study on the Chelating Ability of Etidronate and EDTA Using a Comparative Single-tooth Model. *J. Endod.* **2008**, *34*, 71–75. [CrossRef]
27. Paqué, F.; Rechenberg, D.K.; Zehnder, M. Reduction of Hard-tissue Debris Accumulation during Rotary Root Canal Instrumentation by Etidronic Acid in a Sodium Hypochlorite irrigant. *J. Endod.* **2012**, *38*, 692–695. [CrossRef]
28. Ulusoy, Ö.I.; Savur, I.G.; Alaçam, T.; Çelik, B. The effectiveness of various irrigation protocols on organic tissue removal from simulated internal resorption defects. *Int. Endod. J.* **2018**, *51*, 1030–1036. [CrossRef]
29. Arias-Moliz, M.T.; Ordinola-Zapata, R.; Baca, P.; Ruiz-Linares, M.; García García, M.A.; Duarte, M.A.H.; Bramante, C.M.; Ferrer-Luque, C.M. Antimicrobial activity of chlorhexidine, peracetic acid and sodium hypochlorite/et. *Int. Endod. J.* **2015**, *48*, 1188–1193. [CrossRef]
30. Violich, D.R.; Chandler, N.P. The smear-layer in endodontics—A review. *Int. Endod. J.* **2010**, *43*, 2–15. [CrossRef]
31. Emekli, G.E.; Kaptan, R.F.; Tanalp, J. Evaluation of the effects of traditional irrigation solutions and etidronic acid on the bond strength of endodontic sealers. *BMC Oral Health.* **2025**, *25*, 364. [CrossRef]
32. Fernandes Zancan, R.F.; Hadis, M.; Burgess, D.; Zhang, Z.J.; Maio, A.d.; Tomson, P.; Duarte, M.A.H.; Camilleri, J. A matched irrigation and obturation strategy for root canal therapy. *Sci. Rep.* **2021**, *11*, 4666. [CrossRef]
33. Carvalho, N.K.; Prado, M.C.; Senna, P.M.; Neves, A.A.; Souza, E.M.; Fidel, S.R.; Sassone, L.M.; Silva, E.J.N.L. Do smear layer removal agents affect the push-out bond strength of calcium silicate-based endodontic sealers? *Int. Endod. J.* **2017**, *50*, 612–619. [CrossRef]
34. Lopes, G.R.C.; Dotto, M.E.P.; Nomura, L.H.; Schuldt, D.P.V.; Garcia, L.F.R.; Teixeira, C.S. Impact of Heating Exposure on the Micro-Push-Out Bond Strength of Bioceramic Sealers. *Int. J. Dent.* **2023**, *1*, 3327275.
35. Milanovic, I.; Miletic, V.; Dzeletovic, B.; Antonijevic, D.; Savic Stankovic, T.; Pavlovic, D.; Despotovic, A.; Petrovic, V. Physicochemical properties and push-out bond strength to root dentine of calcium silicate-based sealers. *J. Funct. Biomater.* **2025**, *16*, 131. [CrossRef]
36. Lee, K.W.; Williams, M.C.; Camps, J.J.; Pashley, D.H. Adhesion of Endodontic Sealers to Dentin and Gutta-Percha. *J. Endod.* **2002**, *28*, 684–688. [CrossRef]
37. Sarkar, N.K.; Caicedo, R.; Ritwik, P.; Mooiseyeva, R.; Kawashima, I. Physicochemical Basis of the Biologic Properties of Mineral Trioxide Aggregate. *J. Endod.* **2005**, *31*, 97. [CrossRef]
38. Viapiana, R.; Moinzadeh, A.T.; Camilleri, L.; Wesselink, P.R.; Tanomaru Filho, M.; Camilleri, J. Porosity and sealing ability of root fillings with gutta-percha and BioRoot RCS or AH Plus sealers. Evaluation by three ex vivo methods. *Int. J. Endod.* **2016**, *49*, 774–782. [CrossRef] [PubMed]
39. Benezra, M.K.; Wismayer, P.S.; Camilleri, J. Interfacial Characteristics and Cytocompatibility of Hydraulic Sealer Cements. *J Endod.* **2018**, *44*, 1007. [CrossRef] [PubMed]
40. De-Deus, G.; Ferreira, C.B.; Oliveira DdA, S.; de Queiroz, T.F.; Souza, E.M.; De Gouvêa, C.V.D.; Silva, E.J. Ressistance of Hydraulic Calcium Silicate Cements to Dislogment in Short- and long-term Assessment. *J. Adhes. Dent.* **2016**, *18*, 157–160.
41. Abu Zeid, S.T.; Alnoury, A.S. Impact of Bioactivity on Push-Out Bond Strength of AH Plus Bioceramic versus BC Bioceramic Root Canal Sealers. *Appl. Sci.* **2024**, *14*, 9366. [CrossRef]

42. Creazzo, G.; de Barros Ciribelli Alves, B.M.; de Assis, H.C.; Villamayor, K.G.G.; de Sousa-Neto, M.D.; Mazzi-Chaves, J.F.; Lopes-Olhê, F.C. Bond Strength and Adhesive Interface Quality of new pre-mixed bioceramic sealer. *Microsc. Res. Tech.* **2025**, *88*, 1989–2000. [CrossRef]
43. Chen, J.H.; Raman, V.; Kuehne, S.A.; Camilleri, J.; Hirschfeld, J. Chemical, Antibacterial, and Cytotoxic Properties of Four Different Endodontic Sealer Leachates Over Time. *J. Endod.* **2024**, *50*, 1612–1621. [CrossRef] [PubMed]

applied sciences

MDPI

Article

Patterns and Practices in the Use of Endodontic Materials: Insights from Romanian Dental Practices

Diana Marian [1], Ramona Amina Popovici [2], Iustin Olariu [1,*], Dana Emanuela Pitic (Cot) [2], Maria-Monica Marta [3] and Ioana Veja (Ilyes) [1]

1 Department of Dentistry, Faculty of Dentistry, "Vasile Goldiș" Western University of Arad, 310025 Arad, Romania

2 Management and Communication in Dental Medicine Department I, Faculty of Dental Medicine, Victor Babes University of Medicine and Pharmacy, 300041 Timisoara, Romania; dana.emanuela@gmail.com (D.E.P.)

3 Faculty of Pharmacy, Carol Davila University of Medicine and Pharmacy Bucharest, Street Dionisie Lupu Nr. 37, 020956 Bucharest, Romania; marta_m_monica@yahoo.com

* Correspondence: olariu.iustin@uvvg.ro

Abstract

The success of endodontic treatment depends on the correct use of materials during the cleaning and filling of the root canal system. The field of endodontics is constantly evolving with the introduction of new procedures and materials. Despite the continuous development of a wide range of chemical solutions and the introduction of new materials in endodontics, driven by the advances in state-of-the-art technologies, there is still a lack of data on how these advances are adapted to the daily practice of Romanian dentists in this field. The aim of this cross-sectional questionnaire-based study was the evaluation of current trends in endodontic practice, focusing on the materials used by dentists throughout Romania, performed by a number of dentists who graduated from universities in the Northern, Southern, Eastern, Western, and Central zones of Romania. The questions were about the irrigants used, the interim medication, the type of sealant, the filling technique, and the number of endodontic treatment sessions. The majority of participants in the research were general practitioners and endodontists, with some dentists of different specialties performing endodontic treatments in their practices. Statistical analyses were performed using DATAtab version 2024 software. The results obtained from this study provide a valuable resource and database for researchers to access a wide range of information and an apparent trend towards high-performance endodontic materials used in Romania.

Keywords: cross-sectional study; endodontic irrigant; sealer; interim medication

1. Introduction

The main goal of root canal therapy is to prevent future infections and to control the current infection within the root canal system [1]. The field of endodontics is constantly evolving with the introduction of new procedures and materials, and there is great potential for further advancements. The exponential expansion of endodontics is significantly influenced by the scientific advances in endodontic materials. The optimal approach to debridement, cleaning, shaping, and root canal filling remains a topic of discussion. Indeed, several innovative concepts, techniques, and instruments have been developed and put into practice. It is currently impossible to eradicate intraradicular infections with mechanical instrumentation alone. Therefore, irrigants are essential as a crucial supplement in the disinfection process of root canal therapy [2,3]. Modern root canal treatment recommends comprehensive root canal debridement through mechanical preparation and chemical irrigation, following advancements in technology and knowledge. As a result, traditional root canal dressing agents have gradually become less prevalent, leading to significant changes in the medications and administration techniques used today. However, more standardization is required in root canal treatment protocols [4]. In addition to preparation and irrigation, root canal filling is a key aspect of endodontic treatment. The ultimate goal is to seal the main root canal and its accessory canals. This final step in endodontic intervention is not merely a mechanical act of hermetically sealing the root canal system; it must also exhibit marked biological characteristics. The primary objectives of filling include achieving optimal sealant levels, biocompatibility, and hermeticity. In the pursuit of the ideal endodontic filling, clinicians have developed various materials, instruments, and techniques. Therefore, a high-quality coronal filling that ensures the adhesive interface between the dental structure and the composite material is essential for protecting the tooth structure, maintaining its integrity, and enhancing the success rate of endodontic therapy [5,6]. The longevity of composite restorations also depends on excellent oral hygiene, which implies effective plaque control through appropriate techniques proven to be highly effective in removing plaque deposits [7].

In 1958, Professor Dr. Louis I. Grossman, regarded as the father of contemporary endodontics, remarked, "I seriously doubt whether there is any other space in the human body, outside the root canal, into which such a diversity of materials has been introduced over the ages" [8]. Despite continuous research and the development of new materials and techniques for achieving a "three-dimensional filling", perfect and long-lasting sealing of the complex endodontic space remains elusive [9].

Bioceramics and epoxy resin sealers are two commonly used materials in endodontic filling. Comparative clinical investigations have yielded inconsistent findings regarding their sealing efficacy, treatment outcomes, and the occurrence of postoperative issues such as leakage, periapical inflammation, and root resorption. The performance of these sealers can be influenced by various factors, including the application technique, root canal anatomy, and the operator's skill.

Despite the ongoing advancements in state-of-the-art technologies, the availability of a wide range of chemical solutions, and the market introduction of new materials in endodontics, more data is necessary regarding how these advances align with the daily endodontic practices of Romanian dentists. The aim of this study is to analyze and document the patterns and practices employed by Romanian dentists in selecting and utilizing endodontic materials during clinical procedures. By identifying preferences, influencing factors, and trends, the research aims to contribute to a better understanding of regional practices and provide insights that can inform international collaboration, foster innovation, and bring about significant improvement in endodontic care. The study focuses on the patterns and practices of Romanian dentists while utilizing endodontic materials, providing significant insights into trends and decision-making variables. These findings advance understanding of endodontic materials, encouraging collaboration and innovation in order to improve therapeutic outcomes worldwide.

Advanced endodontic materials and techniques have been well documented in many countries [10,11], reflecting a shift towards more efficient and predictable treatment outcomes. However, there is limited evidence regarding how these advancements are implemented in daily clinical practice in Romania. This gap in data makes it challenging to evaluate the quality and consistency of endodontic care in the country and identify areas that may require additional training or resources. Although global research highlights the widespread adoption of new techniques in endodontics, studies on Romanian dental practices are scarce and do not offer a comprehensive overview of the materials and methods currently in use. For instance, bioceramic sealers and warm-filling techniques are widely adopted worldwide [12–15]. In Romania, the integration of bioceramic sealers into routine practice is limited by issues related to cost and accessibility. This study aims to assess how these global advancements are reflected in Romania's current trends in endodontic practice.

2. Materials and Methods

This observational cross-sectional study was conducted from August 2023 to January 2024 among licensed dentists practicing in Romania. It aimed to identify the materials most frequently used in endodontic therapy by dental professionals who graduated from universities in Romania's Northern, Southern, Eastern, Western, and Central regions. The sample was stratified to ensure proportional representation from Romania's five geographical regions. Dentists were randomly selected from a digital platform designed for the Romanian dental community.

The sample size was determined using the Id Survey Sample Size Calculator (https://www.idsurvey.com/en/sample-size-calculator/, accessed on 1 August 2023). A questionnaire-based survey was emailed to 900 Romanian dentists, of whom 862 responded correctly, resulting in a response rate of 95.77%. Experts in the field reviewed the questionnaire to ensure content validity. The questionnaire was pilot-tested on a small group of dentists to assess its clarity and comprehensibility. Based on feedback from the pilot, we refined the wording to minimize ambiguity and improve question clarity. The survey included eleven open-ended questions on endodontic practice: types of irrigants used, interim medications applied, types of sealants employed, techniques used for filling, number of endodontic treatment sessions performed, and general data about the respondents. The open-ended questions were carefully worded to align with the specific aims of the research and to gather in-depth information about practitioners' experiences and opinions. In addition, to reduce the variability of interpretation, responses to these questions were categorized into themes through a systematic qualitative analysis process. This allowed us to identify common trends and avoid inconsistencies in interpreting responses.

In order to be included in the study, dentists had to be graduates from a Romanian university after 1990, practice clinically in Romania, and perform more than ten endodontic treatments per month, considering in the study only practitioners who are regularly involved in endodontic procedures, as they are likely to provide the most relevant and up-to-date information.

All participants in this study were fully informed about the study's objective, and their consent was obtained before participation. The participants' informed consent and agreement to the handling and use of their personal information were important steps in ensuring the ethical conduct of this study.

2.1. Statistical Analysis

Descriptive analysis was performed, and frequencies of distribution were calculated in percentages; proportions were compared using chi-squared tests, with p-values < 0.05 accepted as statistically significant. Statistical analyses were performed using the software DATAtab version 2024 [16].

2.2. Demographical Data

A total of 862 dentists responded to the survey. Of the respondents, 572 were female and 290 were male. The data were recorded according to the year of graduation. Data were divided into four groups, each representing a different graduation year: Group A (1991–1998), Group B (1999–2006), Group C (2007–2014), and Group D (2015–2023). Table 1 illustrates the distribution of data between graduation year and sex. Figure 1 shows the distribution of data between sex and regional center, with the data divided into five categories: Northern, Southern, Eastern, Western, and Central zones in Romania.

Table 1. Data distribution by sex and graduation year.

	A		B		C		D		Total	
	n	%	n	%	n	%	N	%	n	%
F	42	4.87%	168	19.49%	178	20.65%	184	21.35%	572	66.36%
M	20	2.32%	68	7.89%	98	11.37%	104	12.06%	290	33.64%
Total	62	7.19%	236	27.38%	276	32.02%	288	33.41%	862	100%

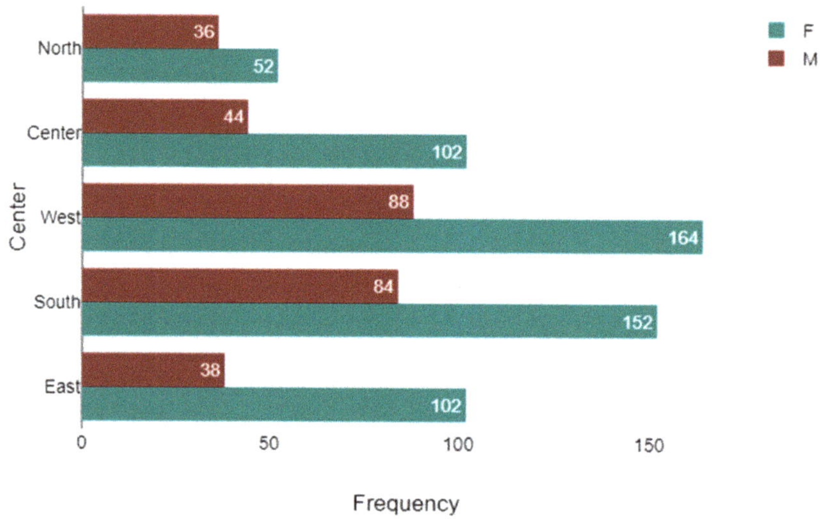

Figure 1. Data distribution by sex and regional center of graduation.

The distribution of data by regional center of graduation and year of graduation is presented in Table 2.

Table 2. Data distribution by graduation year and regional center of graduation.

	Graduation Year									
	A		B		C		D		Total	
	N	%	n	%	n	%	N	%	n	%
East	10	1.16%	36	4.18%	56	6.5%	38	4.41%	140	16.24%
South	16	1.86%	62	7.19%	82	9.51%	76	8.82%	236	27.38%
West	24	2.78%	76	8.82%	74	8.58%	78	9.05%	252	29.23%
Center	10	1.16%	34	3.94%	36	4.18%	66	7.66%	146	16.94%
North	2	0.23%	28	3.25%	28	3.25%	30	3.48%	88	10.21%
Total	62	7.19%	236	27.38%	276	32.02%	288	33.41%	862	100%

The majority of healthcare professionals who participated in the study were general practitioners (91%) and endodontists (3%), with a presence of doctors from various other specialties as well (6%). This data is presented in Figure 2.

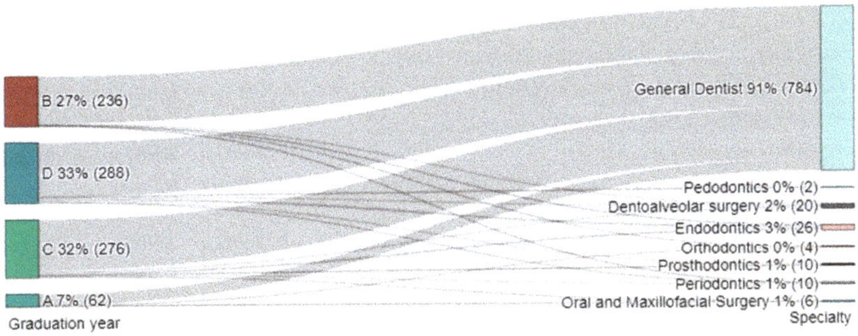

Figure 2. Data distribution by specialty and graduation year.

3. Results

The most frequently utilized endodontic irrigants were sodium hypochlorite (NaOCl), hydrogen peroxide (H_2O_2), chlorhexidine (CHX), ethylenediaminetetraacetic acid (EDTA), citric acid, and MTAD. The chi-square test demonstrated a statistically significant difference between the categories of the independent variable and the dependent variable graduation year ($p < 0.001$). This p-value is less than 0.05, indicating that the groups were significantly different in pairs in favor of NaOCl. The observed differences between groups are statistically significant at the conventional level of 0.05 (Table 3 and Figure 3).

Table 3. Irrigants used according to the year of graduation.

	Graduation Year				
	A	B	C	D	Total
	n	n	n	n	n
NaOCl	20	172	218	254	664
H_2O_2	32	22	14	8	76
CHX	6	16	16	14	52
EDTA	4	16	18	12	50
Acid citric	0	6	2	0	8
MTAD	0	2	0	0	2
Other	0	2	8	0	10
Total	62	236	276	288	862

Chi-square test; $p < 0.001$.

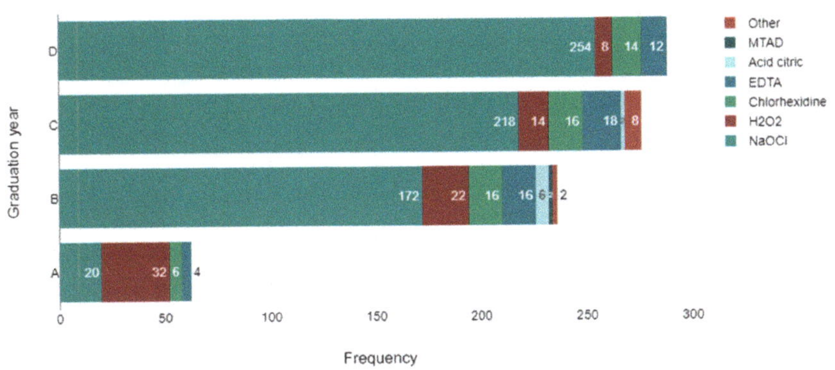

Figure 3. Endodontic irrigants utilized according to the year of graduation.

The most commonly used interim medications were calcium hydroxide ($Ca(OH)_2$), antibiotic paste, and iodoform (CHI_3). A p-value of 0.006 indicates a 0.6% probability of observing the data or something more extreme if there were no actual association between the graduation year and the intracanal medications used. Since the *p*-value is smaller than the common threshold for a significance of 0.05, this suggests that the observed association is unlikely to have occurred by chance. Therefore, there is a significant association between the graduation year and the types of intracanal medications used, as confirmed at the traditional 5% significance level (see Table 4 and Figure 4).

Table 4. Association between graduation year and intracanal medication used.

	Graduation Year									
	A		B		C		D		Total	
	n	%	n	%	n	%	n	%	n	%
Other	6	0.7%	36	4.18%	60	6.96%	40	4.64%	142	16.47%
Antibiotic paste	24	2.78%	26	3.02%	24	2.78%	14	1.62%	88	10.21%
$Ca(OH)_2$	25	2.9%	158	18.33%	178	20.65%	216	25.06%	577	66.94%
CHI_3	7	0.81%	16	1.86%	14	1.62%	18	2.09%	55	6.38%
Total	62	7.19%	236	27.38%	276	32.02%	288	33.41%	862	100%

Chi-square test; $p < 0.001$.

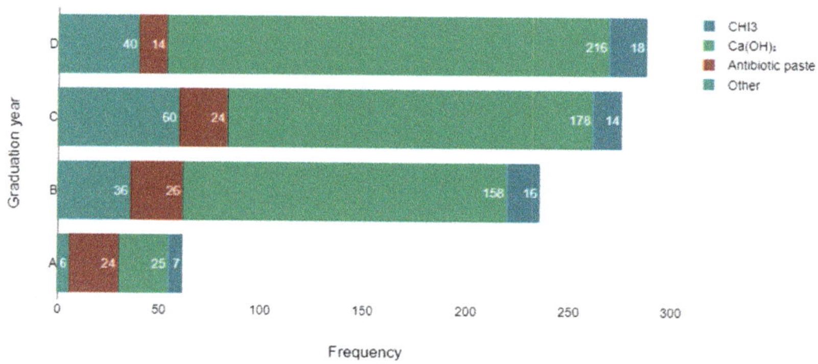

Figure 4. Association between graduation year and intracanal medication used.

Table 5 and Figure 5 demonstrate a correlation between the filling technique used and the year of graduation. The calculated *p*-value of 0.001 indicates a significant association. Since this *p*-value is well below the common significance threshold of 0.05, it suggests that the choice of filling technique is unlikely to have occurred by chance. Thus, there is a statistically significant association between the year of graduation and the filling technique chosen at the traditional 5% significance level (see Table 5 and Figure 5).

The most commonly used endodontic sealers, in descending order of usage, were sealers based on epoxy resins, calcium hydroxide, zinc oxide eugenol, and bioceramics. Table 6 and Figure 6 illustrate a correlation between the type of sealer used and the year of graduation. The calculated *p*-value of 0.001 indicates a significant association. Since this *p*-value is well below the common significance threshold of 0.05, it suggests that the sealer choice is unlikely to be due to chance. Therefore, there is a statistically significant association between the year of graduation and the type of sealer used, as confirmed at the traditional 5% significance level (see Table 6 and Figure 6).

Table 5. Filling techniques used according to graduation year.

	Graduation Year									
	A		B		C		D		Total	
	n	%	n	%	n	%	N	%	n	%
Cold techniques	47	5.45%	66	7.66%	76	8.82%	34	3.94%	223	25.87%
Warm techniques	15	1.74%	170	19.72%	200	23.2%	254	29.47%	639	74.13%
Total	62	7.19%	236	27.38%	276	32.02%	288	33.41%	862	100%

Chi-square test, $p < 0.001$.

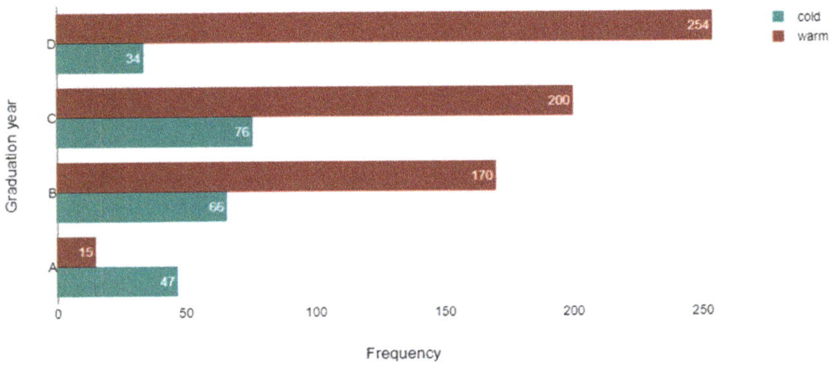

Figure 5. Association between graduation year and filling techniques.

Table 6. Sealer used by graduation year.

	Graduation Year									
	A		B		C		D		Total	
	n	%	n	%	n	%	N	%	n	%
Zinc oxide eugenol	22	2.55%	52	6.03%	56	6.5%	42	4.87%	172	19.95%
Epoxy resin	10	1.16%	94	10.9%	100	11.6%	102	11.83%	306	35.5%
$Ca(OH)_2$	21	2.44%	52	6.03%	56	6.5%	74	8.58%	203	23.55%
Other	8	0.93%	14	1.62%	26	3.02%	18	2.09%	66	7.66%
Bioceramic sealer	1	0.12%	24	2.78%	38	4.41%	52	6.03%	115	13.34%
Total	62	7.19%	236	27.38%	276	32.02%	288	33.41%	862	100%

Chi-square test, $p < 0.001$.

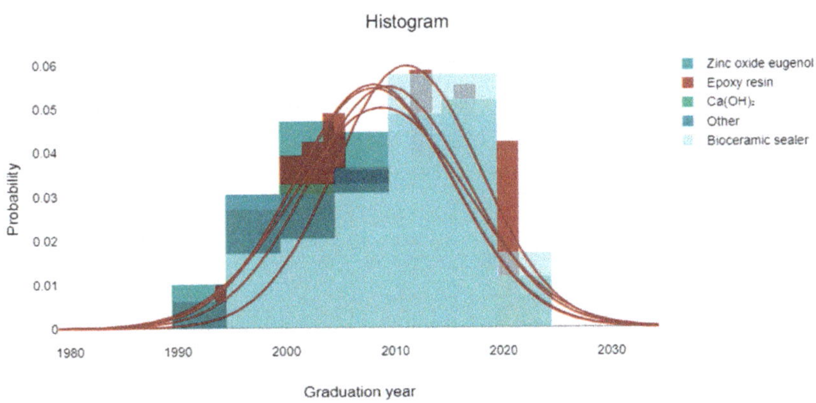

Figure 6. Sealer used by graduation year.

Table 7 and Figure 7 show the number of treatments and retreatments performed by practitioners over the course of one month. The data reveals that the number of retreatments compared to treatments is inversely proportional to the year of graduation. Specifically,

- Practitioners who graduated before 2006 performed about three times fewer retreatments than treatments.
- Those who graduated between 2007 and 2014 performed about four times fewer retreatments than treatments.
- Practitioners who graduated between 2015 and 2023 performed about six times fewer retreatments than treatments.

Table 7. Number of treatments and retreatments performed per month by practitioners.

		Frequency	Mean	Std. Deviation	Maximum
Number of endodontic treatments per month	D	288	24.7	22.26	150
	C	276	33.96	36.77	250
	B	236	28.72	31.87	200
	A	62	24.65	26.48	120
Number of endodontic retreatments per month	D	288	8.17	12.98	100
	C	276	11.57	16.01	100
	B	236	7.22	9.12	50
	A	62	4.23	4.56	20

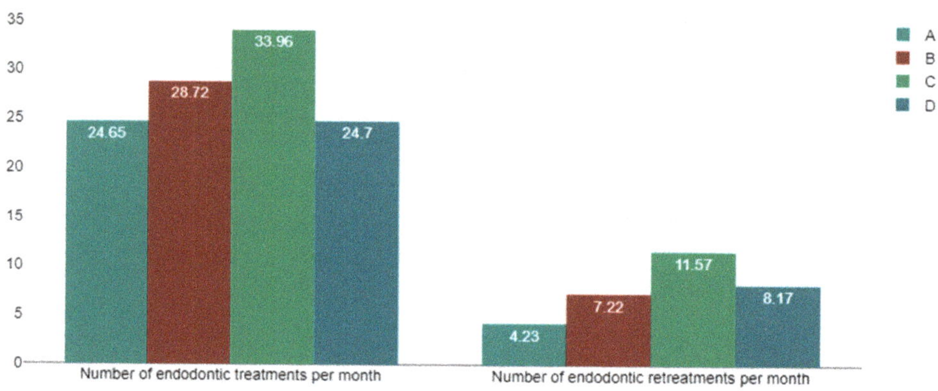

Figure 7. Number of treatments and retreatments performed per month by practitioners.

Table 8 indicates that more than half of the study participants performed endodontic treatment in two sessions.

Table 8. Single-visit/multiple-visit endodontic treatments.

	Graduation Year				
Number of Visits	A	B	C	D	Total
1	24	84	126	138	372
2	32	132	134	142	440
3	6	20	16	8	50
Total	62	236	276	288	862

4. Discussions

In the past decade, the field of endodontics has undergone significant developments, resulting in notable advancements in both endodontic procedures and materials. The objective of this study was to utilize a questionnaire-based survey in order to ascertain the materials most frequently employed in contemporary endodontic therapy by a diverse range of dental professionals who graduated from universities in Romania's Northern, Southern, Eastern, Western, and Central zones.

The ideal irrigant for disinfection of the root canal system should be a substance that is both bactericidal and biocompatible. It should dissolve tissue, lubricate, and remove smear layers effectively, while also removing debris, providing long-lasting results, and not altering the physical characteristics of dentin. In this study, the most commonly used irrigant was sodium hypochlorite (77%), followed by hydrogen peroxide (8.8%), ethylenediaminetetraacetic acid (EDTA) (6%), and chlorhexidine (5.8%). Citric acid and MTAD were used in very low percentages.

Historically, hydrogen peroxide was used for endodontic irrigation, but it has largely been replaced by more effective and safer solutions. Despite this, the study shows that a significant percentage (8.8%) of Romanian dentists still use hydrogen peroxide, particularly those who graduated before 2006. Hydrogen peroxide can have adverse effects, such as forming oxygen bubbles in the root canal, interfering with canal sealing, or leading to gas emboli [17]. There is limited research on the efficacy and risks of using hydrogen peroxide for endodontic irrigation.

The study results indicate that since 2015, very few Romanian dentists have used hydrogen peroxide. This decline may be due to its cytotoxic nature and its reduced effectiveness against *Enterococcus faecalis*. Research on the cytotoxicity of iron oxide nanoparticles combined with hydrogen peroxide as an endodontic irrigant has shown moderate cytotoxic effects at higher concentrations (4 and 8 mg/mL) on cultured human dermal fibroblasts (HDFn) cells [18]. Additionally, hydrogen peroxide (1.5%) has demonstrated lower efficacy against *Enterococcus faecalis* than sodium hypochlorite and chlorhexidine, which are more effective in reducing bacterial counts [19,20].

Worldwide surveys have consistently reported sodium hypochlorite (NaOCl) is the most commonly used irrigating solution in endodontics [21,22]. Research findings provide insights into the safety and efficacy of NaOCl in endodontic procedures, as it is widely regarded for its bactericidal properties and unique ability to dissolve organic tissues [23], especially when using techniques such as the activation of irrigants or negative pressure irrigation to minimize the formation of air bubbles during endodontic therapy [24].

The results of this study reflect similar findings, with NaOCl being used by 77.03% of practitioners, showing a notable increase in its use, especially after 1999. Furthermore, a study by Diaconu et al. on the practices of Romanian dentists revealed that 82.1% of the participants use NaOCl at a 5.25% concentration. In contrast, the remaining dentists opt for lower concentrations [25]. NaOCl dissolves organic substances through three primary reactions: saponification, neutralization of amino acids producing water and salts, and interference with microbial cell metabolism by reacting with chlorine and amino groups through chlorination [26]. Organic tissues can be effectively dissolved in solutions containing more than 2.5% NaOCl. While higher concentrations, temperatures, volumes, and longer durations enhance its bactericidal and tissue dissolution abilities, they also increase its causticity and cytotoxicity, potentially causing periapical tissue damage if accidentally extruded from the apical foramen [27]. Despite its antimicrobial and tissue-dissolving characteristics, NaOCl should be used cautiously to avoid adverse effects caused by its cytotoxicity and its unfavorable impact on dentin qualities [28].

Studies have compared different concentrations of NaOCl with other irrigants like chlorhexidine and peracetic acid, highlighting varying effects on cytotoxicity and antimicrobial efficacy, with cytocompatibility being a critical aspect in developing materials used in dentistry [29–31].

Alternative irrigants, such as chlorhexidine (CHX) and EDTA, address some limitations. CHX is less cytotoxic and offers long-lasting antimicrobial action through substantivity [32], but it lacks the tissue-dissolving properties of NaOCl. EDTA, conversely, is effective at removing the smear layer and enhancing canal cleanliness but does not eliminate bacteria as effectively [33].

A more comprehensive perspective involves exploring protocols that combine sequentially these irrigants to balance their strengths and weaknesses. For example, using NaOCl for its tissue-dissolving ability and CHX for its antimicrobial substantivity can enhance disinfection while reducing risks associated with over-reliance on a single agent [34]. Understanding the interplay between different irrigants and tailoring their use to patient-specific needs can optimize clinical outcomes and minimize adverse effects.

Chlorhexidine (CHX) belongs to the category of cationic antimicrobial agents and exhibits broad-spectrum antibacterial activity. It effectively eliminates *E. faecalis* biofilm at a concentration of 2% and reduces bacterial types and quantities in initially infected root canals [35]. Chlorhexidine gluconate penetrates bacterial cells, inducing leakage of intracellular components and leading to cell death. Gram-positive bacteria are particularly susceptible due to their negatively charged nature [36]. Chlorhexidine is less favored among Romanian dentists, beginning to be used after 1999 and ranking third in preference after hypochlorite and hydrogen peroxide.

EDTA (ethylenediaminetetraacetic acid) ranks fourth in preference among Romanian dentists. It functions as a calcium chelator, removing minerals from the smear layer of root canal walls. Nevertheless, it is essential to consider the risk of dentin erosion in the study of Monea et al., who warned that the chelating agents, particularly EDTA, exhibited a significant decalcifying effect [37]. The smear layer can impede the penetration of chemical irrigants and serve as a bacterial habitat. EDTA is commonly used with NaOCl (2.5%) to eliminate the smear layer in clinical practice [38].

MTAD (a mixture of tetracycline, acid, and detergent) is used by a small percentage (0.23%) of practitioners in this study as an endodontic irrigant.

As for interim medication, calcium hydroxide ($Ca(OH)_2$) is widely used in root canals for its disinfectant properties, achieved by releasing hydroxyl ions in water, creating an alkaline environment. Additionally, it neutralizes bacterial endotoxins on root dentin and promotes tissue repair by reducing inflammatory acidic chemicals [39,40]. $Ca(OH)_2$ also supports the healing of periapical hard tissues and the development of mineralized tissues [41,42]. However, its effectiveness as an intracanal medication is limited against specific pathogens such as *E. faecalis* and *Candida albicans* [43]. As for interim medication, calcium hydroxide remains the most commonly used (67%), with antibiotic paste ranking second, utilized more than six times less frequently by dentists in the study (10%). Other studies also indicate that antibiotics as interim endodontic medication are not widely employed due to their limited effectiveness and the potential for bacterial resistance. Triple antibiotic paste, combining metronidazole, minocycline, and ciprofloxacin, is recognized for its effective antimicrobial treatment and is commonly used in regenerative endodontic procedures [44,45].

According to this study, iodoform is used significantly less frequently than calcium hydroxide as interim medication (6.4%). Literature on this subject is scarce, with few references, particularly regarding Vitapex paste, a mixture of calcium hydroxide, iodoform, and polysiloxane oil. Vitapex possesses antibacterial properties and inhibits the reproduction of residual bacteria in the endodontic system. It promotes the healing of periapical lesions with a minimal inflammatory response in surrounding tissues [46,47].

Regarding sealants used for endodontic filling, epoxy resin-based sealers are preferred by the dentists participating in the study because of their performance in root canal treatments (35.5%). Comparative trials have demonstrated that epoxy resin-based sealers exhibit superior sealing properties, leading to better clinical outcomes for patients with chronic apical periodontitis [48]. Epoxy sealers also demonstrate effective penetration into dentinal tubules, crucial for successful endodontic treatment [49]. Despite various sealants available on the market, epoxy resin sealers maintain their physical and bioactive properties, making them a preferred choice in endodontic procedures [50].

Calcium hydroxide-based sealants rank second in this study (23.5%). These sealers are widely used in root canal treatments due to their antimicrobial properties [51]. Resinous endodontic sealers containing calcium hydroxide have shown promising results in biocompatibility, antibacterial effects, and promotion of biomineralization and collagen maturation. They are effective against *Enterococcus faecalis* [52]. Furthermore, compared with bioceramic sealers, calcium hydroxide sealers have demonstrated superior pH, calcium ion release, and antibacterial effects against *E. faecalis* [52]. Zinc oxide eugenol sealers rank third among the preferences of doctors participating in the study (19.9%), approximately half as often as epoxy resin and nearly equal to calcium hydroxide-based sealers. Sealers utilizing zinc oxide eugenol (ZOE) have been widely and successfully used for many years. Various brands and formulations exist, with zinc oxide as the primary component. Originally, eugenol served as the liquid component in Grossman's original composition, alongside sodium borate (anhydrous), bismuth subcarbonate, hydrogenated resin, zinc oxide, and barium sulfate [53,54]. Even today, new zinc oxide eugenol sealers like EssenSeal have emerged, described by Gaeta et al. as a reliable alternative for root canal sealing [55].

In many developed countries, bioceramic sealers have become standard in endodontics due to their superior properties that enhance the success of root canal treatments. These sealers are known for their biocompatibility, excellent sealing ability, and potential to improve root strength post-filling [56]. They also exhibit antibacterial properties, which are crucial in preventing reinfection of the root canal system [57]. Moreover, bioceramic sealers can augment the bioactivity of the dentin interface, facilitating hydroxyapatite production and enhancing the sealing and integration properties of the material [58]. Their use is also gaining momentum in developing regions, where improvements in dental technology and materials are becoming more accessible. However, cost and availability remain limiting factors in some areas. The global trend towards bioceramic sealers reflects a shift towards more predictable and efficient treatment outcomes in endodontics, with these materials being widely regarded as a key innovation in modern root canal therapy [13,59,60]. The use of bioceramic sealers in clinical practice varies among studies. This study shows that endodontic sealers are used on a much smaller scale than global trends, despite their proven advantages in improving treatment outcomes. Only 13.3% of participants preferred bioceramic sealers, ranking last. A survey in Bulgaria indicated that most dentists do not find bioceramic sealers necessary for endodontic treatments [61]. However, clinical studies have reported a high success rate of 99% when using bioceramic sealers with warm gutta-percha filling techniques [15]. An online questionnaire revealed that 51.70% of dentists use bioceramic sealers, citing improved properties as the primary reason [62]. The study also highlighted differences in bioceramic sealer application between general dental practitioners and endodontic specialists, underscoring the need for standardized usage guidelines [12]. In Diaconu et al.'s study [25], another study on the current practices of dentists in Romania, it is mentioned that when questioned about the use of bioceramics in their daily practice, 61% of respondents with postgraduate training in endodontics preferred the use of bioceramics for filling root canals [25]; however, in our study, the percentage of dentists with practice limited to endodontics is very small. Although it belongs to the category of biomaterials, being biologically compatible, mechanical, functional, and corrosion-resistant and quickly adapting to clinical and laboratory technologies [5], clinicians face challenges with bioceramic sealers due to difficulties in removal during nonsurgical retreatments, variable clinical practices, and limited evidence supporting their use [63–65].

Regarding filling techniques, participants in the study overwhelmingly prefer warm techniques (74.13%) over cold techniques (25.87%). This preference aligns with literature findings, as warm thermoplastic filling materials offer superior dentinal adaptation and a more uniform seal than traditional cold lateral condensation methods [66]. Warm gutta-percha techniques also result in fewer voids during filling and superior outcomes in apical sealing, adaptation to root canal morphology, and reduced void formation [67].

There is no conclusive evidence in endodontics favoring single-visit versus multiple-visit root canal treatments. Both approaches demonstrate similar effectiveness and complication rates [68]. Single-visit endodontics can be particularly effective for cases of irreversible pulpitis when carefully selected and following established protocols [69]. If periodontal pathology is also present, the treatment could be extended as needed, combining nonsurgical periodontal therapy with a 7-day course of antibiotics [70]. The decision between single or multiple visits should consider factors such as case complexity, patient comfort, and treatment success rates, emphasizing the importance of individualized treatment planning in Romanian endodontic practices. More than half of the participants in this study were observed to perform endodontic treatment in two separate sessions.

This study complements the findings of the endodontic materials research by showcasing the broader trends in material selection across the endodontic field. By identifying preferences, influencing factors, and trends, this research and the study of Olariu et al. [71] and Diaconu et al. [25] seek to contribute to a better understanding of regional practices and provide insights that can improve international collaboration and significantly innovate and advance dental care. These studies contribute to the growing shift towards more advanced materials, providing valuable data for manufacturers, educators, and policymakers in the dental field. They underscore the evolving landscape of dental materials in Romania, pointing to challenges and opportunities for improving treatment outcomes and reflecting global trends in dental material innovation [25,71].

The study's limitations include the potential for sample bias; when analyzing the results, it is essential to recognize the limitations inherent in cross-sectional surveys, such as possible biases arising from questionnaires. One key aspect to consider is the need for diverse representation in the sample, which can help ensure a comprehensive understanding of contemporary dental practices. Emerging trends, such as the increasing reliance on CBCT (Cone Beam Computed Tomography) examination and the use of magnification tools, hold significant potential for advancing the precision and scope of endodontic procedures. These developments could form the basis of a broader study, allowing for a detailed exploration of their impact on diagnostic accuracy and clinical outcomes. Despite these constraints, such surveys offer valuable insights, enabling professionals to keep pace with evolving endodontic materials and techniques.

5. Conclusions

This study concludes a trend towards high-performance endodontic materials in Romania, mirroring global preferences. Sodium hypochlorite is the preferred irrigant, while chlorhexidine is less frequently used. Epoxy resin sealers dominate endodontic procedures, whereas bioceramic sealers are currently employed in a minority of root canal fillings, which contrasts with international trends. Thermoplasticized gutta-percha is favored for filling techniques. Calcium hydroxide remains the primary choice for interim medication.

The findings from this research provide a valuable repository of data on preferred endodontic materials in Romania, for further use by researchers. This study offers valuable insights into current preferences of Romanian dentists regarding endodontic materials, highlighting trends in using various sealers, irrigants, and filling techniques. The findings can inform future research and guide clinicians in selecting the most suitable materials for effective root canal treatments. Additionally, these insights can be applied in educational settings to enhance training programs and help dental practitioners stay updated with evolving trends in endodontics. These programs could bridge the gap between research findings and clinical application, empowering practitioners to adopt innovative techniques confidently and effectively. Furthermore, the data could help manufacturers and suppliers to better understand market needs and refine their product offerings. To strengthen the evidence base, longitudinal studies should be conducted to evaluate various materials' long-term durability and biocompatibility. Furthermore, comparative studies on contemporary materials would provide essential insights to assist clinicians in selecting the most appropriate options for diverse clinical scenarios.

Author Contributions: Conceptualization, D.M., I.V. and M.-M.M.; methodology, I.O.; software, I.V.; validation, R.A.P. and D.E.P.; formal analysis, R.A.P. and D.E.P.; investigation, D.M., I.V. and I.O.; resources, M.-M.M., D.M. and I.O.; data curation, I.O.; writing—original draft preparation, D.M. and I.V.; writing—review and editing, R.A.P. and D.E.P.; visualization, I.O.; supervision, D.M. and R.A.P.; project administration, D.M. All authors have read and agreed to the published version of the manuscript.

Funding: This research received no external funding.

Institutional Review Board Statement: This study was conducted by the Declaration of Helsinki. The study has been approved by the Ethics Committee of Victor Babes University of Medicine and Pharmacy in Timisoara, Romania, approval code: No. 73/02.10.2023.

Informed Consent Statement: Informed consent was obtained from all subjects involved in the study.

Data Availability Statement: The data presented in this study are available on request from the corresponding author. The data are not publicly available due to privacy and ethical reasons.

Conflicts of Interest: The authors declare no conflicts of interest.

References

1. Yue, L.; Wang, X.Y. *Cariology and Endodontics*, 3rd ed.; Peking University Medical Press: Beijing, China, 2020.
2. Mensudar, R.; Sukumaran, V.G.; Julius, A. Evaluation of current trends in endodontic treatment procedure among the dental practitioners. *Int. J. Dent. Health Sci.* **2014**, *1*, 861–868.
3. De Souza, R.A.; De Castro, P.F.L.; Pires, O.J. Research of the major methods and clinical outcomes of irrigation in endodontics: A systematic review. *MedNEXT J. Med. Health Sci.* **2022**, *3* (Suppl. S3). [CrossRef]
4. Zou, X.; Zheng, X.; Liang, Y.; Zhang, C.; Fan, B.; Liang, J.; Ling, J.; Bian, Z.; Yu, Q.; Hou, B.; et al. Expert consensus on irrigation and intracanal medication in root canal therapy. *Int. J. Oral Sci.* **2024**, *16*, 23. [CrossRef]
5. Tofan, S.A.; Olteanu, C.; Szuhanek, C.; Popovici, R.A.; Luca, M.M.; Iftode, A.; Pavel, I.Z.; Bonta, D.F. Synthesis and comparative characterization of different microparticles used as biomaterials in dentistry. *Mater. Plast.* **2021**, *58*, 192–200. [CrossRef]
6. Caussin, E.; Izart, M.; Ceinos, R.; Attal, J.-P.; Beres, F.; François, P. Advanced Material Strategy for Restoring Damaged Endodontically Treated Teeth: A Comprehensive Review. *Materials* **2024**, *17*, 3736. [CrossRef] [PubMed]
7. Lile, I.E.; Osser, G.; Negruțiu, B.M.; Valea, C.N.; Vaida, L.L.; Marian, D.; Dulceanu, R.C.; Bulzan, C.O.; Herlo, J.N.; Gag, O.L.; et al. The Structures–Reactivity Relationship on Dental Plaque and Natural Products. *Appl. Sci.* **2023**, *13*, 9111. [CrossRef]
8. Ford, T.R.P.; Rhodes, J.S.; Ford, H.E.P. *Endodontics: Problem-Solving in Clinical Practice*; Taylor & Francis: Oxford, UK, 2002; ISBN 9780323068888.
9. Dobrzańska, J.; Dobrzański, L.B.; Dobrzański, L.A.; Gołombek, K.; Dobrzańska-Danikiewicz, A.D. Is Gutta-Percha Still the "Gold Standard" among Filling Materials in Endodontic Treatment? *Processes* **2021**, *9*, 1467. [CrossRef]

10. Cheung, M.C.; Parashos, P. Current Endodontic Practice and Use of Newer Technologies in Australia and New Zealand. *Aust. Dent. J.* **2023**, *68*, 186–196. [CrossRef] [PubMed]
11. Sasidharan, R. Knowledge, Materials, Methods, and Attitudes Employed during Endodontic Treatment by Dentists to Evaluate and Improve the Quality of Practice of Endodontic Treatment. *Int. J. Prev. Clin. Dent. Res.* **2022**, *9*, 91–94. [CrossRef]
12. Guivarc'h, M.; Jeanneau, C.; Giraud, T.; Pommel, L.; About, I.; Azim, A.A.; Bukiet, F. An International Survey on the Use of Calcium Silicate-Based Sealers in Non-Surgical Endodontic Treatment. *Clin. Oral Investig.* **2020**, *24*, 417–424. [CrossRef]
13. Pendse, G.; Misra, R.; Vandekar, M.; Shah, A.; Hegde, P.; Hulyal, S. Bioceramic Sealers in Endodontics: A Literature Review. *Glob. J. Res. Anal.* **2024**, *13*, 56–59. [CrossRef]
14. Zanza, A.; Reda, R.; Pagnoni, F.; Patil, S. Future Trends in Endodontics: How Could Materials Increase the Long-Term Outcome of Root Canal Therapies? *Materials* **2022**, *15*, 3473. [CrossRef] [PubMed]
15. Zamparini, F.; Spinelli, A.; Cardinali, F.; Ausiello, P.; Gandolfi, M.G.; Prati, C. The Use of Premixed Calcium Silicate Bioceramic Sealer with Warm Carrier-Based Technique: A 2-Year Study for Patients Treated in a Master Program. *J. Funct. Biomater.* **2023**, *14*, 164. [CrossRef] [PubMed]
16. Team DATAtab e.U. Graz, Austria. Available online: https://datatab.net (accessed on 14 April 2024).
17. Zhu, M.; Dang, J.; Dong, F.; Zhong, R.; Zhang, J.; Pan, J.; Li, Y. Antimicrobial and cleaning effects of ultrasonic-mediated plasma-loaded microbubbles on Enterococcus faecalis biofilm: An in vitro study. *BMC Oral Health* **2023**, *23*, 133. [CrossRef]
18. Al-Mallah, S.; Al-Naimi, M.A. An Evaluation of Cytotoxicity of Iron Oxide Nanoparticles with Hydrogen Peroxide Endodontic Irrigant. *Al-Rafidain Dent. J.* **2021**, *23*, 1–8. [CrossRef]
19. Láng, O.; Nagy, K.S.; Láng, J.; Perczel-Kovách, K.; Herczegh, A.; Lohinai, Z.; Varga, G. Comparative study of hyperpure chlorine dioxide with two other irrigants regarding the viability of periodontal ligament stem cells. *Clin. Oral Investig.* **2021**, *25*, 2981–2992. [CrossRef] [PubMed]
20. Parisay, I.; Talebi, M.; Asadi, S.; Sharif, M.A.; Nikbakht, M.H. Antimicrobial Efficacy of 2.5% Sodium Hypochlorite, 2% Chlorhexidine, and 1.5% Hydrogen Peroxide on Enterococcus Faecalis in Pulpectomy of Necrotic Primary Teeth. *J. Dent. Mater. Tech.* **2021**, *10*, 94–101. [CrossRef]
21. Dutner, J.; Mines, P.; Anderson, A. Irrigation trends.among American Association of Endodontists members:.a web-based survey. *J. Endod.* **2012**, *38*, 37–40. [CrossRef] [PubMed]
22. Willershausen, I.; Wolf, T.G.; Schmidtmann, I.; Berger, C.; Ehlers, V.; Willershausen, B.; Briseño, B. Survey of rootcanal irrigating solutions used in dental practiceswithin Germany. *Int. Endod. J.* **2014**, *48*, 654–660. [CrossRef] [PubMed]
23. Boutsioukis, C.; Arias-Moliz, M.T. Present status and future directions—Irrigants and irrigation methods. *Int. Endod. J.* **2022**, *55*, 588–612. [CrossRef]
24. Puleio, F.; Lizio, A.S.; Coppini, V.; Lo Giudice, R.; Lo Giudice, G. CBCT-Based Assessment of Vapor Lock Effects on Endodontic Disinfection. *Appl. Sci.* **2023**, *13*, 9542. [CrossRef]
25. Diaconu, C.T.; Gheorghiță, L.M.; Diaconu, A.E.; Țuculină, M.J.; Gliga, A.; Gaeta, C.; Grandini, S.; Marinescu, I.R.; Amărăscu, M.O.; Diaconu, O.A. Current Endodontic Practices among Romanian Dental Practitioners: A Cross-Sectional Study. *Dent. J.* **2024**, *12*, 283. [CrossRef] [PubMed]
26. Estrela, C.; Estrela, C.R.; Barbin, E.L.; Spanó, J.C.; Marchesan, M.A.; Pécora, J.D. Mechanism of action of sodium hypochlorite. *Braz. Dent. J.* **2002**, *13*, 113–117. [CrossRef] [PubMed]
27. Basrani, B. *Endodontic Irrigation: Chemical Disinfection of the Root Canal System*; Springer: Cham, Switzerland, 2015; ISBN 3319164554.
28. Cai, C.; Chen, X.; Li, Y.; Jiang, Q. Advances in the Role of Sodium Hypochlorite Irrigant in Chemical Preparation of Root Canal Treatment. *BioMed Res. Int.* **2023**, *2023*, 8858283. [CrossRef]
29. Shirdar, M.R.; Taheri, M.M.; Qi, M.-L.; Gohery, S.; Farajpour, N.; Narayanan, S.; Foroozan, T.; Sharifi-Asl, S.; Shahbazian-Yassar, R.; Shokuhfar, T. Optimization of the Mechanical Properties and the Cytocompatibility for the PMMA Nanocomposites Reinforced with the Hydroxyapatite Nanofibers and the Magnesium Phosphate Nanosheets. *Materials* **2021**, *14*, 5893. [CrossRef]
30. Brandão-Neto, D.; Mello, J.; Marceliano-Alves, M.; Carvalho, C.T.; Marceliano, E.; Galhardi, M.; Tavares, V.; Muzy, D.A.; Lins, R. Final Endodontic Irrigation with 2% Peracetic Acid: Antimicrobial Activity and Cytotoxicity. *Eur. J. Dent.* **2021**, *15*, 533–538. [CrossRef]
31. Mostafa, M.; El-Shrief, Y.; Anous, W.; Hassan, M.; Salamah, F.; El Boghdadi, R.; El-Bayoumi, M.; Seyam, R.; Abd-El-Kader, K.; Amin, S. Postoperative pain following endodontic irrigation using 1.3% versus 5.25% sodium hypochlorite in mandibular molars with necrotic pulps: A randomized double-blind clinical trial. *Int. Endod. J.* **2020**, *53*, 154–166. [CrossRef]
32. Sebbane, N.; Abramovitz, I.; Kot-Limon, N.; Steinberg, D. Mechanistic Insight into the Anti-Bacterial/Anti-Biofilm Effects of Low Chlorhexidine Concentrations on Enterococcus faecalis—In Vitro Study. *Microorganisms* **2024**, *12*, 2297. [CrossRef]
33. Baruwa, A.O.; Martins, J.N.R.; Maravic, T.; Mazzitelli, C.; Mazzoni, A.; Ginjeira, A. Effect of Endodontic Irrigating Solutions on Radicular Dentine Structure and Matrix Metalloproteinases—A Comprehensive Review. *Dent. J.* **2022**, *10*, 219. [CrossRef] [PubMed]

34. Czopik, B.; Woźniakiewicz, A.; Świętoniowska, N.; Zarzecka, J.; Woźniakiewicz, M. Quantitative Insight into PCA Formation following Different Chlorhexidine Activation Methods in Endodontic Treatment. *Molecules* **2023**, *28*, 6159. [CrossRef]
35. Ferreira, N.S.; Martinho, F.C.; Cardoso, F.G.R.; Nascimento, G.G.; Carvalho, C.A.T.; Valera, M.C. Microbiological profile resistant to different intracanal medications in primary endodontic infections. *J. Endod.* **2015**, *41*, 824–830. [CrossRef] [PubMed]
36. Cintra, L.T.A.; Watanabe, S.; Samuel, R.O.; da Silva Facundo, A.C.; de Azevedo Queiroz, I.O.; Dezan-Júnior, E.; Gomes-Filho, J.E. The use of NaOCl in combination with CHX produces cytotoxic product. *Clin. Oral Investig.* **2014**, *18*, 935–940. [CrossRef]
37. Monea, M.D.; Olah, P.; Cerghizan, D.; Earar, K.; Budacu, C.; Bică, C. The effectiveness of endodontic irrigating solutions on smear layer removal from radicular dentin a scanning electron microscopic study. *Mater. Plast.* **2016**, *53*, 339–341.
38. Topbas, C.; Adiguzel, O. Endodontic Irrigation Solutions: A Review. *Int. Dent. Res.* **2017**, *7*, 54–61. [CrossRef]
39. Siqueira, J.F.; Lopes, H.P. Mechanisms of antimicrobial activity of calcium hydroxide: A critical review. *Int. Endod. J.* **1999**, *32*, 361–369. [CrossRef]
40. Mohammadi, Z.; Dummer, P.M.H. Properties and applications of calciumhydroxide in endodontics and dental traumatology. *Int. Endod. J.* **2011**, *44*, 697–730. [CrossRef]
41. Alfadda, S.; Alquria, T.; Karaismailoglu, E.; Aksel, H.; AZIM, A.A. Antibacterial effect and bioactivity of innovative and currently used intracanal medicaments in regenerative endodontics. *J. Endod.* **2021**, *47*, 1294–1300. [CrossRef]
42. Lu, J.; Liu, H.; Lu, Z.; Kahler, B.; Lin, L.M. Regenerative endodontic procedures for traumatized immature permanent teeth with severe external root resorption and root perforation. *J. Endod.* **2020**, *46*, 1610–1615. [CrossRef] [PubMed]
43. Van Der Waal, S.V.; Connert, T.; Crielaard, W.; De Soet, J.J. In mixed biofilms Enterococcus faecalis benefits from a calcium hydroxide challenge and culturing. *Int. Endod. J.* **2016**, *49*, 865–873. [CrossRef]
44. Ordinola-Zapata, R.; Bramante, C.M.; Minotti, P.G.; Cavenago, B.C.; Garcia, R.B.; Bernardineli, N.; Jaramillo, D.E.; Duarte, M.A.H. Antimicrobial activity of triantibiotic paste, 2% chlorhexidine gel, and calcium hydroxide on an intraoral-infected dentin biofilm model. *J. Endod.* **2013**, *39*, 115–118.
45. Wei, X.; Yang, M.; Yue, L.; Huang, D.; Zhou, X.; Wang, X.; Zhang, Q.; Qiu, L.; Huang, Z.; Wang, H.; et al. Expert consensus on regenerative endodontic procedures. *Int. J. Oral Sci.* **2022**, *14*, 55. [CrossRef] [PubMed]
46. Agarwal, S.R.; Bendgude, V.D.; Kakodkar, P. Evaluation of success rate of lesion sterilization and tissue repair compared to Vitapex in pulpally involved primary teeth: A systematic review. *J. Conserv. Dent.* **2019**, *22*, 510–515. [CrossRef]
47. Han, J.L.; He, H.; Xu, Z.; Gu, T.; Zhang, L.D.; Zhu, Y.Q. Clinical study on prevention root absorption after teeth replantation with Vitapex paste. *Shanghai Kou Qiang Yi Xue* **2010**, *19*, 346–348. [PubMed]
48. Horhat, R.M.; Bumbu, B.A.; Orel, L.; Velea-Barta, O.; Cirligeriu, L.; Chicin, G.N.; Pricop, M.; Rivis, M.; Dinu, S.; Horhat, D.I.; et al. Assessing the Sealing Performance and Clinical Outcomes of Endodontic Treatment in Patients with Chronic Apical Periodontitis Using Epoxy Resin and Calcium Salicylate Seals. *Medicina* **2023**, *59*, 1137. [CrossRef] [PubMed]
49. Wilkoński, W.; Krupiński, M.; Jamróz-Wilkońska, L.; Kepczynski, M.; Zapotoczny, S.; Maziarz, U.; Opiła, J.; Wychowański, P.; Brus-Sawczuk, K. The Influence of Irrigating Solutions on the Penetration of Epoxy AH Plus Sealer in Dentinal Tubules—In Vitro Confocal Microscopy Study. *Appl. Sci.* **2023**, *13*, 7714. [CrossRef]
50. Moraes, T.G.; Menezes, A.S.; Grazziotin-Soares, R.; Moraes, R.; Ferreira, P.V.C.; Carvalho, C.N.; Bauer, J.; Carvalho, E.M. Impact of Immersion Media on Physical Properties and Bioactivity of Epoxy Resin-Based and Bioceramic Endodontic Sealers. *Polymers* **2022**, *14*, 729. [CrossRef]
51. Suwartini, T.; Santoso, J.; Widyarman, A.S.; Ratnasari, D. Efficacy of Bioceramic and Calcium Hydroxide-Based Root Canal Sealers against Pathogenic Endodontic Biofilms: An In vitro Study. *Contemp. Clin. Dent.* **2022**, *13*, 322–330. [CrossRef] [PubMed]
52. Bueno, C.R.E.; Benetti, F.; Cury, M.T.S.; Vasques, A.M.V.; Cosme-Silva, L.; Queiroz, Í.O.A.; Da Silva, A.C.R.; Jacinto, R.C.; Cintra, L.T.A.; Dezan-Junior, E. Biological investigation of resinous endodontic sealers containing calcium hydroxide. *PLoS ONE* **2023**, *18*, e0287890. [CrossRef]
53. Hauman, C.H.; Love, R.M. Biocompatibility of dental materials used in contemporary endodontic therapy: A review. Part Root canal filling materials. *Int. Endod. J.* **2003**, *36*, 147–160. [CrossRef]
54. Grossman, L.I. *Endodontic Practice*, 10th ed.; Lea & Febiger: Philadelphia, PA, USA, 1982; p. 297.
55. Gaeta, C.; Marruganti, C.; Mignosa, E.; Malvicini, G.; Verniani, G.; Tonini, R.; Grandini, S. Comparison of physico-chemical properties of zinc oxide eugenol cement and a bioceramic sealer. *Aust. Endod. J.* **2022**, *49*, 187–193. [CrossRef]
56. Haji, T.H.; Selivany, B.J.; Suliman, A.A. Sealing Ability: In Vitro Study and Biocompatibility: In Vivo Animal Study of Different Bioceramic-Based Sealers. *Clin. Exp. Dent. Res.* **2022**, *8*, 1582–1590. [CrossRef]
57. Dong, X.; Xu, X. Bioceramics in Endodontics: Updates and Future Perspectives. *Bioengineering* **2023**, *10*, 354. [CrossRef] [PubMed]
58. Marta, M.-M.; Chivu, O.R.; Marian, D.; Enache, I.-C.; Veja, I.; Pitic, D.E.; Flueras, R.; Popovici, R.A.; Stana, A.H.; Cojocariu, C.; et al. Elemental Composition and Dentin Bioactivity at the Interface with AH Plus Bioceramic Sealer: An Energy-Dispersive X-Ray Spectroscopy Study. *Appl. Sci.* **2024**, *14*, 11867. [CrossRef]

59. Marques Ferreira, M.; Martinho, J.P.; Duarte, I.; Mendonça, D.; Craveiro, A.C.; Botelho, M.F.; Carrilho, E.; Miguel Marto, C.; Coelho, A.; Paula, A.; et al. Evaluation of the Sealing Ability and Bond Strength of Two Endodontic Root Canal Sealers: An In Vitro Study. *Dent. J.* **2022**, *10*, 201. [CrossRef] [PubMed]
60. Estivalet, M.S.; de Araújo, L.P.; Immich, F.; da Silva, A.F.; Ferreira, N.d.S.; da Rosa, W.L.d.O.; Piva, E. Bioactivity Potential of Bioceramic-Based Root Canal Sealers: A Scoping Review. *Life* **2022**, *12*, 1853. [CrossRef]
61. Stefanova, V.; Zhekov, K.; Raycheva, R. Application of bioceramic endodontic sealers in clinical practice. *J. Pak. Med. Assoc.* **2023**, *73*, 816–820. [CrossRef] [PubMed]
62. Pontoriero, D.I.K.; Ferrari Cagidiaco, E.; Maccagnola, V.; Manfredini, D.; Ferrari, M. Outcomes of Endodontic-Treated Teeth Obturated with Bioceramic Sealers in Combination with Warm Gutta-Percha Obturation Techniques: A Prospective Clinical Study. *J. Clin. Med.* **2023**, *12*, 2867. [CrossRef]
63. Al-Haddad, A.; Che, A.B.; Aziz, Z.A. Bioceramic-Based Root Canal Sealers: A Review. *Int. J. Biomater.* **2016**, *2016*, 9753210. [CrossRef]
64. Oltra, E.; Cox, T.C.; Lacourse, M.R.; Johnson, J.D.; Paranjpe, A. Retreatability of two endodontic sealers, endosequence BC sealer and AH plus: A micro-computed tomographic comparison. *Restor. Dent. Endod.* **2017**, *42*, 19–26. [CrossRef] [PubMed]
65. Washio, A.; Morotomi, T.; Yoshii, S.; Kitamura, C. Bioactive Glass-Based Endodontic Sealer as a Promising Root Canal Filling Material without Semisolid Core Materials. *Materials* **2019**, *12*, 3967. [CrossRef] [PubMed]
66. Raghuwanshi, S.; Jain, P.; Patni, P.M.; Pandey, S.H.; Hiremath, H.; Baghel, S. Dentinal Adaptation of Warm Thermoplastic Obturating Material and Cold Thermoplastic Obturating Material: An In Vitro Study. *Contemp. Clin. Dent.* **2019**, *10*, 64–68. [CrossRef] [PubMed]
67. Bhandi, S.; Mashyakhy, M.; Abumelha, A.S.; Alkahtany, M.F.; Jamal, M.; Chohan, H.; Raj, A.T.; Testarelli, L.; Reda, R.; Patil, S. Complete Obturation—Cold Lateral Condensation vs. Thermoplastic Techniques: A Systematic Review of Micro-CT Studies. *Materials* **2021**, *14*, 4013. [CrossRef]
68. Mergoni, G.; Ganim, M.; Lodi, G.; Figini, L.; Gagliani, M.; Manfredi, M. Single versus multiple visits for endodontic treatment of permanent teeth. *Cochrane Database Syst. Rev.* **2022**, *12*. [CrossRef]
69. Ahmed, F.; Thosar, N.; Baliga, M.S.; Rathi, N. Single visit endodontic therapy: A review. *Austin J. Dent.* **2016**, *3*, 1035.
70. Boia, S.; Boariu, M.; Baderca, F.; Rusu, D.; Muntean, D.; Horhat, F.; Boia, E.R.; Borza, C.; Anghel, A.; Stratul, Ş.I. Clinical, microbiological and oxidative stress evaluation of periodontitis patients treated with two regimens of systemic antibiotics, adjunctive to non-surgical therapy: A placebo-controlled randomized clinical trial. *Exp. Ther. Med.* **2019**, *18*, 5001–5015. [CrossRef] [PubMed]
71. Olariu, I.; Marian, D.; Veja, I.; Flueras, R.; Popovici, R.A.; Pitic, D.E.; Stana, H.A.; Vaida, L.L.; Lile, I.E. Exploring Dentists' Preferences in Selecting Adhesive Systems: A Survey Analysis. *Appl. Sci.* **2024**, *14*, 10119. [CrossRef]

applied sciences

MDPI

Systematic Review

Effect of the Incorporation of Compounds into Digitally Manufactured Dental Materials—A Systematic Review

Ana Bettencourt [1], Catarina Jorge [2], Vitor Anes [3,4,*] and Cristina Bettencourt Neves [5,*]

1 Research Institute for Medicines (iMed.ULisboa), Faculdade de Farmácia, Universidade de Lisboa, 1649-003 Lisbon, Portugal; abettencourt@edu.ulisboa.pt
2 Faculdade de Farmácia, Universidade de Lisboa, 1649-003 Lisbon, Portugal
3 Instituto Superior de Engenharia de Lisboa, 1959-007 Lisbon, Portugal
4 Mechanical Engineering Institute (IDMEC), Instituto Superior Técnico, Universidade de Lisboa, 1049-001 Lisbon, Portugal
5 Dental Biomaterials Research Group (BIOMAT), Biomedical and Oral Sciences Research Unit (UICOB), Faculdade de Medicina Dentária, Universidade de Lisboa, 1600-277 Lisbon, Portugal
* Correspondence: vitor.anes@isel.pt (V.A.); mneves@edu.ulisboa.pt (C.B.N.)

Abstract: The aim of this review was to evaluate if the properties of digitally produced dental acrylic resins improved when reinforced with compounds. A literature search was conducted in PubMed, Web of Science, and Scopus databases for the past 10 years. Combinations of keywords were chosen to reflect the PICO question: Do digitally produced dental acrylic resins loaded with compounds have better mechanical, surface and/or biological properties than resins without compounds? The selection was carried out by two independent researchers according to the PRISMA flowchart and specific eligibility criteria. Results: The 19 in vitro studies included dealt with incorporated compounds such as zirconium dioxide nanoparticles, graphene nanoplatelets, and zwitterionic compounds. It was found that some compounds had a negative impact on the mechanical and surface properties, while others showed improvements. Most of the loaded resins had more effective antimicrobial activity compared to the controls. There were also differences in biocompatibility depending on the type of compound incorporated. The compounds affect the mechanical and surface properties of loaded acrylic resins, depending on the type and concentration of the compound. In the case of antimicrobial activity and biocompatibility, the results depended on other factors than the chemical composition of the compound included in the resin.

Keywords: dental materials; incorporation; CAD-CAM resin; mechanical properties; antimicrobial activity; biocompatibility

1. Introduction

The geriatric population is increasing due to scientific and technological advances in healthcare, which increase the average life expectancy of the population [1]. Tooth loss is a very common dental problem in this population and has an impact on food swallowing, appearance, and quality of life [2]. Rehabilitation of partial or complete tooth loss can be achieved with a fixed or removable dental prosthesis that improves functional and aesthetic performance [1,3].

Complete dentures for edentulous people were fabricated using conventional methods that involved several clinical and laboratory steps, such as making impressions and plaster models, testing, and selecting the most suitable prosthesis [4]. With the introduction of digital manufacturing technology, the production of prostheses should be optimized and accelerated compared to conventional methods, which means fewer clinical appointments, faster laboratory processes, and less material waste [5].

The use of computer-aided design (CAD) and computer-aided manufacturing (CAM) for the digital fabrication of structures is becoming increasingly common in dentistry, particularly in the fabrication of removable dentures, and this fabrication process involves methods of subtraction and addition [5]. The most common CAD-CAM manufacturing technique in the addition method is rapid prototyping, and in the subtraction method, it is milling. Rapid prototyping uses 3D printing techniques in which the resin is applied layer by layer and then polymerized with various light sources such as visible, ultraviolet and laser light. CAD-CAM milling, on the other hand, is a manufacturing process in which a pre-polymerized resin plate is subtracted [6].

Three-dimensional printing, especially stereolithography (SLA) and the digital light process (DLP), are widely used techniques. SLA is an additive manufacturing technique used for both polymeric and ceramic materials, especially for personalized orthodontic appliances. Compared to the other 3D printing techniques, the SLA process provides better results in terms of surface finish, higher mechanical strength, and greater geometric precision [6]. However, this method also has some disadvantages, as it cannot be sterilized by heat and is a very expensive technology used only for light-cured liquid polymers [7]. The advantages of DLP technology include high precision, smooth surface, fast execution, and lower cost, but it has the same disadvantages as stereolithography [8,9].

Polymethyl methacrylate (PMMA) is a synthetic polymer that is part of most acrylic resins. PMMA has long been used for the fabrication of dentures as it has numerous advantages: Ease of fabrication and repair, good patient acceptance, low cost, biocompatibility, odor and taste neutrality, and good esthetic properties [5]. However, it also has some disadvantages, such as low wear resistance, allergic reactions due to the release of monomers into the oral cavity, and, above all, a high susceptibility to microbial and fungal contamination [4,10–12].

In view of these problems associated with the use of PMMA, the incorporation of compounds into CAD-CAM dental materials is increasingly being investigated to improve the mechanical properties and, above all, to prevent the development of microorganisms. Some examples of compounds with antimicrobial properties are zinc dioxide nanoparticles [13], graphene nanoplatelets [14], silver-reinforced mesoporous silica nanoparticles [15], titanium dioxide [16], cellulose-silver nanocrystals [17], ceramic nitrides [18], zwitterionic materials [19], chlorhexidine [20–24], and tocopherol [25].

In dentistry, new CAD-CAM materials have also been developed that combine the properties of ceramics with those of resins. One example of this type of material is the infiltrated polymeric ceramic network [10]. Examples of other materials currently under investigation are nano-ceramic resins, which consist of 80% zirconia and silica clusters, and lithium disilicate ceramics, which consist of 40% lithium metasilicate crystals [26].

The aim of this systematic review was to analyze whether the compounds incorporated into the acrylic resins produced by CAD-CAM can improve their performance, i.e., surface and mechanical properties; their effectiveness of antimicrobial activity; and to ensure safety through cytotoxicity and genotoxicity tests.

2. Materials and Methods

2.1. PICO Question

A systematic literature search was conducted according to the PRISMA (Preferred Reporting Items for Systematic Reviews and Meta-analyses) guidelines [27,28] to answer the following PICO question: Do acrylic resins used in dentistry that are produced using CAD-CAM procedures with incorporated compounds have better mechanical, surface, and/or biological properties than resins without these compounds? (Problem: Acrylic resins produced using the CAD-CAM process; intervention: Incorporation of compounds; comparison: No incorporation of compounds; result: Mechanical and surface properties as well as antimicrobial and biocompatible properties of the resins) (Table S1). The proposal for the study was registered on the National Institute for Health Research, International Prospective Register of Systematic Reviews (PROSPERO) platform with the number CRD42024514141.

2.2. Inclusion and Exclusion Criteria

Inclusion and exclusion criteria were used in this systematic review. The inclusion criteria were articles incorporating compounds in acrylic resins, dealing with CAD-CAM technology in dental medicine, published in the last 10 years, describing in vitro experimental studies, and articles presenting the full version (full text). The exclusion criteria were systematic and narrative reviews; case studies; population studies (case-control and cohort studies); clinical studies; records written in languages other than English or Portuguese; other materials than acrylic resins; not dental materials; grey literature.

2.3. Bibliographical Research

From January to March 2023, a search was conducted in a primary database with MEDLINE, via the search engine PubMed, Web of science and Scopus with the following search equation ("dent*" OR "oral" OR "buccal") AND ("3D" OR "three-dimensional*" OR "print*" OR "CAD-CAM") AND ("acrylic resin" OR "polymethyl methacrylate" OR "poly-methyl methacrylate" OR "PMMA") AND ("incorporate" OR "compound" OR "nano*" OR "particle") AND ("mechanical*" OR toxicity* OR "biological" OR "antibacterial*" OR "antimicrobial" OR "antifungal").

After verification using an EndNote version 21 and exclusion of duplicates articles were assessed by two independent reviewers (CJ, CBN) based on their title and abstract. These reviewers analyzed the titles and abstracts of the selected articles against the inclusion and exclusion criteria. Discussions involving a third reviewer (AB) addressed any disparities in assessments regarding the appropriateness of the study. Subsequently, the full articles and the bibliographic references of each article were analyzed to find relevant articles in this field through a manual search.

2.4. Data Extraction

Extracted data was deposited in an Excel version 2021 sheet and included the characteristics of each study, such as the type of resin, the manufacturing process, the incorporated compound, and the analyzed properties of each study: surface properties, mechanical properties, antimicrobial activity, and biocompatibility.

2.5. Assessment of the Quality of Articles

To assess the quality of the articles that were included in the systematic review, a modified version of the "Guideline for Reporting Pre-clinical In Vitro Studies on Dental Materials" [29] was used. This guideline includes several evaluation items such as: Item 1: abstract, item 2: introduction (2a—background and 2b—objectives), methods (item 3—intervention, item 4—outcomes, item 5—sample size, item 6–9—various types of randomization, item 10—statistical methods), item 11—results, item 12—discussion (limitations), and other information (item 13—financing, item 14—protocols). Then, a total score of 15 points was used to classify each article, depending on the number of positive item assessments, with a score of 0–5 referring to an article with a low overall quality, 6–10 an article with an average overall quality, and a score of 11–15 being considered an article with a high overall quality.

3. Results

3.1. Results of the Bibliographical Research

A PRISMA-FLOW diagram was created to illustrate the results of this systematic review (Figure 1). The results of the bibliographic search in the databases yielded a total of 139 articles: 31 articles from PubMed, 53 articles from Web of Science, and 55 articles from Scopus. After excluding 49 duplicates, 90 articles remained and were evaluated based on their title and abstract according to the inclusion and exclusion criteria. In this phase, 68 articles were excluded: 36 articles did not include compounds, 5 did not mention CAD-CAM techniques, 11 were not acrylic resins, 7 were systematic reviews, 1 was a clinical study, 2 were grey literature, 1 article was written in Mandarin, and 5 articles did not discuss dental materials.

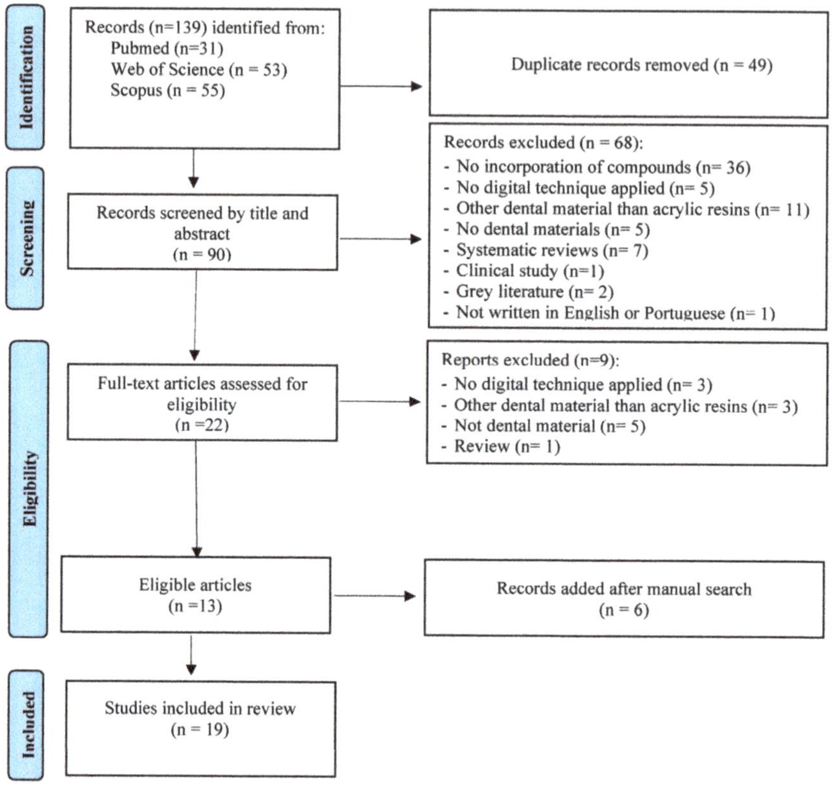

Figure 1. PRISMA-FLOW diagram used for the bibliographic search.

Thus, 22 articles were independently evaluated according to their full-text version to determine whether they met the previously defined criteria. In addition, a search was carried out in the bibliography of the selected articles to analyze which articles could be added manually. Six articles were added through the manual search. A total of 28 articles were analyzed, 9 of which were subsequently excluded because they did not meet the defined criteria. This left a total of 19 articles that could be included in the systematic review for data extraction.

3.2. Main Characteristics of the Studies Included in the Systematic Review

This systematic review includes articles on dental materials fabricated with CAD-CAM whose mechanical and biological properties were possibly modified by the incorporation of composite materials. Thus, 8 articles were analyzed in which the materials were printed using the additive SLA technique, 2 articles referred to fabrication by milling, 8 articles to DLP printing, and 1 article to daylight polymer printing (DPP).

The different compounds incorporated into the CAD-CAM-fabricated dental materials were zirconia nanoparticles (ZrO_2 NPs) [13,30,31], graphene [25], graphene oxide [32], graphene nanoplatelets (GNPs) [14,33], silver-reinforced mesoporous silica nanoparticles (Ag-MSN) [15], aluminum nitride [34], bioactive glasses [35], ceramic nitrides [18], zwitterionic particles [19], nanodiamonds [36], aminated nanodiamonds (A-ND) [37], titanium dioxide (TiO_2) nanoparticles [16,38–40], and silver-reinforced cellulose nanocrystals (Ag-CNCs) [17].

Another piece of information described in most studies is related to the size and distribution of the particles incorporated in the materials. The distribution is often referred to as uniform in the resin matrix [15,31] or forms regular agglomerates [17,37,38,40]. Particle size varied from 4–6 nm of aminated nanodiamonds [37] to 56–170 nm for TiO_2 nanoparticles [40] and 100–150 nm for ZrO_2 NPs [31] (Table 1).

Table 1. Main characteristics of the studies.

Study	Chemical Composition		Manufacturer	Manufacturing Technique	Distribution and Size of Particles	Quality Assessment Score
	Resin	Compound				
Khattar et al., 2023 [13]	PMMA-based resin	Zirconium dioxide nanoparticles (ZrO_2 NPs)	Denture 3D+, NextDent BV, Soesterberg, The Netherlands	SLA printing	Not determined	8 average
Selva-Otaolaurruchi et al., 2023 [32]	PMMA	Graphene oxide	Huge PMMA blocks, Huge Dental Material, Co., Beijing, China	Milling	Not determined	8 average
Salgado et al., 2023 [33]	PMMA-based resin	Graphene nanoplatelets (GNPs) 0%, 0.25%, 0.5%	Dental Sans, Harz Labs, Riga, Latvia	SLA printing	Not determined	8 average
Aati et al., 2022 [14]	PMMA-based resin	Graphene nanoplatelets (GNPs) 0.025%, 0.1%, 0.25%	Denture 3D+, NextDent BV, The Netherlands	DLP printing	Not determined	7 average
Aati et al., 2022 [15]	PMMA-based resin	Silver-reinforced mesoporous silica nanoparticles (Ag-MSN) 0.025%, 0.05%, 0.5%, 1.0%, 2.0%	Denture 3D+, NextDent BV, The Netherlands	DLP printing	Uniform distribution; size 10–20 nm.	7 average
Alshaikh et al., 2022 [30]	PMMA-based resin	Zirconium dioxide nanoparticles (ZrO_2 NPs) 1%, 5%	Denture 3D+, NextDent BV, The Netherlands	DLP printing	Not determined	9 average
Hada et al., 2022 [31]	PMMA-based resin	Zirconium dioxide nanoparticles (ZrO_2 NPs)	Photopolymer resin (Clear V4 resin) (Nagase ChemteX Corporation, Delaware, OH, USA)	SLA printing	Uniform distribution; average size 206 μm; particle size = 100–150 nm.	8 average
Marin et al., 2022 [34]	PMMA-based resin	Aluminum nitride; Barium titanate	Clear photoreactive resin, Formlabs, Somerville, MA, USA	SLA printing	Barium titanate better dispersion than aluminum nitride	6 average
Raszewski et al., 2022 [35]	PMMA-based resin	Bioactive glasses	FotoDent splint, Dreve, Unna, Germany	DPP printing	Not determined	8 average

Table 1. *Cont.*

Study	Chemical Composition		Manufacturer	Manufacturing Technique	Distribution and Size of Particles	Quality Assessment Score
	Resin	Compound				
Marin et al., 2021 [18]	PMMA-based resin	Ceramic nitrides	Clear photoreactive resin, Formlabs, USA	SLA printing	Not determined	4 low
Kwon et al., 2021 [19]	PMMA-based resin	Zwitterionic materials	Orthorigid, NextDent BV, The Netherlands	DLP printing	Not determined	8 average
Mangal et al., 2020 [36]	PMMA-based resin	Nanodiamonds	Orthorigid, NextDent BV, The Netherlands	DLP printing	Not determined	7 average
Mangal et al., 2020 [37]	PMMA-based resin	Aminated nanodiamonds	Orthorigid, NextDent BV, The Netherlands	DLP printing	Particle size 4–6 nm; more agglomerates of nanodiamonds than aminated nanodiamonds	8 average
Mubarak et al., 2020 [38]	Urethane-acrylate resin	Silver-reinforced titanium dioxide nanoparticles (Ag-TNP) 1%, 1.2%	Resin based on urethane-acrylate (Sartomer America, Exton, PA, USA)	SLA printing	Titanium dioxide = 30–40 nm; silver nanoparticles = 5–10 nm	7 average
Agarwalla et al., 2019 [26]	PMMA	Graphene	PMMA, Zotion, Chongqing, China	Milling	Not determined	5 low
Chen et al., 2019 [16]	PMMA-based resin	Titanium dioxide (TiO_2)-polyether ether ketone (PEEK) nanoparticles TiO_2-1%-PEEK-1%, TiO_2-1%-PEEK-2%	Orthorigid, NextDent BV, The Netherlands	DLP printing	TiO_2 nanoparticles = 40 nm; PEEK = 10 µm (irregular)	6 average
Chen et al., 2018 [17]	PMMA-based resin	Silver-reinforced cellulose nanocrystals (Ag-CNCs) 0.05, 0.1%, 0.25%	Denture 3D+, NextDent BV, The Netherlands	DLP printing	Particle size 80 nm, agglomerates due to the high hydroxyl bonding	8 average
Totu et al., 2018 [39]	PMMA-based resin	Titanium dioxide (TiO_2) nanoparticles	E-Dent 100; E-Denture, EnvisionTec GmbH, Gladbeck, Germany	SLA printing	Not determined	5 low
Totu et al., 2017 [40]	PMMA-based resin	Titanium dioxide (TiO_2) nanoparticles	E-Dent 100, EnvisionTec GmbH, Germany	SLA printing	Spherical structure; diameter 56–170 nm	5 low

Legend: PMMA—poly(methylmethacrylate), PEEK—polyether ether ketone; SLA—stereolithography; DLP—digital light processing; DPP—daylight polymer printing.

The studies showed testing of the surface properties (7 articles), mechanical properties (15 articles), antimicrobial properties (11 articles), cytotoxicity (7 articles), and genotoxicity (1 article).

3.3. Surface Properties (Roughness, Topography and Wettability)

Regarding surface roughness, it was found that this parameter depends on the concentration of the compounds. In general, the incorporation of zirconia nanoparticles increased the surface roughness of resins [13,14,30,33], making this effect more evident with increasing concentration [14,33] and subjected them to aging [14,15]. Also, the surface topography changed from flat in the non-loaded resins to having peaks after the incorporation of 0.25% of graphene nanoparticles [14] and 2% of silver-enhanced mesoporous silica nanoparticles (Ag/MSN) [15]. Nevertheless, there were no statistically significant differences in surface roughness between the control group and the groups with nanodiamonds [36] (Table 2).

Table 2. Comparation of outcomes reflecting the relation of incorporated resins with compounds and the control group without compound loading.

Study	Surface Properties	Mechanical Properties	Antimicrobial Properties	Biocompatibility
Khattar et al., 2023 [13] ZrO_2 NPs	Roughness: increased	--------------------	CFU number: decreased	Cell proliferation: increased
Selva-Otaolaurruchi et al., 2023 [32] Graphene oxide	--------------------	Fracture strength: increased	--------------------	--------------------
Salgado et al., 2023 [33] GNPs	Roughness: increased as concentration increased	Hardness: decreased as concentration increased Flexural strength: decreased as concentration increased	--------------------	--------------------
Aati et al., 2022 [14] GNPs	Roughness: increased as concentration increased Topography: control = flat; 0.25% of graphene nanoplatelets = peaks of about 1 µm	Hardness: 0.25% graphene NPs = increased hardness Elastic modulus: decreased as concentration increased Flexural strength: decreased as concentration increased and after aging Fracture strength: decreased as concentration increased and after aging	Adhesion of *C. albicans*: decreased	Biocompatibility: no differences
Aati et al., 2022 [15] Ag/MSN	Roughness: increased as concentration increased Topography: control = flat, Ag/MSN 2% = irregularity	Flexural strength: decreased as concentration increased and after aging Fracture toughness: increased as concentration increased, decreased after aging	*C. albicans* biofilm mass: decreased as concentration increased	FCell viability: increased with 0.025% and 0.05% Ag/MSN, decreased with 1.0% and 2.0% Ag/MSN
Alshaikh et al., 2022 [30] ZrO_2 NPs	Roughness: increased	Hardness: decreased Elastic modulus and flexural strength: dependent on the resin Impact strength: dependent on the resin	--------------------	--------------------

Table 2. *Cont.*

Study	Surface Properties	Mechanical Properties	Antimicrobial Properties	Biocompatibility
Hada et al., 2022 [31] ZrO_2 NPs		Hardness: increased as concentration increased Flexural strength: dependent on the printing direction	-------------------	-------------------
Marin et al., 2022 [34] aluminum nitride, barium titanate	Roughness: increased as concentration increased	-------------------	CFU number: decreased	-------------------
Raszewski et al., 2022 [35] bioactive glasses	-------------------	Flexural strength: decreased	-------------------	Cell viability: 24 h incubation = no differences, 96 h incubation = decreased
Marin et al., 2021 [18] ceramic nitrides	-------------------	-------------------	Antimicrobial activity: increased for *E. coli* and *Staphylococcus epidermidis*	-------------------
Kwon et al., 2021 [19] zwitterionic materials	Wettability: decreased contact angle, with and without aging	Hardness: decreased Elastic modulus and flexural strength: decreased, with and without aging	Bacterial adhesion: decreased for *S. mutans*, *S. aureus*, *Klebsiella oxytoca*, *Klebsiella pneumoniae*	Adsorption of proteins: decreased
Mangal et al., 2020 [36] nanodiamonds	Roughness: no differences	Hardness: increased (18.71 ± 1.25 kg/mm^2) vs. (15.91 ± 1.27 kg/mm^2) Friction coefficient: increased Wear resistance: increased	Bacterial growth: decreased *S. mutans*	-------------------
Mangal et al., 2020 [37] aminated nanodiamonds	Wettability: decreased contact angle	Hardness: increased Flexural strength: increased	-------------------	-------------------
Mubarak et al., 2020 [38] Ag/TNP	-------------------	Hardness: increased as concentration increased Elastic modulus: decreased as concentration increased Flexural strength: increased as concentration increased Tensile strength: increased up to a concentration of 1% Ag; decreased in the group with Ag/TNF-1.2%	-------------------	-------------------
Agarwalla et al., 2019 [26] Graphene	-------------------	Hardness: decreased Flexural Strength: decreased	-------------------	-------------------
Chen et al., 2019 [16] TiO_2-PEEK	-------------------	Flexural Strength: increased Impact Strength: increased	CFU number: decreased in *S. aureus* and *E. coli*	Cytotoxicity (CCK-8 assay): adequate Blood compatibility test: good blood tolerance

Table 2. *Cont.*

Study	Surface Properties	Mechanical Properties	Antimicrobial Properties	Biocompatibility
Chen et al., 2018 [17] CNCs-Ag	--------------------	Flexural Strength: increased but decreased as concentration increased;	Bacterial growth: decreased *S. aureus* and *E. coli*	Cytotoxicity: no differences
Totu et al., 2018 [39] TiO_2 nanoparticles	--------------------	--------------------	Antimicrobial activity: increase for *S. aureus*	Cytotoxicity: no differences DNA damage: no differences
Totu et al., 2017 [40] TiO_2 nanoparticles	--------------------	--------------------	Bacterial and fungi growth: decreased	--------------------

Legend: ZrO_2—zirconia; NPs nanoparticles; CFU-colony-forming units; G—graphene; Ag/MSN—silver-enhanced mesoporous silica nanoparticles; Ag/TNP-titanium dioxide nanoparticles reinforced with silver; TiO_2—titanium dioxide; PEEK—polyether ether ketone; CNCs-Ag—silver-enriched cellulose nanocrystals.

The wettability was assessed by analyzing the contact angle. The contact angle was lower in resins containing nanodiamonds [37] or zwitterionic materials, even after the thermocycling process [19] (Table 2).

3.4. Mechanical Properties

Hardness was evaluated in several articles of the systematic review, and most of the results show that it also depends on the concentration of the compounds. However, when GNPs were incorporated in the resin, one study showed that the groups with higher concentrations (0.25%, 0.5%) showed lower hardness values [33], and another showed that the group with the highest concentration of GNP resin (0.25%) had the highest hardness. After being subjected to an aging process, the hardness of specimens decreased by 6–18% [14]. The addition of zwitterionic materials also decreased the hardness of the resins, even after they were subjected to a thermocycling process. When ZrO_2 NPs were incorporated into NextDent Denture 3D+ and ASIGA DentaBase resins, the resins with this compound showed lower hardness values than the control group [30]. In another study, the group with the highest zirconia concentration was also the one with the highest hardness [31]. For resins containing nanodiamonds, the hardness was higher (18.71 ± 1.25 kg/mm^2) than in the control group (15.91 ± 1.27 kg/mm^2) [36], and the same occurred when aminated nanodiamonds were incorporated [37] (Table 2).

In terms of elastic modulus, the groups with the highest values were the least concentrated resins, and a reduction of about 2–6% was observed after aging [14].

When TiO_2 nanoparticles reinforced with silver were incorporated, the hardness was found to increase with increasing concentration of the compound, except in the group with the highest concentration of nanoparticles in the resins (1.2%), where the hardness decreased [38].

The elastic modulus showed statistically significant differences in the NextDent Denture 3D+ resin group, with the control group showing the highest value (1909.4 ± 679.3 MPa). In the group with ASIGA DentaBase, there were no significant differences in the values, with the group with 5% nanoparticles showing the highest modulus (2031.2 ± 77.2 MPa) [30]. The addition of zwitterionic materials also decreased the elastic modulus [19]. When titanium dioxide nanoparticles reinforced with silver were incorporated, the modulus of elasticity was found to increase with increasing concentrations of the compound [38] (Table 2).

The flexural strength was investigated in several studies. The incorporation of GNPs had a negative effect on this parameter, as the groups with 0.25% and 0.5% had a lower value compared to the control group [26,33]. After 3 months of storage in artificial saliva, all groups showed lower values [14]. When Ag-MSN were incorporated, the flexural strength decreased with increasing silver concentration, and it was also found that all groups showed lower values after 3 months under aging conditions [15]. In the studies on the incorporation of TiO_2-PEEK [17], ZrO_2 NP [30,31], A-ND [37], and Ag-TNP [38], it was found that the group with the highest flexural strength was the more concentrated resin. When bioactive glasses [35], zwitterionic materials [19], or Ag-CNCs [17] were incorporated into acrylic resins, a decrease in flexural strength was observed, even after undergoing the thermocycling process (Table 2).

To compare the fracture strength between the CAD-CAM-fabricated resins with and without graphene oxide, the materials were subjected to several load cycles. It was found that the PMMA + graphene group had better fracture strength values compared to the control group [32]. Another study used GNP, and the group with 0.025% GNP showed the highest value, while the group with the highest GNP concentration showed the lowest fracture strength. After aging, all groups showed lower values [14]. The fracture toughness was also investigated for resins with Ag/MSN, and the higher the concentration of nanoparticles, the higher the fracture strength value compared to the control group [15] (Table 2).

When analyzing the wear rate, the control group showed higher values compared to the other groups, both for stainless steel and titanium, suggesting that the incorporation of these compounds improves wear resistance [36,37] (Table 2).

In the study on the incorporation of zirconia nanoparticles, impact strength was also evaluated, and it was found that the NextDent resin group had higher values compared to the control group, in contrast to the ASIGA resin group, in which all resins with nanoparticles had lower values compared to the control group [30]. This parameter was also examined when using titanium dioxide nanoparticles and PEEK, with the groups with PEEK achieving higher values than the other groups [16] (Table 2).

To complete the evaluation of the mechanical properties in one article, the tensile strength was evaluated in the case of the incorporation of silver reinforced titanium dioxide nanoparticles (Ag-TNP), and it was found that the tensile strength increased up to a concentration of 1% Ag-TNP in the resin. This parameter decreased in the group with Ag-TNF-1.2% [38] (Table 2).

3.5. Antimicrobial Properties

In the studies included in the systematic review, the antimicrobial properties were also analyzed. Most of the dental resins produced with CAD-CAM showed better antimicrobial properties when combined with the investigated compounds. It was found that the incorporation of zirconia nanoparticles [14], aluminum nitride and barium titanate [34], titanium dioxide nanoparticles and PEEK [16], nanodiamonds [36], zwitterionic materials [19], and nitrides [18] into the PMMA resin resulted in a lower number of bacterial colony-forming units (CFU) than the control group. The incorporation of graphene nanoplatelets [14] and Ag-MSN [15] into 3D-printed PMMA resin reduced the adhesion of *Candida albicans* to the resin surface (Table 2).

The incorporation of silver-enriched cellulose nanocrystals [17] and titanium dioxide [39] into the PMMA resin also showed a decrease in the concentration of Staphylococcus aureus bacterial cells, proving that these nanomaterials have an antimicrobial effect.

The titanium dioxide also inhibited the growth of the strain Candida scotti, demonstrating that titanium dioxide nanoparticles have a broad spectrum of activity against Gram-positive and Gram-negative microorganisms and fungi [16,40]. The antimicrobial activity of ceramic nitrides was also investigated in an in vitro test against *E. coli* and *Staphylococcus epidermidis* (Table 2).

3.6. Biocompatibility

Biocompatibility was also assessed in some of the articles selected for this systematic review. Cytotoxicity was assessed in six articles using human oral fibroblasts. Protein adsorption test was investigated in one article [19], the blood compatibility test in one article [16], and genotoxicity [39].

In the case of the incorporation of zirconia nanoparticles (ZrO_2 NPs), the group with the highest cell proliferation was the one with 5% ZrO_2 NPs in the acrylic resin [13]. When graphene nanoplatelets were incorporated, the viability of cells showed no significant differences between the tested groups and the control group [14]. For the Ag/MSN, cell viability was found to be dependent on their concentration in the PMMA resin, as high cell viability was observed in the groups with 0.025% and 0.05% Ag/MSN compared to the other groups [15] (Table 2).

To analyze the effects of the bioactive glasses on PMMA resin, the growth of fibroblasts was examined after 24 h with the PrestoBlue assay and after 96 h with methylthiazolyl diphenyl tetrazolium bromide. It was found that cell viability was not affected after 24 h of incubation, but after 96 h of incubation, cell viability decreased in all groups with bioactive glasses compared to the control group [35]. The adsorption of proteins was also investigated in conjunction with the zwitterionic materials. The analysis of the results showed that the adsorption decreased and was lower in the groups with this compound than in the control group [19] (Table 2).

For the titanium dioxide and PEEK nanoparticles, the cytotoxicity of the groups was analyzed using the CCK-8 assay. This parameter was evaluated for 7 days, and it was found that the groups showed adequate cytocompatibility with these compounds. Blood compatibility was also tested in this study, including hemolysis and analysis of blood coagulation parameters such as activated partial thromboplastin time (APTT) and prothrombin time (PT). The APPT was approx. 36.5 s, and the PT approx. 13.5 s, thus within the normal range. It was concluded that the groups, both the control group and the groups with the nanoparticles, had good blood tolerance [16] (Table 2).

Regarding the incorporation of cellulose nanocrystals reinforced with silver, they show that these exhibit no significant toxicity in L929 fibroblasts compared to the control group. The survival rate of the cells was more than 85% in all groups studied [17]. In the case of titanium dioxide nanoparticles in acrylic resin, cytotoxicity was investigated in two acrylic resins, E-Dent 100 (dent-PMMA) and E-Denture (base-PMMA). In the case of the dent-PMMA material, the extract test was used for the different groups studied (control group, 1% nanoparticles, and 4% nanoparticles), and it was found that the group with the highest viability was the control group, followed by the group with 1% nanoparticles. In the case of the PMMA base matrix, it was evaluated with the XTT method, and there were no differences in the cytotoxic effect between the groups studied [39]. Genotoxicity was evaluated using the micronucleus test (Mtvit) for the two groups, base PMMA without titanium dioxide nanoparticles and base PMMA + 0.4% TiO_2 nanoparticles, and it was found that the TiO_2 nanoparticles caused hardly any DNA damage compared to the negative control group [39] (Table 2).

3.7. Quality Assessment of the Studies

From the 19 included studies, four were considered to have low quality since they scored above six points, and the remaining 15 scored between six and nine points, having average quality (Table 3).

Table 3. Quality assessment of the included studies.

	Items															
Study	**1**	**2a**	**2b**	**3**	**4**	**5**	**6**	**7**	**8**	**9**	**10**	**11**	**12**	**13**	**14**	**Score**
Khattar et al., 2023 [13]	yes	yes	yes	yes	yes	no	no	no	no	no	yes	yes	yes	no	no	8 average
Selva-Otaolaurr uchi et al., 2023 [32]	yes	yes	yes	yes	yes	no	no	no	no	no	yes	yes	yes	no	no	8 average
Salgado et al., 2023 [33]	yes	yes	yes	yes	yes	no	no	no	no	no	yes	yes	yes	no	no	8 average

Table 3. *Cont.*

	Items															
Study	**1**	**2a**	**2b**	**3**	**4**	**5**	**6**	**7**	**8**	**9**	**10**	**11**	**12**	**13**	**14**	**Score**
Aati et al., 2022 [14]	yes	yes	yes	yes	yes	no	no	no	no	no	yes	yes	no	no	no	7 average
Aati et al., 2022 [15]	no	yes	yes	yes	yes	no	no	no	no	no	yes	yes	yes	no	no	7 average
Alshaik h et al., 2022 [30]	yes	yes	yes	yes	yes	no	no	no	no	no	yes	yes	yes	yes	no	9 average
Hada et al., 2022 [31]	no	yes	yes	yes	yes	no	no	no	no	no	yes	yes	yes	yes	no	8 average
Marin et al., 2022 [34]	no	yes	no	yes	yes	no	no	no	no	no	yes	yes	no	yes	no	6 average
Raszewsk i et al., 2022 [35]	yes	yes	yes	yes	yes	no	no	no	no	no	yes	yes	no	yes	no	8 average
Marin et al., 2021 [18]	no	yes	no	yes	yes	no	no	no	no	no	yes	no	no	no	no	4 low
Kwon et al., 2021 [19]	no	yes	yes	yes	yes	no	no	no	no	no	yes	yes	yes	yes	no	8 average
Manga l et al., 2020 [36]	yes	yes	yes	yes	yes	no	no	no	no	no	yes	yes	no	no	no	7 average
Manga l et al., 2020 [37]	yes	yes	yes	yes	yes	no	no	no	no	no	yes	yes	no	yes	no	8 average
Mubar ak et al. [38]	yes	yes	yes	yes	yes	no	no	no	no	no	no	no	no	yes	yes	7 average
Chen et al., 2019 [16]	no	yes	yes	yes	yes	no	no	no	no	no	no	no	no	yes	no	5 low
Agarw alla et al. [26]	no	yes	yes	yes	yes	no	no	no	no	no	yes	no	yes	no	no	6 average
Chen et al., 2018 [17]	no	yes	yes	yes	yes	no	no	no	no	no	yes	yes	no	yes	yes	8 average
Totu et al., 2018 [39]	no	yes	yes	yes	yes	no	no	no	no	no	no	yes	no	no	no	5 low
Totu et al. [40]	yes	yes	yes	yes	yes	no	no	no	no	no	no	no	no	no	no	5 low

4. Discussion

In this systematic review, it was found that there are differences in the parameters analyzed depending on the type of compound studied.

4.1. Surface Properties (Roughness, Topography and Wettability)

Regarding surface roughness, it was found that this parameter depends on the concentration of the compound incorporated into the resin. Surface roughness is a parameter that influences both the esthetics and the mechanical properties of the restoration [14]. It has been described that rough materials are more susceptible to the adhesion of microorganisms, which can lead to diseases in the oral cavity such as stomatitis [13,30]. It is influenced by various factors, e.g., the manufacturing method, the type of resin used, and the monomer elution [13]. However, if the surface roughness of the investigated resins is below the recommended limit for dental materials (Sa $\leq$ 0.2 μm), this may not have a major impact on debris accumulation or biofilm adhesion [14]. The compounds incorporated into the resins that showed values below the limit were GNPs [14] and Ag-MSN [15], while in the case of ZrO_2 NPs [13,30] and nanodiamonds [36], the surface roughness values were above the established limit. Although the roughness values are above the limit, the article states that the incorporation of zirconia nanoparticles did not have a major impact on microbial adhesion [13]. The article with the nanodiamonds described that roughness values above 2 μm would increase the possibility of bacterial colonization of the resin surface, which was not observed in the groups studied [36]. It can be concluded that even if the roughness of the tooth material is above the recommended limit, this does not mean that bacterial adhesion will occur. It is necessary to analyze the properties of the individual materials.

4.2. Mechanical Properties

Subsequently, the mechanical properties, antimicrobial activity, and biocompatibility of the resin-containing compounds were analyzed. Some articles describe that the degree of conversion of a resin material is a critical factor because if the polymerization is not performed properly, the mechanical properties and biocompatibility are compromised. The conversion of the polymer monomer is influenced by the layer thickness, the light source, the polymerization method, and the composition of the material [14,15].

The hardness of the material is related to the degree of resistance that a material has to plastic deformation, e.g., due to the abrasive effects that dental material may be subjected to [33], both by medical procedures and by mechanical abrasion during tooth brushing [14]. Dentures made of materials with low hardness can be attacked by tooth brushing, leading to a change in color and the accumulation of bacterial plaque [30]. Therefore, hardness is related to the wear resistance of the prosthesis and is influenced by the composition of the dental material and the polymerization rate [14]. In the case of GNPs incorporated into the Dental Sans resin, there was a decrease in hardness [33], while the incorporation of this compound into the NextDent resin resulted in an increase in hardness the higher the concentration. However, after NextDent resins are aged, their hardness decreases, possibly due to the degradation that occurs [14]. In this way, it can be concluded that this difference in results is due to the different types of resins produced with different manufacturing processes [33]. It has also been reported that the hardness values of 3D-printed resins are lower than those of thermopolymerized PMMA resin, which was also the case when ZrO_2 NPs were incorporated [30]. When zwitterionic materials are added, the hardness also decreases as high doses deteriorate the mechanical properties [19]. PMMA resins with graphene also exhibited lower hardness than the other groups, as some studies have already shown that PMMA-based materials have lower hardness values than other materials investigated in this study [26].

When Ag-TNP were incorporated into urethane acrylate-based resins, the hardness increased with the increase in nanoparticle concentration, except when the concentration was above 1%, as there were problems with printing in this case. When zirconia was incorporated, the hardness increased [31], as did nanodiamonds, which showed a low wear rate compared to the control group [36,37].

The flexural strength of a material is related to the flexibility of the material before it reaches its limit. The bending forces to which the materials are subjected are related to the forces that occur in clinical situations, i.e., the ability of the materials to withstand bending and torsion. Therefore, when dental materials are subjected to permanent deformation, it is important that they have high flexural strength [41]. When analyzing the articles included in this systematic review, it was found that there were differences in the values of this parameter due to the different compounds contained in the resins. In most of the articles, the flexural strength decreased when the compounds were incorporated into the resins.

When graphene nanoplatelets were added, the flexural strength was found to decrease at concentrations above 0.1%. This has also been shown in other articles [33], as when the graphene concentration is above 0.1%, zones of force concentration are created, which affect flexural strength and ultimate strength [14]. Thus, it was described that at lower graphene concentrations, such as 0.01% graphene, the flexural strength of the resin becomes more similar to that of the resin without incorporation [33]. The same occurred when mesoporous silica nanoparticles reinforced with silver were incorporated into the acrylic resin: As the concentration increased, the flexural strength decreased because clusters of these compounds formed in the polymer network. Although the flexural strength of the resin with nanoparticles was impaired, the flexural strength value corresponded to that for dental restorations (ISO 20795-1) [15]. In terms of fracture strength, the resins with this compound showed higher values than the control group, as the nanoparticles impaired the propagation of cracks and fissures in the resin [15].

In the case of zwitterionic materials in resins, some studies have already reported that their high dose in dental materials may negatively affect the mechanical properties, which is related to the gelation process of zwitterionic materials in high concentrations, which affects the polymerization process of the resin. However, it is important to note that the results presented in this article are in accordance with ISO 20795-1 [19]. For the zirconia nanoparticles (ZrO_2-NP), the increase in flexural strength in the ASIGA resins depends on the concentration of ZrO_2-NP, as this parameter also increases with increasing concentration [42]. In the NextDent resins, however, the flexural strength is higher in the group with 1% ZrO_2-NP, while it decreases in the other groups, so that the difference in the flexural strength values could be due to the different compositions of the resins tested. This article also described that the 3D-printed resins fulfill the ISO recommendations (65 MPa) as the minimum value for the flexural strength of this type of material [30]. When zirconia was incorporated into the resin, the printing direction affected the flexural strength values, as in the 0° printing direction, the control group showed a higher flexural strength, while in the 90° printing direction, the group with 3% zirconia showed the highest value. This study showed that the flexural strength value of the resin with 3% zirconia printed at 90° was in line with the ISO10477 recommendation [31]. The introduction of bioactive glasses reduces flexural strength and fracture resistance [35].

When aminated nanodiamonds were incorporated into the resin, their incorporation was found to increase flexural strength, as it has already been described in several studies that their addition increases mechanical strength due to their strong covalent bonds and the fact that they are evenly distributed in the polymer [37]. When investigating the incorporation of graphene into PMMA resins, it was found that nano-ceramic resins (LU) and lithium disilicate ceramics (EX) had higher flexural strength values than the other materials, namely polyurethane resins. PMMA, which contained graphene. In the LU group, the higher flexural strength was due to the formation of zirconia/silica agglomerates; in the EX group, the high flexural strength was related to the homogeneity of the crystals in the ceramic. It was also described that further clinical studies on flexural strength after the incorporation of graphene into PMMA resins are needed [26].

Finally, the flexural strength of titanium dioxide and PEEK nanoparticles and silver-reinforced titanium dioxide nanoparticles in acrylic resins was also investigated. For the silver-reinforced titanium dioxide nanoparticles, the flexural strength was only impaired when the concentration of this compound was greater than 1% because agglomerates formed, resulting in poor dispersion of this compound in the resin matrix [38]. In the case of titanium dioxide and PEEK nanoparticles, their incorporation into the PMMA resin leads to an increase in flexural strength compared to the control group. However, in group 2 (TiO_2-1%-PEEK-0%), problems occurred during the printing process as agglomerates of TiO_2 nanoparticles formed, especially in the polymerization phase of the resin, which affected the flexural strength value and impaired the polymerization phase of the resin [13]. It was also reported that the incorporation of PEEK reduced the agglomeration of the nanoparticles and thus improved mechanical properties [16]. When cellulose nanocrystals reinforced with silver were incorporated, it was found that their concentration was a critical factor because, although the nanocrystals were well incorporated into the resin matrix, their agglomeration on the surface could affect the flexural strength [17].

The accidental fall of dentures is one of the most common causes of fractures. It is therefore important that dental materials have good impact resistance [30]. The impact strength of resins with zirconia nanoparticles has increased because they are evenly distributed in the acrylic resin matrix. However, as with flexural strength, there were also differences in impact strength between the two resin types. The NextDent resin showed an increase in impact strength, while the ASIGA resin did not, which could be related to the printing process [30].

When titanium dioxide and PEEK nanoparticles were incorporated into the resins, it was found that the groups with higher concentrations of these compounds achieved higher impact strength values than the control group. These results could be related to the fact that the compounds incorporated into the resin matrix are able to absorb large amounts of fracture force and prevent the absorption of energy through the destructive cracks present in the material. However, to observe this behavior, it is important that the nanoparticles do not aggregate in the polymer matrix [16]. When graphene oxide was incorporated into PMMA acrylic resin, it was found that the fracture strength in these groups was improved by the compound compared to the control group. The good homogenization of graphene oxide in the acrylic resin influenced this parameter, and the study described that this compound has good properties for incorporation into dental and orthopedic prostheses [32].

Friction and wear resistance has been studied in the incorporation of nanodiamonds [36,37] and is a parameter that must be considered in dental materials, as wear and friction in the oral cavity depend on several factors, e.g., the wetting properties of saliva and the concentration of salivary proteins [36].

Tensile strength is a parameter often used to measure the ductility of a material [40,41]. When Ag-TNP were incorporated into the acrylic resin, an increase in tensile strength was observed, except at a concentration of 1.2% [38].

4.3. Antimicrobial Properties and Biocompatibility

Finally, antimicrobial activity and biocompatibility were also examined as parameters in this systematic review. The biocompatibility of dental materials is a factor that must be considered in their manufacture, as it is important to avoid adverse reactions during treatment. The toxicity of acrylate-based resins is related to the possibility of unpolymerized monomers migrating and subsequently penetrating the oral cavity [15]. Therefore, it is important that this polymerization process of acrylate resins be carried out completely. It is also important to wash the dental materials in alcoholic solutions to remove unpolymerized monomers [35].

Regarding zirconia nanoparticles in resins, it has been described that their antimicrobial effect is related to the production of reactive oxygen species that inhibit the activity of microorganisms by forming pores in the cell wall, which increases cell permeability and causes cell death [13]. This article also described that the incorporation of zirconia nanoparticles, the type of resin, and the hydrophobicity of the resin affect the adhesion of *C. albicans* [13]. Regarding cell proliferation, it has been described that the cell counting method (CCK-8/WST-8) is a reliable, accurate, and practical method to determine the amount of biofilm for the studied microorganisms [13].

Several mechanisms involved in the inhibition of antimicrobial activity have been identified in the context of graphene nanoplatelet incorporation. In terms of physical damage to the microorganisms [14,15], the graphene nanoplatelets rupture the cell membrane and cause cell death. Another proposed mechanism is the entrapment of microorganisms in the graphene layers, preventing cell nutrition. Finally, it has been described that the antifungal effect of graphene is due to the formation of oxygen radicals, which increase cytotoxicity. However, in vitro studies investigating the viability of the oral biofilm revealed that no toxicity occurred in oral cells, possibly due to the low concentration of incorporated graphene nanoparticles as well as the presence of the polycarboxylate functional group, which improves the biocompatibility of graphene [14].

With respect to silver-enriched mesoporous silica nanoparticles (Ag/MSN), it has been described that the toxicity of silver is related to the release of large amounts of ions that ultimately affect the release of oxygen radicals. Therefore, it is important to incorporate silver into mesoporous silica nanoparticles to reduce their toxicity. In this case, it was found that the cell viability of the groups with 1–2% Ag/MSN decreased compared to the others, possibly due to the release of monomers by the resin and silver ions. However, all species achieved a cell viability of greater than 75%, which is not considered a toxic effect according to ISO 10993-5 [15]. Regarding the mechanism of antimicrobial activity of Ag/MSN, it was mentioned that the amine group shows antimicrobial activity due to the interaction between the positive charge of the amine group and the negative charge of the cell membranes of the microorganisms. On the other hand, the amine group increases the hydrophobicity of the surface, which ultimately prevents the adhesion of microorganisms. The penetration of silver ions also leads to cell death because the cell membranes rupture [15].

For the ceramic nitrides Si3N4, Hf3N4, Zr3N4, and AIN contained in acrylic resins, the antibacterial activity of silicon and aluminum nitrides has been associated with the release of ammonia at the surface, while the mechanism for hafnium and zirconium nitrides has not yet been described, as further studies are needed to understand the mechanism of their antimicrobial activity [18]. The zwitterionic materials in the resins have a similar morphology to the lipid bilayers of cell membranes, with a hydrophilic head and a hydrophobic tail. When resins containing zwitterionic substances are exposed to the oral environment, they repel the proteins in human saliva through their interaction with water molecules, thus preventing the adhesion of microorganisms in the oral cavity. It has been described that groups of zwitterionic substances have the ability to inhibit bacterial adhesion even after being exposed to hydrothermal fatigue through a thermocycling process, but it is not clear which mechanism of action causes the antimicrobial activity [19].

Regarding the nanodiamonds investigated, it was found that surface hydrophobicity is a parameter that influences the formation of biofilms on dental materials. Due to their antimicrobial activity and the high hydrophobicity of acrylic resins with nanodiamonds and nanodiamond aminates, these materials are able to resist the formation of biofilms and thus exhibit high antimicrobial activity [36]. The incorporation of zirconia and PEEK nanoparticles into PMMA resins does not alter cytocompatibility, as shown by the analysis of L929 fibroblast survival rates and blood compatibility. Several studies have already mentioned that dental materials can damage the cellular integrity of red blood cells if they have a hemolysis rate greater than 20%. The APTT is a sensitive test for the coagulation system, while the PT refers to hemostasis, with acceptable values ranging between 27–40 s and 11–14 s. In this case, it was found that all groups had values within the acceptable range, showing that zirconia and PEEK nanoparticles have good blood compatibility [16].

Regarding the cellulose nanocrystals reinforced with silver, the article did not describe the mechanism of action, but only what is described in the results [17]. Therefore, further studies are needed to analyze the mechanism of action of nanocrystals that exhibit antimicrobial activity and biocompatibility. [43] Finally, the titanium dioxide nanoparticles incorporated into the resins also have an antimicrobial effect by deactivating the cellular enzymes, which leads to the disintegration of the cell wall and thus to cell death. The article also states that a concentration of 0.4% titanium dioxide nanoparticles prevents the colonization of microorganisms [39,40]. Preliminary studies on cytotoxicity and genotoxicity tests have shown that a concentration of 0.4% titanium dioxide nanoparticles shows positive results when this compound is incorporated into acrylic resins [39].

5. Conclusions

In this systematic review, the surface properties of acrylic resins with incorporated compounds were analyzed, and it was found that the concentration of the compound incorporated into the acrylic resin and the manufacturing process influence this parameter. It was also described that there is a threshold value for the roughness of dental materials and that some of the investigated compounds have higher roughness values. However, further studies are needed to determine whether this parameter can also be influenced by the physiological conditions in the mouth, such as pH, as the selected articles, which are only in vitro studies, are not exposed to the same loading conditions as in the oral cavity.

In terms of mechanical properties, the results showed that there is a wide range of results depending on the different compounds contained in the resins, as there are several factors that influence the determination of these parameters. Therefore, it was concluded that there is no significant scientific evidence that all compounds contained in acrylic resins improve mechanical properties compared to control groups. The studies analyzed in this systematic review have some limitations, as only in vitro studies were analyzed. For future work, it is suggested that more studies be conducted, including studies that adequately evaluate the mechanical properties of dental materials under mechanical and thermal loading conditions such as those in the oral cavity, using different concentrations of nanomaterials, different resins, and different manufacturing techniques with CAD-CAM. Some articles also pointed out the need to conduct long-term studies to analyze the properties of dental materials in a clinical environment.

Finally, regarding the antimicrobial activity of the resins with the incorporated compounds, an improvement in antimicrobial activity was observed compared to the control group. In terms of biocompatibility, not all resins containing compounds were found to have better biocompatibility than resins without compounds. One of the limitations in the articles used for the systematic review was the fact that the groups studied were not exposed to the pH conditions characteristic of the oral cavity, and this parameter has an influence on bacterial adhesion. Therefore, in order to make a clearer statement about antimicrobial activity and biocompatibility, more studies need to be conducted in which resins with and without compounds are exposed to intraoral conditions, and longitudinal studies need to be conducted to determine whether the incorporation of these compounds into acrylic resins actually has an impact on clinical practice.

Supplementary Materials: The following supporting information can be downloaded at: https://www.mdpi.com/article/10.3390/app14072931/s1, Table S1: PRISMA 2020 checklist.

Author Contributions: Conceptualization, A.B., C.J. and C.B.N.; methodology, A.B. and C.J.; software, V.A.; validation, A.B., C.B.N. and V.A.; formal analysis, C.J.; investigation, C.J.; resources, A.B.; data curation, C.B.N.; writing—original draft preparation, C.J.; writing—review and editing, V.A.; visualization, V.A.; supervision, A.B.; project administration, A.B.; funding acquisition, A.B. All authors have read and agreed to the published version of the manuscript.

Funding: The authors gratefully acknowledge the support from FCT–Fundação para a Ciência e Tecnologia (Portuguese Foundation for Science and Technology), through IDMEC, under LAETA, project UIDB/50022/2020.

Institutional Review Board Statement: Not applicable.

Informed Consent Statement: Not applicable.

Data Availability Statement: The original contributions presented in the study are included in the article and Supplementary Material, further inquiries can be directed to the corresponding authors.

Conflicts of Interest: The authors declare no conflicts of interest.

References

1. Lee, D.J.; Saponaro, P.C. Management of edentulous patients. *Dent. Clin. N. Am.* **2019**, *63*, 249–261. [CrossRef] [PubMed]
2. Krausch-Hofmann, S.; Cuypers, L.; Ivanova, A.; Duyck, J. Predictors of Patient Satisfaction with Removable Denture Renewal: A Pilot Study. *J. Prosthodont.* **2018**, *27*, 509–516. [CrossRef] [PubMed]
3. Conceição, P.; Franco, M.; Alves, N.; Portugal, J.; Neves, C.B. Fit accuracy of removable partial denture metal frameworks produced by CAD-CAM—A clinical study. *Rev. Port. Estomatol. Med. Dentária E Cir. Maxilofac.* **2021**, *62*, 194–200. [CrossRef]
4. Batisse, C.; Nicolas, E. Comparison of CAD/CAM and Conventional Denture Base Resins: A Systematic Review. *Appl. Sci.* **2021**, *11*, 5990. [CrossRef]
5. Janeva, N.M.; Kovacevska, G.; Elencevski, S.; Panchevska, S.; Mijoska, A.; Lazarevska, B. Advantages of CAD/CAM versus Conventional Complete Dentures-a Review. *Open Access Maced. J. Med. Sci.* **2018**, *6*, 1498. [CrossRef] [PubMed]
6. Srinivasan, M.; Gjengedal, H.; Cattani-Lorente, M.; Moussa, M.; Durual, S.; Schimmel, M.; Müller, F. CAD/CAM Milled Complete Removable Dental Prostheses: An in Vitro Evaluation of Biocompatibility, Mechanical Properties, and Surface Roughness. *Dent. Mater. J.* **2018**, *37*, 526–533. [CrossRef] [PubMed]
7. Dawood, A.; Marti, B.M.; Sauret-Jackson, V.; Darwood, A. 3D Printing in Dentistry. *Br. Dent. J.* **2015**, *219*, 521–529. [CrossRef] [PubMed]
8. De Armentia, S.L.; Fernández-Villamarín, S.; Ballesteros, Y.; Del Real, J.C.; Dunne, N.; Paz, E. 3D Printing of a Graphene-Modified Photopolymer Using Stereolithography for Biomedical Applications: A Study of the Polymerization Reaction. *Int. J. Bioprinting* **2022**, *8*, 182–197. [CrossRef] [PubMed]
9. Kamonkhantikul, K.; Arksornnukit, M.; Takahashi, H. Antifungal, optical, and mechanical properties of polymethylmethacrylate material incorporated with silanized zinc oxide nanoparticles. *Int. J. Nanomed.* **2017**, *12*, 2353–2360. [CrossRef] [PubMed]
10. Awada, A.; Nathanson, D. Mechanical Properties of Resin-Ceramic CAD/CAM Restorative Materials. *J. Prosthet. Dent.* **2015**, *114*, 587–593. [CrossRef] [PubMed]
11. Alghazzawi, T.F. Advancements in CAD/CAM Technology: Options for Practical Implementation. *J. Prosthodont. Res.* **2016**, *60*, 72–84. [CrossRef] [PubMed]
12. Zafar, M.S. Prosthodontic Applications of Polymethyl Methacrylate (PMMA): An Update. *Polymers* **2020**, *12*, 2299. [CrossRef] [PubMed]

13. Khattar, A.; Alghafli, J.A.; Muheef, M.A.; Alsalem, A.M.; Al-Dubays, M.A.; AlHussain, H.M.; AlShoalah, H.M.; Khan, S.Q.; AlEraky, D.M.; Gad, M.M. Antibiofilm Activity of 3D-Printed Nanocomposite Resin: Impact of ZrO2 Nanoparticles. *Nanomaterials* **2023**, *13*, 591. [CrossRef] [PubMed]
14. Aati, S.; Chauhan, A.; Shrestha, B.; Rajan, S.M.; Aati, H.; Fawzy, A. Development of 3D Printed Dental Resin Nanocomposite with Graphene Nanoplatelets Enhanced Mechanical Properties and Induced Drug-Free Antimicrobial Activity. *Dent. Mater.* **2022**, *38*, 1921–1933. [CrossRef] [PubMed]
15. Aati, S.; Aneja, S.; Kassar, M.; Leung, R.; Nguyen, A.; Tran, S.; Shrestha, B.; Fawzy, A. Silver-Loaded Mesoporous Silica Nanoparticles Enhanced the Mechanical and Antimicrobial Properties of 3D Printed Denture Base Resin. *J. Mech. Behav. Biomed. Mater.* **2022**, *134*, 105421. [CrossRef] [PubMed]
16. Chen, S.-G.; Yang, J.; Jia, Y.-G.; Lu, B.; Ren, L. TiO2 and PEEK Reinforced 3D Printing PMMA Composite Resin for Dental Denture Base Applications. *Nanomaterials* **2019**, *9*, 1049. [CrossRef] [PubMed]
17. Chen, S.; Yang, J.; Jia, Y.-G.; Lu, B.; Ren, L. A Study of 3D-Printable Reinforced Composite Resin: PMMA Modified with Silver Nanoparticles Loaded Cellulose Nanocrystal. *Materials* **2018**, *11*, 2444. [CrossRef] [PubMed]
18. Marin, E.; Boschetto, F.; Zanocco, M.; Honma, T.; Zhu, W.; Pezzotti, G. Explorative Study on the Antibacterial Effects of 3D-Printed PMMA/Nitrides Composites. *Mater. Des.* **2021**, *206*, 109788. [CrossRef]
19. Kwon, J.-S.; Kim, J.-Y.; Mangal, U.; Seo, J.-Y.; Lee, M.-J.; Jin, J.; Yu, J.-H.; Choi, S.-H. Durable Oral Biofilm Resistance of 3D-Printed Dental Base Polymers Containing Zwitterionic Materials. *Int. J. Mol. Sci.* **2021**, *22*, 417. [CrossRef] [PubMed]
20. Bettencourt, A.F.; Costa, J.; Ribeiro, I.A.C.; Gonçalves, L.; Arias-Moliz, M.T.; Dias, J.R.; Franco, M.; Alves, N.M.; Portugal, J.; Neves, C.B. Development of a chlorhexidine delivery system based on dental reline acrylic resins. *Int. J. Pharm.* **2023**, *631*, 122470. [CrossRef] [PubMed]
21. Costa, J.; Bettencourt, A.; Madeira, A.; Nepomuceno, L.S.; Portugal, J.; Neves, C.B. Surface Properties after Chemical Aging of Chlorhexidine Delivery Systems Based on Acrylic Resin. *Rev. Port. Estomatol. Med. Dent. E Cir. Maxilofac.* **2019**, *60*, 155–162. [CrossRef]
22. Neves, C.B.; Costa, J.; Nepomuceno, L.; Madeira, A.; Portugal, J.; Bettencourt, A. Microhardness and Flexural Strength after Chemical Aging of chlorhexidine delivery systems based on acrylic resin. *Rev. Port. Estomatol. Med. Dentária E Cir. Maxilofac.* **2019**, *60*, 104–110. [CrossRef]
23. Montoya, C.; Roldan, L.; Yu, M.; Valliani, S.; Ta, C.; Yang, M.; Orrego, S. Smart dental materials for antimicrobial applications. *Bioact. Mater.* **2022**, *24*, 1–19. [CrossRef] [PubMed]
24. Neves, C.B.; Costa, J.; Portugal, J.; Bettencourt, A.F. Understanding the Mechanical, Surface, and Color Behavior of Oral Bioactive Prosthetic Polymers under Biodegradation Processes. *Polymers* **2023**, *15*, 2549. [CrossRef] [PubMed]
25. Bettencourt, A.; Florindo, H.F.; Ferreira, I.F.S.; Matos, A.; Monteiro, J.; Neves, C.; Lopes, L.P.; Calado, A.; Castro, M.; Almeida, A.J. Incorporation of tocopherol acetate-containing particles in acrylic bone cement. *J. Microencapsul.* **2010**, *27*, 533–541. [CrossRef] [PubMed]
26. Agarwalla, S.V.; Malhotra, R.; Rosa, V. Translucency, Hardness and Strength Parameters of PMMA Resin Containing Graphene-like Material for CAD/CAM Restorations. *J. Mech. Behav. Biomed. Mater.* **2019**, *100*, 103388. [CrossRef] [PubMed]
27. Moher, D. Preferred Reporting Items for Systematic Reviews and Meta-Analyses: The PRISMA Statement. *Ann. Intern. Med.* **2009**, *151*, 264. [CrossRef]
28. Page, M.J.; McKenzie, J.E.; Bossuyt, P.M.; Boutron, I.; Hoffmann, T.C.; Mulrow, C.D.; Shamseer, L.; Tetzlaff, J.M.; Akl, E.A.; Brennan, S.E.; et al. The PRISMA 2020 statement: An updated guideline for reporting systematic reviews. *BMJ* **2021**, *372*, 71. [CrossRef] [PubMed]
29. Faggion, C.M., Jr. Guidelines for Reporting Pre-Clinical in Vitro Studies on Dental Materials. *J. Evid. Based Dent. Pract.* **2012**, *12*, 182–189. [CrossRef] [PubMed]
30. Alshaikh, A.A.; Khattar, A.; Almindil, I.A.; Alsaif, M.H.; Akhtar, S.; Khan, S.Q.; Gad, M.M. 3D-Printed Nanocomposite Denture-Base Resins: Effect of ZrO2 Nanoparticles on the Mechanical and Surface Properties in Vitro. *Nanomaterials* **2022**, *12*, 2451. [CrossRef] [PubMed]
31. Hada, T.; Kanazawa, M.; Miyamoto, N.; Liu, H.; Iwaki, M.; Komagamine, Y.; Minakuchi, S. Effect of Different Filler Contents and Printing Directions on the Mechanical Properties for Photopolymer Resins. *Int. J. Mol. Sci.* **2022**, *23*, 2296. [CrossRef] [PubMed]
32. Selva-Otaolaurruchi, E.J.; Fernández-Estevan, L.; Solá-Ruiz, M.F.; García-Sala-Bonmati, F.; Selva-Ribera, I.; Agustín-Panadero, R. Graphene-Doped Polymethyl Methacrylate (PMMA) as a New Restorative Material in Implant-Prosthetics: In Vitro Analysis of Resistance to Mechanical Fatigue. *J. Clin. Med.* **2023**, *12*, 1269. [CrossRef] [PubMed]
33. Salgado, H.; Fialho, J.; Marques, M.; Vaz, M.; Figueiral, M.H.; Mesquita, P. Mechanical and Surface Properties of a 3D-Printed Dental Resin Reinforced with Graphene. *Rev. Port. Estomatol. Med. Dent. Cir. Maxilofac.* **2023**, *64*, 12–19. [CrossRef]
34. Marin, E.; Mukai, M.; Boschetto, F.; Sunthar, T.P.; Adachi, T.; Zhu, W.; Rondinella, A.; Lanzutti, A.; Kanamura, N.; Yamamoto, T. Production of Antibacterial PMMA-Based Composites through Stereolithography. *Mater. Today Commun.* **2022**, *32*, 103943. [CrossRef]
35. Raszewski, Z.; Kulbacka, J.; Nowakowska-Toporowska, A. Mechanical Properties, Cytotoxicity, and Fluoride Ion Release Capacity of Bioactive Glass-Modified Methacrylate Resin Used in Three-Dimensional Printing Technology. *Materials* **2022**, *15*, 1133. [CrossRef]

36. Mangal, U.; Min, Y.J.; Seo, J.-Y.; Kim, D.-E.; Cha, J.-Y.; Lee, K.-J.; Kwon, J.-S.; Choi, S.-H. Changes in Tribological and Antibacterial Properties of Poly (Methyl Methacrylate)-Based 3D-Printed Intra-Oral Appliances by Incorporating Nanodiamonds. *J. Mech. Behav. Biomed. Mater.* **2020**, *110*, 103992. [CrossRef] [PubMed]
37. Mangal, U.; Seo, J.-Y.; Yu, J.; Kwon, J.-S.; Choi, S.-H. Incorporating Aminated Nanodiamonds to Improve the Mechanical Properties of 3D-Printed Resin-Based Biomedical Appliances. *Nanomaterials* **2020**, *10*, 827. [CrossRef] [PubMed]
38. Mubarak, S.; Dhamodharan, D.B.; Kale, M.; Divakaran, N.; Senthil, T.P.S.; Wu, L.; Wang, J. A Novel Approach to Enhance Mechanical and Thermal Properties of SLA 3D Printed Structure by Incorporation of Metal–Metal Oxide Nanoparticles. *Nanomaterials* **2020**, *10*, 217. [CrossRef] [PubMed]
39. Totu, E.; Cristache, C.; Isildak, İ.; Yildirim, R.; Burlibasa, M.; Nigde, M.; Burlibasa, L. Preliminary Studies on Citotoxicity and Genotoxicity Assessment of the PMMA-TiO2 Nanocompozites for Stereolithographic Complete Dentures Manufacturing. *Rev. De Chim.* **2018**, *69*, 1160–1165. [CrossRef]
40. Totu, E.E.; Nechifor, A.C.; Nechifor, G.; Aboul-Enein, H.Y.; Cristache, C.M. Poly (Methyl Methacrylate) with TiO_2 Nanoparticles Inclusion for Stereolitographic Complete Denture Manufacturing- the Fututre in Dental Care for Elderly Edentulous Patients? *J. Dent.* **2017**, *59*, 68–77. [CrossRef] [PubMed]
41. Wang, L.; D'Alpino, P.H.P.; Lopes, L.G.; Pereira, J.C. Mechanical Properties of Dental Restorative Materials: Relative Contribution of Laboratory Tests. *J. Appl. Oral Sci.* **2003**, *11*, 162–167. [CrossRef] [PubMed]
42. Albero, A.; Pascual, A.; Camps, I.; Grau-Benitez, M. Comparative Characterization of a Novel Cad-Cam Polymer-Infiltrated-Ceramic-Network. *J. Clin. Exp. Dent.* **2015**, *7*, e495–e500. [CrossRef] [PubMed]
43. Pratap, B.; Gupta, R.; Bhardwaj, B.; Nag, M. Resin based restorative dental materials: Characteristics and future perspectives. *Jpn. Dent. Sci. Rev.* **2019**, *55*, 126–138. [CrossRef] [PubMed]

applied sciences

MDPI

Article

In Vitro Evaluation of Surface Roughness and Color Variation after Two Brushing Protocols with Toothpastes Containing Different Whitening Technologies

Angel Lobito [1,*], Catarina Colaço [1], Joana Costa [1], Jorge Caldeira [1,2], Luís Proença [1] and José João Mendes [1]

[1] Clinical Research Unit (CRU), Egas Moniz Center for Interdisciplinary Research (CiiEM), Egas Moniz School of Health & Science, 2829-511 Almada, Portugal; ccolaco@egasmoniz.edu.pt (C.C.); jcosta@egasmoniz.edu.pt (J.C.); jcaldeira@egasmoniz.edu.pt (J.C.); lproenca@egasmoniz.edu.pt (L.P.); jmendes@egasmoniz.edu.pt (J.J.M.)

[2] LAQV Requimte, Faculdade de Ciências e Tecnologias, Universidade Nova de Lisboa, 2829-516 Almada, Portugal

* Correspondence: alobito@egasmoniz.edu.pt

Abstract: The aim was to evaluate the effect of different whitening toothpastes on the enamel surface roughness and color variation. Twenty-four molars were sectioned and divided into eight groups ($n = 3$) considering the following two factors under study: toothpaste type (Colgate® Total Original, Oral B® 3D White Luxe Perfection, Curaprox® Black is White, and Signal® White Now) and brushing protocol (short- and long-term). Surface roughness was examined by atomic force microscopy (AFM), and color change (ΔE) was measured using the CIE L*a*b* system. Data were statistically analyzed using comparative parametric tests at a 5% significance level. In the short-term protocol, only the Signal® White Now toothpaste increased surface roughness ($p = 0.038$) compared to the Colgate® Total Original group. No significant differences ($p > 0.05$) were observed in surface roughness in the long-term protocol. Regarding color variation, no statistically significant differences ($p > 0.05$) were observed in either protocol. Overall, the whitening toothpastes did not affect enamel surface roughness or color, except for Signal® White Now, which caused increased roughness in the short-term protocol. However, all toothpastes induced a visual change in color.

Keywords: roughness; color; enamel; whitening; toothpaste; brushing; aesthetics

1. Introduction

Achieving an aesthetically pleasing smile often holds greater significance for patients than prioritizing their oral health [1,2]. Consequently, a considerable number of individuals opt for over-the-counter whitening toothpastes, often without a comprehensive understanding of associated risks or its appropriate usage protocols [3].

Tooth discoloration represents a prevalent concern among the population; its origins derive often from dental pigmentation, characterized by the deposition of pigments within the tooth structure. The pigmentation can be of intrinsic and/or extrinsic origin, the latter being the most predominant type that can be removed prophylactically through daily oral hygiene practices and with the use of toothpastes. This discoloration occurs when chromogenic substances adhere to the enamel surface and change its original color [4,5].

Whitening toothpastes have been observed to effectively remove and manage the deposition of chromophores responsible for extrinsic pigmentation [6–9] and the color of teeth is altered by increasing the brightness of the tooth structure, through a combination of mechanical and chemical reactions [10]. These toothpastes commonly contain abrasive particles, optical agents, and/or chemical agents [11].

Whitening toothpastes incorporating abrasive microspheres rely on a mechanical mechanism for pigment removal targeting biofilm and extrinsic pigmentation. Among the abrasives commonly employed in these formulations are calcium carbonate, hydrated silica, dicalcium phosphate, aluminum oxide, and sodium bicarbonate [8,9,12–15].

Activated charcoal toothpastes typically incorporate various abrasives, with silica as the most prevalent. The more abrasive the formulation, the more effective it is at removing extrinsic pigmentation; however, prolonged use may lead to the removal of tooth surface, which can lead to changes in surface roughness [12,13]. Activated charcoal operates by binding to the deposits, bacteria, and pigments (hydrophobic) present on the tooth surface, facilitated by its high surface area, porous nature, and high hydrophobicity. This high adsorption capacity can counteract the effects of fluoride ions, which are typically present in lower concentrations (950 ppm) compared to those found in conventional toothpaste formulations [9,12].

Recently introduced to the market, blue covarine-based whitening toothpastes incorporate a whitening agent that has an optical effect on the color of the tooth surface, altering its perceived shade [7,8]. This optical operates by altering the apparent color of the tooth surface through a uniform deposition of a thin, semi-transparent layer of bluish pigment uniformly on it, with the intensity of the effect correlating with pigment concentration. Examining the additional constituents of whitening toothpastes that include blue covarine reveals the presence of modified silica particles that have an abrasive action on enamel. This coating immediately modifies the interaction and perception of incident light, which is an advantage of this agent and results in yellowed teeth that convey the effect of being whiter and brighter due to the change in the b* axis of the CIE L*a*b* [7,8,14].

In 2019, Vaz et al. conducted a study to evaluate a range of whitening toothpastes with different mechanisms of action, including activated charcoal, blue covarine, hydrogen peroxide, and microbeads [8]. However, this study was limited to the evaluation of color and used a visual assessment method, which is highly subjective. Visual assessments of color variation have a high risk of bias and cannot accurately correlate to the in vivo performance. In an attempt to achieve a more realistic assessment, in our study a colorimeter (Optishade Style Italiano, Smile Line, St-Imier, Switzerland) was used. However, there is a lack of scientific support for this type of instrument [16].

While the efficacy of the whitening toothpastes is often only evaluated based on color changes alone [8], there is a notable gap in understanding their effects on enamel surface roughness. A systematic review was performed in 2022, assessing the effect of whitening toothpaste on the surface roughness of human teeth, including seven studies from which four were included in a meta-analysis [17]. Therefore, more studies are needed to perform a systematic review with more power to evaluate multiple parameters [18].

Understanding the impact of these toothpastes on enamel roughness and color appearance is crucial for offering both professionals and patients valuable insights into balancing desired dental aesthetics with the maintenance of tooth structural integrity. Thus, the objective of this study was to assess the influence of various whitening toothpastes containing different active agents on enamel surface roughness and color variation. This investigation involved two parallel studies, evaluating the effects over both short- and long-term periods using distinct mechanical brushing protocols.

2. Materials and Methods

2.1. Tooth Preparation

This in vitro experimental study was performed on twenty-four permanent human molars, without caries or any type of restoration, obtained from the biobank of the Egas Moniz Dental Clinic (approved by the Ethics Committee of the Egas Moniz School of Health and Science, Portugal, n° 1142).

All teeth were cleaned in running water with detergent with the help of a brush/sponge, followed by scraping with a specific Gracey curette for posterior teeth, and an HW-3H scaler (Woodpecker, Guilin, China). Subsequently, polishing of the teeth was carried out with a prophylaxis paste (Henry Schein, Melville, NY, USA) and pumice stone powder in a counter-angle with a prophylactic brush. After this procedure, the teeth were placed in a

0.5% chloramine trihydrate (v/v) solution for one week and then stored in distilled water in a refrigerator at 4 °C (Bosch GmbH, Munich, Germany) and changed weekly [19].

Twenty-four teeth were sectioned in a mesial–distal direction with a single cut, using a hard tissue microtome (Accutom-50, Struers A/S, Ballerup, Denmark), at a cutting speed of 0.350 mm/s and a rotation of 3200 rpm while irrigated with deionized water. With the implementation of this step in the protocol, it was possible to duplicate the sample number by means of obtaining two identical surfaces per tooth sectioned at the buccal and lingual/palatal sections. Pulp remnants were removed from the internal surface and the pulp cavity was sealed with cyanoacrylate glue (Loctite, Bilbao, Barcelona, Spain). Of the forty-eight surfaces obtained, half were used to assess surface roughness and the other half for color variation. Both assessments were classified as independent studies to evaluate the potential interactions between the two independent variables under study (n = 3): toothpaste types and brushing protocol duration.

The twenty-four specimens used for surface roughness evaluation, within each group, were immersed in 13 mL of deionized water in a single sterilized tube (VWR, Matsonford, PA, USA) in a refrigerator (Bosch GmbH, Munich, Germany) at 4 °C, where they remained until the first roughness evaluation. As of the start of the brushing protocols, all specimens were transferred to an incubator at 37 °C (Memmert, Schwabach, Germany) and immersed in artificial saliva (Table A1, Appendix A).

The remaining twenty-four specimens used to evaluate surface color variation were subjected to a staining protocol that consisted of the placement of each specimen in a 15 mL single sterilized tube (VWR, Matsonford, PA, USA), containing a concentrated coffee solution prepared by mixing 120 mL of boiling water with 2.4 g of instant coffee (Delta Cafés, Campo Maior, Portugal), so that each specimen remained immersed in 5 mL of the solution [20]. The staining protocol consisted of four cycles of 18 h immersion in the staining solution followed by 6 h of drying [8,21]. Throughout the cycles, the samples remained in the incubator at 37 °C (Memmert, Schwabach, Germany). After the staining protocol and before the initial color evaluation, the samples remained in the same conditions as the specimens used for the surface roughness evaluation.

2.2. Brushing Protocols

In both the surface roughness and color variation studies, the specimens were randomly divided into eight different experimental groups based on potential interactions between the two independent variables studies (n = 3): toothpaste types and brushing protocol duration.

Within each protocol, four groups were assigned to different toothpastes:

- Control group (CTO): Colgate® Total Original (Colgate, Palmolive, Porto Salvo, Portugal) conventional toothpaste;
- Group 1 (OB3D): Oral B® 3D White Luxe Perfection (Procter & Gamble, Schwalbach am Taunus, Germany) based on abrasive microsphere whitening technology;
- Group 2 (CBW): Curaprox® Black is White (Curaden Swiss Headquarters, Kriens, Switzerland) based on the activated charcoal whitening technology;
- Group 3 (SWN): Signal® White Now (Unilever RA, Rueil-Malmaison, France) based on blue covarine whitening technology.

These four types of toothpaste (one control and three whitening) share several ingredients with each other (Table A2, Appendix A).

Two different brushing protocols (S and L) were designed to obtain short- and long-term results. Protocol S aimed to mimic human behavior by performing one cycle (5 s), three times a day for 15 days. Protocol L replicated intense brushing, consisting of 30 cycles, 6 times a day, for 3 days, simulating the number of cycles the tooth surface would receive if brushed one cycle three times a day for 6 months, totaling 540 cycles. Both of the mechanical brushing protocols S and L were each carried out with an electric toothbrush Oral B Pro 3 3700 (Braun GmbH, Frankfurt, Germany) with a pressure sensor, by the same pre-calibrated investigator (A.L.), applying a defined volume of toothpaste (6 × 3 × 2 mm) on the respective Oral B CrossAction brush head with soft bristles (Braun GmbH, Frankfurt, Germany), exclusive for each of the toothpaste group.

After each brushing, the samples were rinsed with deionized water for 10 s and restored in artificial saliva (Table A1, Appendix A), which was renewed daily, and then placed back in the incubator at 37 °C after each brushing procedure (Memmert, Schwabach, Germany).

2.3. Surface Roughness Measurement

Surface roughness measurements (Ra) were performed before the initial brushing and after the final one, using an atomic force microscope (AFM) TT-AFM (AFM Workshop, Signal Hill, CA, USA), with the following formula [22,23]:

$$\text{Ra} = \frac{1}{L}\int_0^L |Z(x)|dx \quad (1)$$

The deflection and height-mode images of the samples were obtained with a scan rate of 0.7 Hz, using a vibration mode with a resolution of 512 × 512 pixels. Within each sample, a region with dimensions of 40 × 40 μm was randomly selected, which, using the Gwyddion 2.63 software (CMI, Brun, Czech Republic), made it possible to obtain 16 observations of 10 × 10 μm, resulting in a total of 48 observations for each group in each protocol (under ideal conditions). Since the AFM is limited to a maximum height variation of 17 μm in the area to be evaluated, and taking into account the irregularity of the enamel surface, there were cases in which it was necessary to 'reject' some of the zones obtained because they had atypical values that did not represent the real condition of the enamel. The Ra values were recorded for all the areas tested, representing the average roughness value, and then the difference between the average final and initial roughness values was carried out.

2.4. Color Variation

Color measurements were conducted at two distinct time points: the initial color, immediately following the staining procedure, and the final color, after the completion of the brushing protocols. These measurements were performed with a colorimeter (Optishade Style Italiano, Smile Line, St-Imier, Switzerland) on the tooth crown surface in three different zones: occlusal, middle and cervical [24,25]. This instrument registered the parameters of the CIE L*a*b* system, and the total overall color change (ΔE) was calculated using the formula [7,8,14,26]:

$$\Delta E = \left[(\Delta L^*)^2 + (\Delta a^*)^2 + (\Delta b^*)^2\right]^{1/2} \quad (2)$$

The National Institute of Standards and Technology recommends converting ΔE to National Bureau of Standards (NBS) units by applying the equation:

$$\text{NBS units} = \Delta E \times 0.92 \quad (3)$$

to assess the color differences as shown in Table 1 [26–28].

Table 1. National Bureau of Standards (NBS) units for expressing color differences.

NBS units	Color Differences
<0.5	Extremely slight change
0.5–1.5	Slight change
1.5–3.0	Perceivable change
3.0–6.0	Marked change
6.0–12	Extremely marked change
≥12	Change to another color

2.5. Statistical Analysis

The statistical analysis program IBM SPSS Statistics version 29.0 (IBM, Armonk, NY, USA) was used to analyze all data obtained in this research, using descriptive and inferential statistical analysis methodologies.

Since normality and homogeneity of variance were verified (Shapiro–Wilk and Levene tests, $p > 0.05$), a one-way ANOVA with post hoc Tukey HSD parametric tests was used. In all statistical tests, the level of significance was set at 5%.

3. Results

3.1. Surface Roughness

Descriptive analysis was performed with the mean and standard deviation values of surface roughness difference shown in Table 2. Higher surface roughness values were obtained in the SWN group in protocol S with an increase of 436.2 (± 141.8) nm. Conversely, lower values were obtained in the CTO group in the same protocol with a decrease of 66.1 (± 139.0) nm.

Table 2. Distribution of surface roughness differences (ΔRa, nm) presented as mean (± standard deviation, SD) among the groups, according to the experimental protocol ($n = 3$).

ΔRa (nm) M (± SD)	Protocol S	Protocol L
CTO	−66.1 (± 139.0) ^{a}	−19.9 (± 301.3) ^{a}
OB3D	150.4 (± 130.8) ^{a}	−51.2 (± 4.5) ^{a}
CBW	400.7 (± 273.5) ^{a}	115.5 (± 259.0) ^{a}
SWN	436.2 (± 141.8) ^{b}	155.2 (± 123.0) ^{a}

M = mean, SD = standard deviation. Different lowercase letters indicate significant differences between means in the same protocol (Tukey HSD post hoc test, $p < 0.05$).

In protocol S, there were statistically significant differences in the surface roughness difference mean values among the four different toothpaste groups ($p = 0.03$, ANOVA). The SWN toothpaste resulted in significantly ($p = 0.038$, Tukey HSD) higher surface roughness differences compared to the control group (CTO group). In the other groups (OB3D and CBW), the surface roughness differences' mean values were not statistically significant compared to the control group ($p > 0.05$, Tukey HSD).

On the other hand, in protocol L, no statistically significant differences were observed among the surface roughness difference mean values from the toothpaste experimental groups ($p = 0.576$, ANOVA).

3.2. Color Variation

Descriptive analysis was performed with the mean and standard deviation values of color variation shown in Table 3. Color difference values ranged between 14.9 (± 2.4), in the OB3D group in protocol S, and 10.7 (± 2.9) in the CTO group in protocol L.

Table 3. Distribution of color variation (ΔE) presented as mean (± standard deviation, SD) among the groups, according to the experimental protocol ($n = 3$).

ΔE M (± SD)	Protocol S	Protocol L
CTO	14.7 (± 3.7)	10.7 (± 2.9)
OB3D	14.9 (± 2.4)	10.9 (± 2.5)
CBW	11.6 (± 3.2)	12.2 (± 2.4)
SWN	11.8 (± 1.1)	11.7 (± 3.9)

M = mean, SD = standard deviation.

For both protocols, there were no statistically significant differences in the color difference values among the four different toothpaste groups ($p > 0.05$, ANOVA).

Table 4 shows the data for NBS. In protocol S, the CTO and OB3D caused a change to another tooth color. The other two groups of protocol S and all four experimental groups of protocol L caused an extremely marked color change to the teeth.

Table 4. Distribution of color perception (NBS units, presented as absolute value, and color differences) among the groups, according to the experimental protocol ($n = 3$).

NBS Units Color Differences	Protocol S	Protocol L
CTO	13.5 Change to another color	6.7 Extremely marked change
OB3D	13.7 Change to another color	7.5 Extremely marked change
CBW	10.7 Extremely marked change	11.2 Extremely marked change
SWN	10.8 Extremely marked change	10.8 Extremely marked change

NBS = National Bureau of Standards.

4. Discussion

One of the most critical aspects of an aesthetically pleasing smile is the color of the teeth, which can affect the patient's self-esteem, social interactions, environmental adaptations, employment opportunities and other important aspects that affect their quality of life. Therefore, whitening toothpastes have gained popularity due to their convenience use and widespread accessibility [29].

An ideal whitening toothpaste should effectively remove extrinsic stains while causing minimal effect on tooth structure, but patients are driven by social media and marketing strategies to purchase whitening toothpastes as a reliable and effective alternative to more efficient but more expensive treatments in order to achieve whiter teeth without really understanding their effects. It is important to clarify that these types of whitening toothpastes lack scientific evidence, and their results are highly manipulated by the industry. Further research with robust methodology that reduces the risk of bias is needed to establish the role of abrasive and whitening components present in these toothpastes and their correlation with alterations in surface roughness and color [6,30].

It is important to understand the effects of the different active agents present in whitening toothpastes and their effect on the enamel surface roughness and color following the application of two different mechanical brushing protocols. Such insights are essential to guide both oral health professionals and patients in the selection of an appropriate whitening toothpaste, balancing the desired aesthetic goals with the preservation of the structural integrity of the teeth.

Surface roughness plays a critical role in the retention and adhesion of substances such as bacteria and pigments to the enamel surface. According to the literature, a surface with an average roughness greater than 200 nm is more likely to accumulate bacteria and pigments, which in turn leads to an increase in bacterial plaque, thereby increasing the risk of dental caries, periodontal disease, and tooth discoloration. In addition, enamel surface roughness is a critical variable, as it can affect not only the aesthetic aspects of the smile, but also the enamel's resistance to erosive processes [31–34].

In protocol S of the present study, only the SWN toothpaste increased the surface roughness values compared to the control group (CTO). This can be explained due to the abrasive components present in the composition of the toothpaste. The manufacturer does not specify the exact amount of the different abrasives, nor the relative dentin/enamel abrasiveness. Having high abrasiveness values could be one of the reasons for the statistically significant values in surface roughness. An experimental technique to quantify the abrasive content of different toothpastes requires further studies. Using a combination of scanning electron microscopy (SEM) and energy-dispersive X-ray spectroscopy (EDS) could aid in the identification of the composition of the abrasive particles and their concentration [35,36]. While the study conducted by Shamel et al. (2019) [27] did not verify this, it is plausible that the methodological choice of mixing the toothpaste with distilled water could have influenced the results.

In the same protocol, OB3D and CBW toothpastes did not show differences in surface roughness. These findings are in line with other studies, such as those by Yaghini et al. (2023) and Shaikh et al. (2021) that also concluded that the use of charcoal whitening toothpastes did not increase enamel surface roughness [18,37]. However, there are differences between the methodology of the studies, with the main one being the usage of bovine teeth in the studies carried out by Shaikh et al. (2021) [37].

Despite this result, the CBW group displayed a tendency to higher average roughness values in comparison to the control group. The observed decrease in values within the control group across both protocols can be attributed to the absence of whitening agents in this toothpaste variant (control group). This validates the study's findings.

In the long-term protocol, none of the three whitening toothpastes resulted in differences in the enamel surface roughness. However, it is noteworthy that the surface roughness value recorded for the OB3D group in protocol L differs from the value reported in the current literature [10], which may have resulted from the inherent limitations of an in vitro study.

Regarding the color evaluation for protocol S and considering the NBS scale, no differences were observed within the groups. However, the CBW and SWN groups exhibited a "extremely marked change", while the CTO and OB3D groups demonstrated a "change to another color". Nevertheless, it would be expected that the control group, which is absent of whitening agents, would exhibit lower scores than any of the other groups. This can be attributed to the fact that this toothpaste, although considered "conventional" and containing no additional whitening agent, also contains abrasive particles that remove extrinsic pigmentation from tooth surfaces. Additionally, the literature suggests that the efficacy of extrinsic pigment removal is also directly related to the level of oral hygiene practices, motivation, and the mechanical action of the toothbrush, which may influence the results regardless of the toothpaste used [30,38]. The outcome was as expected for the three whitening toothpastes, all of which demonstrated a whitening effect on the enamel surface, probably due to the chemical and mechanical combination of the whitening and abrasive agents, respectively.

In the long-term protocol and considering the NBS score, all groups registered a score between 6 and 12, which is considered a "extremely marked change". The control group had the lowest score, followed by the OB3D, SWN, and CBW groups, contrary to what was expected based on the assumption that the effects registered in the S protocol would only intensify in the L protocol [10].

Protocol S was designed to mimic normal daily brushing of three cycles per day for 15 days. Protocol L aimed to simulate, in just three days, the same number of cycles that would be obtained if the samples were brushed three times a day for six months, to try and simulate the long-term effects of different toothpastes. Regarding the results of protocol L, one would anticipate the values to align or potentially exacerbate those recorded in protocol S, given that the aim of protocol L was to simulate extensive use. However, it is important to note that this discrepancy was not the primary focus of the study, nor was it subjected to statistical analysis. We can assume that for protocol L, within each of the 30 brushing cycles, the amount of toothpaste used replicated only the amount used in a single brushing, which may have caused a loss in properties over time within the same cycle, due to the long duration.

The Optishade Style Italiano is a contemporary and underutilized colorimeter, with only one scientific study existing in the field of endodontics [39]. Equipped with red, green, and blue filters to approximate the human eye's spectrum, this colorimeter operates by capturing colors through processing the light reflection via said filters [40].

In every in vitro study, inherent limitations are present during its execution. In this study, the limitations include the size of the sample and the irregularity of the enamel surface, which interact with the small size of the area studied (40 μm × 40 μm × 17 μm). The brushing mechanism utilized also posed a limitation, as it was not possible to employ an automatic brushing apparatus. Instead, an electric toothbrush was used, which hindered the ability to predict and rigorously control various factors such as temperature, revolutions per minute, and the pressure exerted between the different samples. Other limitations may derive from the operator such as fatigue, stress, the angle of the brush bristles, and excessive pressure. Furthermore, inherent flaws in analytical instruments, such as the nanometric probes utilized in the AFM and the calibration card of the colorimeter, may contribute to inaccurate measurements, thereby representing an additional limitation in this study.

Further studies with microhardness, SEM images, and EDS, for example, should be performed to enhance the comprehensiveness of this information and facilitate better clinical application.

5. Conclusions

According to the results obtained and attending to all the limitations associated with an in vitro laboratory study, it was possible to conclude that the different whitening toothpastes did not affect the surface roughness of enamel, either in short- or long-term protocols. However, some caution should be taken regarding toothpastes with blue covarine whitening technology, which showed the highest increase in surface roughness.

In terms of color variation after pigmentation with the coffee solution, and, in accordance with the limitations mentioned above, the whitening toothpastes were effective in changing the color of the tooth surface of the samples studied. However, there were no variations between the four toothpastes, so all were effective in removing extrinsic pigmentation.

Whitening toothpastes are increasingly being used by patients as a quick, inexpensive, and effective solution to remove unwanted pigmentation. However, there remains a lack of studies conducted under comparable conditions for the three whitening technologies examined in this investigation. Dentists play a pivotal role in acquiring current evidence on this subject to confidently recommend suitable whitening toothpaste options and offer well-informed guidance to patients in selecting the most appropriate tooth whitening product, considering not only their efficacy but also to avoid oral health complications.

Author Contributions: Conceptualization, A.L., C.C., J.C. (Joana Costa) and J.J.M.; methodology, A.L. and C.C.; validation, J.C. (Joana Costa) and J.J.M.; investigation, A.L., C.C., J.C. (Joana Costa) and J.C. (Jorge Caldeira); resources, J.J.M.; statistical analysis, J.C. (Joana Costa) and L.P.; data curation, A.L., C.C., J.C. (Joana Costa) and L.P.; writing—original draft preparation, A.L., C.C. and J.C. (Joana Costa); writing—review and editing, J.C. (Joana Costa), J.C. (Jorge Caldeira) and L.P.; supervision, J.J.M. All authors have read and agreed to the published version of the manuscript.

Funding: This research was funded by CiiEM Investiga 2019 Shining Spectroscopic Smile EI19/12.

Institutional Review Board Statement: The study was approved by the Ethics Committee of the Egas Moniz School of Health & Science, Portugal (n° 1142 and date of approval 15/12/2022).

Informed Consent Statement: Not applicable.

Data Availability Statement: The original contributions presented in the study are included in the article and further inquiries can be directed to the corresponding authors.

Conflicts of Interest: The authors declare no conflicts of interest.

Appendix A

Table A1. Composition of artificial saliva (with respective quantification).

Compound	Quantity
NaCl	0.80 g
KCl	0.80 g
$CaCl_2 \bullet 2H_2O$	1.812 g
$NaH_2PO_4 \bullet 2H_2O$	1.38 g
$Na_2S \bullet 9H_2O$	0.01 g
Urea	2 g
Distilled H_2O	2000 mL

Table A2. Toothpastes used in this study.

Toothpaste Name	Tooth Technology	Composition	Manufacturer (Batch Number)
Colgate® Total Original (CTO)	Control non-whitening	Glycerin, Aqua, Hydrated Silica, Sodium Lauryl Sulfate, Arginine, Aroma, Cellulose Gum, Zinc Oxide, Poloxamer 407, Zinc Citrate, Tetrasodium Pyrophosphate, Xanthan Gum, Benzyl Alcohol, Cocamidopropyl Betaine, Sodium Fluoride (1450 ppm F^-), Sodium Saccharin, Phosphoric Acid, Hydroxypropyl Methylcellulose, Sucralose, CI 73360, CI 74160, CI 77891.	Colgate, Palmolive, Porto Salvo, Portugal (3104PL1171)
Oral B® 3D White Luxe Perfection (OB3D)	Abrasive microsphere whitening technology	Glycerin, Hydrated Silica, Sodium Hexametaphosphate, Aqua, PEG-6, Aroma, Trisodium Phosphate, Sodium Lauryl Sulfate, Cocamidopropyl Betaine, Sodium Saccharin, Sodium Fluoride (1450 ppm F^-), Carrageenan, PVP, Xanthan Gum, Limonene, Sucralose, Sodium Benzoate, Sodium Hydroxide, CI 74160, Citric Acid, Sodium Citrate, Potassium Sorbate.	Procter & Gamble, Schwalbach am Taunus, Germany (2306G7)
Curaprox® Black is White (CBW)	Activated charcoal whitening technology	Aqua, Sorbitol, Hydrated Silica, Glycerin, Charcoal Powder, Aroma, Decyl Glucoside, Cocamidopropyl, Betaine, Sodium Monofluorophospate (950 ppm F^-), Tocopherol, Xanthan Gym, Maltodextrin, Mica, Hydroxyapatite (Nano), Potassium Acesulfame, Titanium Dioxide, Micro-Crystalline Cellulose, Sodium Chloride, Potassium Chloride, Citrus Limon Peel Oil, Sodium Hydroxide, Zea Mays Starch, Amyloglucosidase, Glucose Oxidase, Urtica Dioica Leaf Extract, Potassium Thiocyanate, Cetearyl Alchohol, Hydrogenated Lecithin, Menthyl Lactate, Mehtyl Diisopropyl Propionamide, Ethyl Menthane Carboxamide, Stearic Acid, Mannitol, Sodium Bisulfite, Tin Oxide, Lactoperoxidase, Limonene.	Curaden Swiss Headquarters, Kriens, Switzerland (199MHD)
Signal® White Now (SWN)	Blue covarine whitening technology	Aqua, Hydrogenated Starch Hydrolysate, Hydrated Silica, Sodium Lauryl Sulfate, Aroma, Cellulose Gum, Sodium Saccharin, Sodium Fluoride (1450 ppm F^-), PVM/MA Copolymer, Glycerin, CI 42090, CI 74160.	Unilever RA, Rueil-Malmaison, France (2038FCA)

References

1. Goettems, M.L.; Fernandez, M.D.S.; Donassollo, T.A.; Henn Donassollo, S.; Demarco, F.F. Impact of Tooth Bleaching on Oral Health-Related Quality of Life in Adults: A Triple-Blind Randomised Clinical Trial. *J. Dent.* **2021**, *105*, 103564. [CrossRef] [PubMed]
2. Goulart, M.D.A.; Condessa, A.M.; Hilgert, J.B.; Hugo, F.N.; Celeste, R.K. Concerns about Dental Aesthetics Are Associated with Oral Health Related Quality of Life in Southern Brazilian Adults. *Ciênc. Saúde Coletiva* **2018**, *23*, 3957–3964. [CrossRef] [PubMed]
3. Demarco, F.F.; Meireles, S.S.; Masotti, A.S. Over-the-Counter Whitening Agents: A Concise Review. *Braz. Oral Res.* **2009**, *23*, 64–70. [CrossRef] [PubMed]
4. Mortazavi, H.; Baharvand, M.; Khodadoustan, A. Colors in Tooth Discoloration: A New Classification and Literature Review. *Int. J. Clin. Dent.* **2014**, *7*, 17.
5. Schemel-Suaréz, M.; López-López, J.; Chimenos-Kustner, E. Dental Pigmentation and Hemochromatosis: A Case Report. *Quintessence Int.* **2017**, *48*, 155–159. [CrossRef] [PubMed]
6. Joiner, A. Whitening Toothpastes: A Review of the Literature. *J. Dent.* **2010**, *38*, e17–e24. [CrossRef] [PubMed]
7. Tao, D.; Smith, R.N.; Zhang, Q.; Sun, J.N.; Philpotts, C.J.; Ricketts, S.R.; Naeeni, M.; Joiner, A. Tooth Whitening Evaluation of Blue Covarine Containing Toothpastes. *J. Dent.* **2017**, *67*, S20–S24. [CrossRef] [PubMed]
8. Peraro Vaz, V.T.; Jubilato, D.P.; Mendonca de Oliveira, M.R.; Freitas Bortolatto, J.; Floros, M.C.; Dantas, A.A.R.; Batista Oliveira Junior, O.D. Whitening Toothpaste Containing Activated Charcoal, Blue Covarine, Hydrogen Peroxide or Microbeads: Which One Is the Most Effective? *J. Appl. Oral Sci.* **2019**, *27*, e20180051. [CrossRef]
9. Vural, U.K.; Bagdatli, Z.; Yilmaz, A.E.; Yalçın Çakır, F.; Altundaşar, E.; Gurgan, S. Effects of Charcoal-Based Whitening Toothpastes on Human Enamel in Terms of Color, Surface Roughness, and Microhardness: An in Vitro Study. *Clin. Oral Investig.* **2021**, *25*, 5977–5985. [CrossRef]
10. Suriyasangpetch, S.; Sivavong, P.; Niyatiwatchanchai, B.; Osathanon, T.; Gorwong, P.; Pianmee, C.; Nantanapiboon, D. Effect of Whitening Toothpaste on Surface Roughness and Colour Alteration of Artificially Extrinsic Stained Human Enamel: In Vitro Study. *Dent. J.* **2022**, *10*, 191. [CrossRef]
11. Lippert, F. An Introduction to Toothpaste-Its Purpose, History and Ingredients. In *Monographs in Oral Science*; Van Loveren, C., Ed.; S. Karger AG: Basel, Switzerland, 2013; Volume 23, pp. 1–14. ISBN 978-3-318-02206-3.
12. Greenwall, L.H.; Greenwall-Cohen, J.; Wilson, N.H.F. Charcoal-Containing Dentifrices. *Br. Dent. J.* **2019**, *226*, 697–700. [CrossRef] [PubMed]
13. Forouzanfar, A.; Hasanpour, P.; Yazdandoust, Y.; Bagheri, H.; Mohammadipour, H.S. Evaluating the Effect of Active Charcoal-Containing Toothpaste on Color Change, Microhardness, and Surface Roughness of Tooth Enamel and Resin Composite Restorative Materials. *Int. J. Dent.* **2023**, *2023*, 6736623. [CrossRef]
14. Del Mar Pérez, M.; Ghinea, R.; Rivas, M.J.; Yebra, A.; Ionescu, A.M.; Paravina, R.D.; Herrera, L.J. Development of a Customized Whiteness Index for Dentistry Based on CIELAB Color Space. *Dent. Mater.* **2016**, *32*, 461–467. [CrossRef] [PubMed]
15. Epple, M.; Meyer, F.; Enax, J. A Critical Review of Modern Concepts for Teeth Whitening. *Dent. J.* **2019**, *7*, 79. [CrossRef] [PubMed]
16. Cone, M.R.; Choi, J.; Awdaljan, M. Optimized Digital Shade Calibration Technology for the Restoration of a Single Central Incisor. *J. Prosthet. Dent.* **2022**, *128*, 1–3. [CrossRef] [PubMed]
17. Jamwal, N.; Rao, A.; Shenoy, R.; Pai, M.; Ks, A.; Br, A. Effect of Whitening Toothpaste on Surface Roughness and Microhardness of Human Teeth: A Systematic Review and Meta-Analysis. *F1000Research* **2022**, *11*, 22. [CrossRef] [PubMed]
18. Yaghini, J.; Moghareabed, A.; Hatam, F.; Keshani, F. Effect of Two Types of Charcoal Toothpaste on the Enamel Surface Roughness of Permanent Teeth. *Dent. Res. J.* **2023**, *20*, 98.
19. *ISO 11405*; Dental Materials–Testing of Adhesion to Tooth Structure. International Organisation for Standardisation: Geneva, Switzerland, 2015.
20. Bazzi, J.Z.; Bindo, M.J.F.; Rached, R.N.; Mazur, R.F.; Vieira, S.; De Souza, E.M. The Effect of At-Home Bleaching and Toothbrushing on Removal of Coffee and Cigarette Smoke Stains and Color Stability of Enamel. *J. Am. Dent. Assoc.* **2012**, *143*, e1–e7. [CrossRef]
21. ElAziz, R.H.; Gadallah, L.K.; Saleh, R.S. Evaluation of Charcoal and Sea Salt–Lemon-Based Whitening Toothpastes on Color Change and Surface Roughness of Stained Teeth. *J. Contemp. Dent. Pract.* **2022**, *23*, 169–175. [CrossRef]
22. De Oliveira, R.R.L.; Albuquerque, D.A.C.; Cruz, T.G.S.; Yamaji, F.M.; Leite, F.L. Measurement of the Nanoscale Roughness by Atomic Force Microscopy: Basic Principles and Applications. In *Atomic Force Microscopy-Imaging, Measuring and Manipulating Surfaces at the Atomic Scale*; InTech: London, UK, 2012; ISBN 978-953-51-0414-8.
23. Anderson, L.N.; Alsahafi, T.; Clark, W.A.; Felton, D.; Sulaiman, T.A. Evaluation of Surface Roughness of Differently Manufactured Denture Base Materials. *J. Prosthet. Dent.* **2023**, S0022-3913(23)00568-1. [CrossRef]
24. Rutkūnas, V.; Dirsė, J.; Bilius, V. Accuracy of an Intraoral Digital Scanner in Tooth Color Determination. *J. Prosthet. Dent.* **2020**, *123*, 322–329. [CrossRef] [PubMed]
25. Chu, S.J.; Trushkowsky, R.D.; Paravina, R.D. Dental Color Matching Instruments and Systems. Review of Clinical and Research Aspects. *J. Dent.* **2010**, *38*, e2–e16. [CrossRef] [PubMed]
26. Inami, T.; Tanimoto, Y.; Minami, N.; Yamaguchi, M.; Kasai, K. Color Stability of Laboratory Glass-Fiber-Reinforced Plastics for Esthetic Orthodontic Wires. *Korean J. Orthod.* **2015**, *45*, 130. [CrossRef] [PubMed]
27. Neves, C.B.; Costa, J.; Portugal, J.; Bettencourt, A.F. Understanding the Mechanical, Surface, and Color Behavior of Oral Bioactive Prosthetic Polymers under Biodegradation Processes. *Polymers* **2023**, *15*, 2549. [CrossRef] [PubMed]

28. Pero, A.C.; Ignárcio, J.; Giro, G.; Mendoza-Marin, D.O.; Paleari, A.G.; Compagnoni, M.A. Surface Properties and Color Stability of an Acrylic Resin Combined with an Antimicrobial Polymer. *Rev. Odontol. UNESP* **2013**, *42*, 237–242. [CrossRef]
29. Bersezio, C.; Martín, J.; Mayer, C.; Rivera, O.; Estay, J.; Vernal, R.; Haidar, Z.S.; Angel, P.; Oliveira, O.B.; Fernández, E. Quality of Life and Stability of Tooth Color Change at Three Months after Dental Bleaching. *Qual. Life Res.* **2018**, *27*, 3199–3207. [CrossRef]
30. Agustanti, A.; Ramadhani, S.A.; Adiatman, M.; Rahardjo, A.; Callea, M.; Yavuz, I.; Maharani, D.A. Efficacy Test of a Toothpaste in Reducing Extrinsic Dental Stain. *J. Phys. Conf. Ser.* **2017**, *884*, 012135. [CrossRef]
31. Rahardjo, A.; Gracia, E.; Riska, G.; Adiatman, M.; Maharani, D.A. Potential Side Effects of Whitening Toothpaste on Enamel Roughness and Micro Hardness. *Int. J. Clin. Prev. Dent.* **2015**, *11*, 239–242. [CrossRef]
32. Gharechahi, M.; Moosavi, H.; Forghani, M. Effect of Surface Roughness and Materials Composition. *J. Biomater. Nanobiotechnol.* **2012**, *3*, 541–546. [CrossRef]
33. Mullan, F.; Austin, R.S.; Parkinson, C.R.; Bartlett, D.W. An In-Situ Pilot Study to Investigate the Native Clinical Resistance of Enamel to Erosion. *J. Dent.* **2018**, *70*, 124–128. [CrossRef]
34. Teutle-Coyotecatl, B.; Contreras-Bulnes, R.; Rodríguez-Vilchis, L.E.; Scougall-Vilchis, R.J.; Velazquez-Enriquez, U.; Almaguer-Flores, A.; Arenas-Alatorre, J.A. Effect of Surface Roughness of Deciduous and Permanent Tooth Enamel on Bacterial Adhesion. *Microorganisms* **2022**, *10*, 1701. [CrossRef] [PubMed]
35. Hodoroaba, V.-D. Energy-Dispersive X-Ray Spectroscopy (EDS). In *Characterization of Nanoparticles*; Elsevier: Amsterdam, The Netherlands, 2020; pp. 397–417. ISBN 978-0-12-814182-3.
36. Peetsch, A.; Epple, M. Characterization of the Solid Components of Three Desensitizing Toothpastes and a Mouth Wash. *Mater. Werkst.* **2011**, *42*, 131–135. [CrossRef]
37. Shaikh, M.; Sung, H.; Lopez, T.; Andra, R.; McKean, B.; Jesson, J.; Pascal, C.; Pascal, C.; Chavez, A.; Schwieterman, K.; et al. Effect of Charcoal Dentifrices on Tooth Whitening and Enamel Surface Roughness. *Am. J. Dent.* **2021**, *34*, 295–299. [PubMed]
38. Aškinytė, D.; Bendinskaitė, R.; Valeiðaitė, S.; Zekonienė, J. The Effectiveness of Whitening Toothpastes in Reducing Extrinsic Dental Stain. *Sveik. Moksl./Health Sci.* **2011**, *21*, 57–60.
39. Lin, H.-N.; Wang, L.-C.; Chen, M.-S.; Chang, P.-J.; Lin, P.-Y.; Fang, A.; Chen, C.-Y.; Lee, P.-Y.; Lin, C.-K. Discoloration Improvement by Mechanically-Milled Binary Oxides as Radiopacifier for Mineral Trioxide Aggregates. *Materials* **2022**, *15*, 7934. [CrossRef]
40. Snizhko, D. Colorimeter Based on Color Sensor. *Electrotech. Rev.* **2017**, *1*, 98–103. [CrossRef]

applied sciences

MDPI

Article

Does Repolishing Affect the Gloss and Roughness of Lithium Disilicate and Monolithic Zirconia Ceramics?

Cigdem Cebi Tuysuz [1], Necla Demir [1,*] and Emir Yuzbasioglu [2]

1 Department of Prosthodontics, Faculty of Dentistry, Selcuk University, Konya 42090, Turkey; cigdemcebi6195@gmail.com
2 Independent Researcher, Istanbul 34365, Turkey; emiryuzbasioglu@icloud.com
* Correspondence: necladt@gmail.com

Abstract: Purpose: Maintaining the surface quality of ceramic restorations after clinical adjustments is critical for both aesthetic outcomes and long-term oral health, yet the optimal approach to restoring gloss and smoothness remains unclear. The purpose of this study is to investigate the effect of different surface finishing and grinding procedures on the surface gloss and roughness of three different monolithic lithium disilicate ceramics and one monolithic ultra-translucent zirconia ceramic. **Materials and Methods**: A total of 104 specimens (1.5 × 12 × 14 mm) were prepared from four ceramic materials: LiSi CEREC Tessera (CT), GC Initial LiSi (LS), IPS e.max CAD (EC), and zirconia disc (KATANA UTML (KAT)). Each was divided into two subgroups based on surface finishing (mechanical polishing or glazing; $n = 10$). Gloss and surface roughness were measured using a glossmeter and a profilometer, respectively. One specimen per subgroup was analyzed under SEM at ×1000 magnification. **Results**: Gloss and roughness values were analyzed with the two-way robust ANOVA test and multiple comparisons were made with Bonferroni correction. The significance level was set at $p < 0.05$. Mechanical polishing, glazing, and repolishing increased the gloss values of the materials, with the KAT group achieving the highest gloss in the repolishing groups. The lowest gloss values were observed in the grinding groups. Additionally, these surface treatments reduced the roughness of the surface of all the materials. **Conclusions**: Surface finishing procedures significantly influenced the gloss and roughness of monolithic lithium disilicate and zirconia ceramics. Mechanical polishing systems performed similarly or better than glazing. However, selecting an appropriate polishing system for each material is essential.

Keywords: mechanical polishing; monolithic ceramics; surface finishing; surface gloss

1. Introduction

Computer-aided design–computer-aided manufacturing (CAD-CAM) ceramic materials facilitate a fully digital workflow, from impression acquisition to final restoration, offering both clinical reliability and high patient satisfaction [1,2]. Lithium disilicate ceramics are widely favored as monolithic ceramic systems for anterior and posterior single crowns [3]. Although glass ceramics offer aesthetic benefits, there has been a growing demand for stronger ceramic restorations [4]. The utilization of anatomically contoured zirconia restorations, known as monolithic zirconia, without the need for veneer porcelain, is on the rise in dentistry due to its superior optical and mechanical properties [5–7]. To overcome the issue of limited translucency in conventional zirconia, a new high-translucency monolithic zirconia has been developed for practical application in clinical use [7].

The final-stage adjustments made on these ceramic restorations using diamond burs are essential for removing occlusal interferences, optimizing the contours of the restorations, and enhancing their aesthetic appearance [8]. These adjustments remove the glaze layer, increasing surface roughness, reducing reflected light, and affecting the restoration's color and gloss while also raising the risk of external staining [9,10]. Ceramic polishing kits are widely used for smooth-polishing the surfaces of ceramic restorations after adjustment. Studies have explored whether ceramic polishing kits can effectively restore ceramic surfaces to a state similar to the original glazed ceramic surfaces prior to any adjustments [11–13]. It has been strongly emphasized that maintaining a smooth ceramic surface during clinical use is crucial for preventing the initiation and progression of microcracks and minimizing the wear of opposing teeth [14]. Therefore, applying a surface finishing procedure after grinding is crucial to restore and enhance the surface properties of ceramic restorations [15,16].

Most recent studies agree that the glazing procedure can produce a sufficiently smooth surface on ceramic restorations [17–20]. Conversely, the polishing process can yield a surface that closely resembles the properties of a natural tooth [21]. Following adjustments of dental ceramics, the laboratory process for reglazing is a time-consuming process. Moreover, once the restoration has been cemented in the mouth, reglazing is no longer feasible. Consequently, mechanical polishing of the adjusted restoration offers a viable solution to achieve a smooth surface, and it can be conducted both intraorally and extraorally [22]. The search for effective clinical polishing methods after adjusting porcelain restorations is of great importance as it reduces the treatment time and enables cementation to be completed in the same session. Reglazing of the restoration requires multiple visits for the patient, as it is performed by glaze firing in the dental laboratory [23]. Patients' desire for a natural tooth appearance can be attained by achieving the right contour, smoothness, and glossiness [24]. Maintenance of a smooth restoration is essential not only for the health of the tooth and the surrounding periodontal tissues but also for the aesthetic aspect of the restoration [25]. Conversely, rough surfaces create an environment conducive to plaque accumulation and staining, potentially resulting in plaque-induced gingivitis, secondary cavities, and adverse effects on gloss [26,27]. Surface profilometry is convenient for quantitative assessment of surface roughness [28]. Surface roughness of the restorations is an important factor for bacterial adhesion. It was reported that a further reduction in Ra below a threshold level of 0.2 μm had no effect on supra- and subgingival microbiological adhesion or colonization [29].

Gloss is defined as a specific light intensity reflectance on a surface, with the incident angle equal and opposite to the reflectance angle [30]. A value of 0 GU indicates a completely non-reflective surface, while 100 GU corresponds to a polished opal glass with the highest refractive surface [31]. In addition, gloss measurements at a 60° angle are considered to be more clinically reliable [32]. The existing literature lacks clarity on the most effective surface finishing method to smooth rough surfaces that arise during the clinical adjustment of monolithic all-ceramic restorations. Additionally, there is inadequate information regarding the impact of surface finishing protocols on surface roughness and gloss. The main objective of this study was to examine how various surface finishing and grinding procedures influence the surface gloss and surface roughness of different CAD-CAM restorative materials. The null hypotheses were that for each restorative material (1) there was no significant difference in surface roughness and gloss values between specimens that underwent only polishing and those that underwent only glazing, and (2) mechanically polishing glazed samples after grinding with a diamond bur did not affect surface roughness or gloss values.

2. Materials and Methods

Based on the results of the power analysis (G*Power software v3.1.10, Heinrich Heine University, Düsseldorf, Germany), it was determined that at least 5 specimens were required in each group to achieve 95% confidence (1-α), 95% test power (1-β), and an effect size of f = 0.57797. To ensure reliability, 10 specimens were prepared for each subgroup (n = 10). Each ceramic group was divided into two subgroups based on the surface treatment applied—mechanical polishing and glazing. In total, 104 specimens (n = 104) were prepared, comprising 20 samples for each CAD-CAM material for surface treatment protocols and 6 additional samples per material for SEM analysis. The materials used in the study are listed in Table 1.

Table 1. Materials used.

Material	Product	Manufacturer	Lot Number
Lithium disilicate ceramic	IPS e.max CAD (EC)	Ivoclar Vivadent, Schaan, Liechtenstein	YB54FL
Lithium disilicate ceramic	CEREC Tessera (CT)	Dentsply Sirona, York, PA, USA	16012436
Lithium disilicate ceramic	GC Initial LiSi (LS)	GC, Tokyo, Japan	2107161
Monolithic zirconia	KATANA UTML (KAT)	Kuraray Noritake, Tainai City, Japan	EFJTM
Mechanical polishing set used for lithium disilicate ceramics	G&Z Instrumente/ DPLT 14 RA Set	EVE Ernst Vetter GmbH, Birkenfeld, Germany	473021
Mechanical polishing set used for monolithic zirconia	G&Z Instrumente/ DCAT 14 RA Set	EVE Ernst Vetter GmbH, Birkenfeld, Germany	473724
Glaze paste and liquid used for IPS e.max CAD	IPS Ivocolor Glaze Paste IPS Ivocolor Mixing Liquid allround	Ivoclar Vivadent, Schaan, Liechtenstein	Z038YF Z03PP9
Glaze paste and liquid used for CEREC Tessera	Universal Overglaze High Flu Universal Stain and Glaze Liquid	Dentsply Sirona, York, PA, USA	21002882 21002448
Glaze paste and liquid used for GC Initial LiSi Block	GC Initial IQ Lustre Pastes ONE/NF GC Initial IQ Lustre Pastes ONE Diluting Liquid	GC, Tokyo, Japan	2205021 2204111
Glaze paste used for KATANA UTML	Cerabien ZR FC Paste Stain Glaze	Kuraray Noritake, Tainai City, Japan	EJABU
Diamond bur with fine grain (red band) (27–76 µm grain size) used for grinding	Meisinger 881Z3-017-FG	Hager & Meisinger GmbH, Neuss, Germany	R14777

Three different lithium disilicate ceramics were used in the present study: CEREC Tessera blocks (CT) (Dentsply Sirona, York, PA, USA); GC Initial LiSi (LS) Block (GC, Tokyo, Japan); IPS e.max CAD (EC) (Ivoclar Vivadent, Schaan, Liechtenstein); and zirconia disc (KATANA (KAT)). All blocks were selected in A2 color, high translucency (HT), and C14 size. The blocks were cut with a thickness of 1.5 $\pm$ 0.05 mm using a diamond cutting disc (Buehler Diamond Wafering Blade, Series 15 LC, Buehler, IL, USA) with a low-speed sectioning device (Isomet 1000, Buehler, Lake Bluff, IL, USA) and samples were prepared in accordance with the block dimensions (1.5 mm $\times$ 12 mm $\times$ 14 mm). Crystallization for EC was performed using the Programat P310 ceramic furnace (Ivoclar Vivadent, Schaan, Liechtenstein) following the manufacturer's instructions. The lithium disilicate blocks (LS and CT) were also crystallized. KATANA 5Y-PSZ monolithic zirconia (Kuraray Noritake, Tainai City, Japan) was used in this study, with a disc of 18 mm thickness and A2 color selected based on the sample dimensions. The zirconia specimens were designed using the Exocad DentalCAD 3.0 Galway (Darmstadt, Germany) software and milled on a Yenadent D15 milling machine (Yena Makina, Istanbul, Turkey). After milling, the samples were sintered in a Protherm PLF 110/6 dental furnace (Protherm Furnaces, Ankara, Turkey) according to the manufacturer's sintering parameters. The thickness of all lithium disilicate and zirconia samples was checked with an electronic caliper (Absolute Digimatic Caliper, Mitutoyo, Kawasaki, Japan). To standardize the surface quality, the specimens were polished using 600-, 800-, 1000-, and 1200-grit silicon carbide papers (3M ESPE, St. Paul, MN, USA) under running water for 30 s. The samples were cleaned in 100% distilled water for 10 min in an ultrasonic cleaner (Ultrasonic Cleaner Cd 4820, Codyson, Shenzhen, China) before finishing.

Mechanical polishing of the lithium disilicate samples was carried out with the G&Z Instrumente DPLT-14 RA (EVE Ernst Vetter GmbH, Keltern, Germany) set, specially produced for mechanical polishing of feldspathic ceramics and lithium disilicate ceramics; it was used in order according to the grain size and color code. Mechanical polishing of the monolithic zirconia specimens was performed with the G&Z Instrumente DCAT-14 RA set (EVE Ernst Vetter GmbH, Germany), which is specially designed for mechanical polishing of zirconia ceramics. The polishing process was applied with a contra-angle rotary instrument (Contra angle 500, Kavo, Germany) under water cooling at a speed of 12,000 rpm according to the manufacturer's recommendation, and carried out by a single investigator. The specimens were polished for 30 s in one direction and for another 30 s at 90 degrees to the first direction [33–36].

Glazing applications were performed with the glazing pastes and liquids recommended by the manufacturer for each different ceramic group. All samples were fired in the glaze programs recommended by the manufacturers. The glazed specimens in each ceramic group were ground with a red-striped fine-grit (27–76 μm) diamond bur (Meisinger 881Z3-017-FG, Hager & Meisinger GmbH, Neuss, Germany) especially recommended for grinding ceramic restorations [37–39].

Surface roughness measurements of the samples were made using a profilometer device (SJ-210, Mitutoyo, Japan) before the surface finishing procedures (control) and after the mechanical polishing, glazing, and grinding processes were completed. Three parallel readings were performed per sample and the Ra parameter (μm) was evaluated. The surface roughness was further observed by scanning electron microscope analysis (Zeiss, Evo LS10, Jena, Germany) at a $\times 1000$ magnification to investigate the effects of the surface finishing procedures. A glossmeter (Novo Curve Benchtop Glossmeter 60°, Rhopoint, UK) with a 60° angle was used for the gloss evaluation [40–42]. Gloss measurements were made of the samples before the surface finishing (control) and after the completion of mechanical polishing, glazing, and grinding. During the measurement, the samples were covered with a black film container to block the external light. Three gloss unit (GU) values were calculated from each specimen and the average value was calculated.

Statistical Analysis

The datasets were analyzed with statistical software (SPSS V23; IBM Corp, Armonk, NY, USA). The conformity to the normal distribution was examined using the Shapiro–Wilk and Kolmogorov–Smirnov tests. The Pearson correlation coefficient was used to analyze the relationship between normally distributed gloss and roughness values, and the Spearman's rho correlation coefficient was used to analyze the relationship between non-normally distributed gloss and roughness values. The analysis results are presented as mean $\pm$ standard deviation (SD) and median (minimum–maximum). The significance level was set at $p < 0.05$. The descriptive statistics and multiple comparison results of the gloss and roughness values were evaluated according to the interaction of the material and surface treatment in the glazing, grinding, and repolishing groups. Compliance with the normal distribution was analyzed by the Shapiro–Wilk test. Gloss and roughness values that did not conform to the normal distribution according to the ceramic and surface treatment were analyzed with the two-way robust ANOVA test and multiple comparisons were made with Bonferroni correction. The analysis results are presented as the median (minimum–maximum). The significance level was set at $p < 0.05$.

3. Results

3.1. Surface Roughness (Ra)

The mean ± SD and median (minimum–maximum) values of the surface roughness values obtained after mechanical polishing of the monolithic CAD-CAM ceramic materials used in this study are presented in Table 2. After the mechanical polishing process for all ceramic groups, the median roughness values decreased and a statistically significant difference was found compared to the control readings ($p = 0.005$). The median roughness value decreased for CT from 0.18 µm to 0.09 µm; for LS from 0.19 µm to 0.08 µm; for EC from 0.2 µm to 0.08 µm; and for KAT from 0.26 µm to 0.12 µm.

Table 2. Comparison of the roughness values after mechanical polishing for each ceramic.

	Control		Mechanical Polishing		Test Statistic	p
	Mean ± SD	**Median (Min–Max)**	**Mean ± SD**	**Median (Min–Max)**		
CT	0.19 ± 0.04	0.18 (0.15–0.26) [b]	0.09 ± 0.01	0.09 (0.07–0.11) [ab]	Z = −2.803	**0.005**
LS Block	0.2 ± 0.02	0.19 (0.17–0.26) [ab]	0.09 ± 0.02	0.08 (0.06–0.13) [b]	Z = −2.805	**0.005**
EC	0.2 ± 0.01	0.2 (0.18–0.21) [ab]	0.09 ± 0.02	0.08 (0.07–0.13) [b]	Z = −2.805	**0.005**
KAT	0.25 ± 0.05	0.26 (0.18–0.31) [a]	0.11 ± 0.02	0.12 (0.09–0.13) [a]	Z = −2.805	**0.005**
Test Statistic	$\chi^2 = 9.594$		$\chi^2 = 11.744$			
p	**0.022**		**0.008**			

Z: Wilcoxon test; χ^2: Kruskal–Wallis test; mean ± SD (standard deviation); median (minimum–maximum); [a,b]: there is no difference between ceramics with the same letter in each column.

The mean ± SD and median (minimum–maximum) values of the surface roughness values obtained after glazing, grinding, and mechanical polishing (repolishing) of the monolithic CAD-CAM ceramic materials used in this study are presented in Table 3. No significant differences ($p < 0.05$) were observed among the ceramic materials in the control, glazing, and grinding protocols. A statistically significant difference was found between the median roughness values in the repolishing groups according to the ceramics ($p = 0.006$). The value obtained for LS Block was higher and differed from the roughness value obtained from CT and KAT. There was no statistically significant difference ($p < 0.05$) between EC and LS Block. A statistically significant difference was observed in the median surface roughness values across all ceramic materials based on the applied surface treatment protocols ($p < 0.001$). While the highest roughness values were obtained in the grinding process, they differed from the values of the repolishing and glazing groups. No statistically significant difference ($p < 0.05$) was found between the repolishing and glazing groups. The roughness values of the glazing groups were lower than the control readings and showed significant differences. The mean ± SD and median (minimum–maximum) values of the surface roughness values obtained after glazing and mechanical polishing of the materials and the differences between the groups are presented in Table 4. A statistically significant difference was observed in the surface roughness values of all lithium disilicate ceramic groups, depending on whether glazing or polishing was applied ($p < 0.05$). The median surface roughness values in the mechanical polishing groups were lower than those in the glazing groups. No statistically significant difference was found in the surface roughness values of the KAT ceramic following the different surface finishing procedures ($p = 0.677$). Two-way analysis of variance (ANOVA) revealed that neither the ceramic type ($p = 0.766$) nor the interaction between ceramic type and surface treatment ($p = 0.217$) had a statistically significant effect on the surface roughness value. However, the surface treatment protocol itself showed a statistically significant effect on the Ra value ($p < 0.001$).

Table 3. Comparison of the roughness values according to the ceramic and the process applied to each ceramic (glazing, grinding, and repolishing).

	Control	Glazing	Grinding	Repolishing	Test Statistic	p
CT	0.19 ± 0.01	0.13 ± 0.02	0.81 ± 0.08	0.16 ± 0.01	$\chi^{2*} = 29.727$	**<0.001**
	0.18 (0.17–0.21) ^{BC}	0.13 (0.11–0.16) ^{A}	0.82 (0.67–0.93) ^{B}	0.17 (0.15–0.18) $^{AC(a)}$		
LS Block	0.19 ± 0.03	0.12 ± 0.01	0.84 ± 0.08	0.18 ± 0.01	$\chi^{2*} = 27.12$	**<0.001**
	0.19 (0.16–0.24) ^{BC}	0.13 (0.11–0.14) ^{A}	0.84 (0.71–0.96) ^{B}	0.18 (0.17–0.2) $^{AC(b)}$		
EC	0.19 ± 0.02	0.12 ± 0.03	0.77 ± 0.12	0.17 ± 0.02	$\chi^{2*} = 26.04$	**<0.001**
	0.19 (0.15–0.23) ^{BC}	0.13 (0.09–0.18) ^{A}	0.76 (0.61–0.98) ^{B}	0.17 (0.15–0.2) $^{AC(ab)}$		
KAT	0.24 ± 0.05	0.11 ± 0.03	0.72 ± 0.13	0.16 ± 0.02	$\chi^{2*} = 30$	**<0.001**
	0.24 (0.17–0.35) ^{BC}	0.11 (0.07–0.14) ^{A}	0.74 (0.47–0.9) ^{B}	0.17 (0.11–0.18) $^{AC(a)}$		
Test Statistic	$\chi^2 = 8.693$	$\chi^2 = 5.587$	$\chi^2 = 6.461$	$\chi^2 = 12.459$		
p	0.051	0.134	0.091	**0.006**		

χ^{2*}: Friedman test; χ^2: Kruskal–Wallis test; mean ± standard deviation; median (minimum–maximum); ^{a,b}: no difference between ceramics with the same lower case letter within each column; $^{A–C}$: no difference between roughness values with the same upper case letter within each row.

Table 4. Comparison of roughness values according to the ceramic and surface finishing process.

	Glazing		Mechanical Polishing		Test Statistic	p
	Mean ± SD	Median (Min–Max)	Mean ± SD	Mean (Min–Max)		
CT	0.13 ± 0.02	0.13 (0.11–0.16)	0.09 ± 0.01	0.09 (0.07–0.11) ^{ab}	U = 0.000	**<0.001**
LS Block	0.12 ± 0.01	0.13 (0.11–0.14)	0.09 ± 0.02	0.08 (0.06–0.13) ^{b}	U = 5.000	**0.001**
EC	0.12 ± 0.03	0.13 (0.09–0.18)	0.09 ± 0.02	0.08 (0.07–0.13) ^{b}	U = 14.000	**0.006**
KAT	0.11 ± 0.03	0.11 (0.07–0.14)	0.11 ± 0.02	0.12 (0.09–0.13) ^{a}	U = 44.500	0.677
Test Statistic	$\chi^2 = 5.587$		$\chi^2 = 11.744$			
p	0.134		**0.008**			

U: Mann–Whitney U test; χ^2: Kruskal–Wallis test; mean ± SD (standard deviation); median (minimum–maximum); ^{a,b}: there is no difference between ceramics with the same letter within each column.

3.2. Surface Gloss (GU)

The mean ± SD and median (minimum–maximum) values of the gloss values obtained after mechanical polishing of the monolithic CAD-CAM ceramic materials used in this study are presented in Table 5. No statistically significant difference was found in the mean gloss values of the control readings across the different ceramic materials ($p = 0.128$). A statistically significant difference was observed in the mean gloss values after mechanical polishing, depending on the type of ceramic material ($p < 0.001$). Here, the highest average value was obtained in the KAT ceramic and it differs from other ceramics (161.7 GU) (KAT > CT > LS~EC). A statistically significant difference was observed between the average gloss values after mechanical polishing and those of the control readings in all the ceramic groups ($p < 0.001$). Mechanical polishing increased the gloss values of all the ceramic materials.

Table 5. Comparison of the gloss values after mechanical polishing for each ceramic.

	Control		**Mechanical Polishing**		**Test Statistic**	***p***
	Mean ± SD	**Median (Min–Max)**	**Mean ± SD**	**Median (Min–Max)**		
CT	64.37 ± 6.81	64.82 (54.2–75.33)	104.33 ± 3.03 [c]	103.77 (99.97–111.6)	t = −18.555	**<0.001**
LS Block	62.79 ± 6.94	60.15 (55.43–76.47)	102.34 ± 4.27 [bc]	102.6 (94.1–108.17)	t = −12.003	**<0.001**
EC	62.37 ± 5.9	61.03 (54.37–75.9)	95.76 ± 5.66 [b]	95.37 (85.4–103.47)	t = −13.666	**<0.001**
KAT	69.29 ± 8.37	68.25 (56.93–84.73)	161.7 ± 15.72 [a]	167.25 (129.37–179.93)	t = −16.035	**<0.001**
Test Statistic	F = 2.023		F = 48.902			
p	0.128		**<0.001**			

t: Paired two-sample *t* test; F: one-way analysis of variance; mean ± SD (standard deviation); median (minimum–maximum); [a–c]: there is no difference between ceramics with the same letter in each column.

The mean ± SD and median (minimum–maximum) values of the gloss values obtained after glazing, grinding, and mechanical polishing (repolishing) of the monolithic CAD-CAM ceramic materials used in this study are presented in Table 6. A statistically significant difference was observed in the median gloss values of the control readings among the different ceramic materials ($p = 0.004$). The median value obtained in the EC ceramic and the value obtained in the KAT ceramic showed a significant difference. No statistically significant difference was found in the median gloss values of the glaze groups among the different ceramic materials ($p = 0.127$). A statistically significant difference was observed in the median gloss values of the grinding groups across the different ceramic materials ($p < 0.001$). While the highest gloss value was obtained in KAT, it did not differ from the value obtained in EC and LS Block, and there was no difference between KAT and CT. A statistically significant difference was observed in the median gloss values of the repolishing groups among the different ceramic materials ($p < 0.001$). Here, the value obtained in the KAT ceramic was higher than the gloss values obtained from all the other ceramics (104.6 GU). A statistically significant difference was found between the median gloss values obtained from different surface treatments in all ceramic groups ($p < 0.001$). The values of the control readings and glazing groups differed from each other for all lithium disilicate ceramic materials used in this study; gloss median values increased with glaze application. The gloss values in the grinding groups were significantly lower than those in the glazing and repolishing groups. The gloss values, which declined following the grinding process, significantly increased after repolishing. No significant difference was found between the glazing and repolishing groups for any of the ceramic materials.

Table 6. Comparison of the gloss values according to the ceramic and the process applied to each ceramic (glazing, grinding, and repolishing).

	Control	Glazing	Grinding	Repolishing	Test Statistic	p
CT	64.2 ± 5.54	101.98 ± 2.71	14.13 ± 0.35	86.22 ± 3.68	$\chi^{2*} = 30$	**<0.001**
	62.55 (58.83- 75.77) $^{BC(ab)}$	102.95 (96.77–105.07) ^{A}	14.03 (13.8–15) $^{B(ac)}$	84.77 (83.2–94.57) $^{AC(b)}$		
LS Block	67.95 ± 6.7	101.29 ± 2.43	13.46 ± 0.17	84.34 ± 2.15	$\chi^{2*} = 30$	**<0.001**
	68.12 (58.07–76.5) $^{BC(ab)}$	100.37 (97.3–105.87) ^{A}	13.42 (13.23–13.73) $^{B(b)}$	83.7 (81.63–89.07) $^{AC(b)}$		
EC	62.05 ± 5.9	100 ± 1.8	13.92 ± 0.25	87.55 ± 7.56	$\chi^{2*} = 28.92$	**<0.001**
	59.85 (54.23–71.93) $^{BC(b)}$	99.6 (98.07–102.53) ^{A}	13.88 (13.63–14.37) $^{B(bc)}$	85.57 (79.03–102.73) $^{AC(b)}$		
KAT UTML	72.34 ± 3.71	101.84 ± 2.62	15.9 ± 1.75	104.92 ± 9.95	$\chi^{2*} = 27.12$	**<0.001**
	72.38 (66.87–76.9) $^{BC(a)}$	102 (98.2–107.4) ^{AC}	15.3 (13.83–18.53) $^{B(a)}$	104.6 (89.8–122.13) $^{A(a)}$		
Test Statistic	$\chi^2 = 13.537$	$\chi^2 = 5.702$	$\chi^2 = 28.303$	$\chi^2 = 20.75$		
p	**0.004**	0.127	**<0.001**	**<0.001**		

χ^{2*}: Friedman test; χ^2: Kruskal–Wallis test; mean ± standard deviation; median (minimum–maximum); $^{a–c}$: no difference between ceramics with the same lower case letter within each column; $^{A–C}$: no difference between gloss values with the same upper case letter within each row.

The mean ± SD and median (minimum–maximum) values of the gloss values obtained after glazing and mechanical polishing of the materials and the differences between the groups are presented in Table 7. A statistically significant difference was found between the gloss values obtained in the KAT ceramics after glazing (102 GU) and mechanical polishing (167.25 GU) ($p < 0.001$). For CT, LS Block, and EC, no significant difference was found between the groups ($p > 0.050$).

Table 7. Comparison of gloss values according to the ceramic and surface finishing process.

	Glazing		Mechanical Polishing		Test Statistic	p
	Mean ± SD	Median (Min–Max)	Mean ± SD	Median (Min–Max)		
CT	101.98 ± 2.71	102.95 (96.77–105.07)	104.33 ± 3.03	103.77 (99.97–111.6) ^{b}	U = 27.50	0.088
LS Block	101.29 ± 2.43	100.37 (97.3–105.87)	102.34 ± 4.27	102.6 (94.1–108.17) ^{b}	U = 38.00	0.364
EC	100 ± 1.8	99.6 (98.07–102.53)	95.76 ± 5.66	95.37 (85.4–103.47) ^{b}	U = 27.00	0.082
KAT UTML	101.84 ± 2.62	102 (98.2–107.4)	161.7 ± 15.72	167.25 (129.37–179.93) ^{a}	U = 0.00	**<0.001**
Test Statistic	$\chi^2 = 5.702$		$\chi^2 = 28.879$			
p	0.127		**<0.001**			

U: Mann–Whitney U test; χ^2: Kruskal–Wallis test; mean ± SD (standard deviation); median (minimum–maximum); ^{a,b}: there is no difference between ceramics with the same letter within each column.

Two-way ANOVA demonstrated that the effect of ceramic type, surface treatment, and ceramic- surface treatment interaction was statistically significant on the gloss variable ($p < 0.001$).

3.3. Correlation Between Gloss and Surface Roughness

No statistically significant correlation was found between the gloss and roughness values of the control readings ($p = 0.683$). There was no statistically significant correlation between the gloss and roughness values after glazing ($p = 0.539$). There was no statistically significant relationship between the gloss and roughness values after grinding ($p = 0.069$).

A statistically negative correlation was found between the gloss and roughness values after repolishing (r = −0.398; p = 0.011) (Table 8).

Table 8. Correlation between gloss and surface roughness values.

		Control—Gloss
Control—Roughness	r	0.046
	p	0.683
		Glazing—Gloss
Glazing—Roughness	r*	0.070
	p	0.539
		Grinding—Gloss
Grinding—Roughness	r	−0.290
	p	0.069
		Repolishing—Gloss
Repolishing—Roughness	r	−0.398
	p	**0.011**

r: Spearman's rho correlation coefficient; r*: Pearson correlation coefficient.

3.4. SEM Evaluation

Shallow scratches and grooves were clearly visible in the control images for all ceramic types. Mechanical polishing enabled a significant reduction in irregularities and scratches. The glazed specimens had a smooth surface texture with no significant grooves or scratches compared to the control readings, although some small voids were observed. Glazing reduced the surface roughness considerably. The images of the grinding groups showed that the homogeneous structure of the glaze layer was destroyed. Grinding with a diamond bur significantly altered the surface morphology. Morphological changes such as intense cracks, grooves, and scratches parallel to the direction of movement of the bur were clearly visible. By applying repolishing after grinding, the surfaces were gradually smoothed, but some deep grinding grooves could not be completely removed and some streaks were observed. Repolished surfaces were noticeably smoother than the ground surfaces (Figures 1–4).

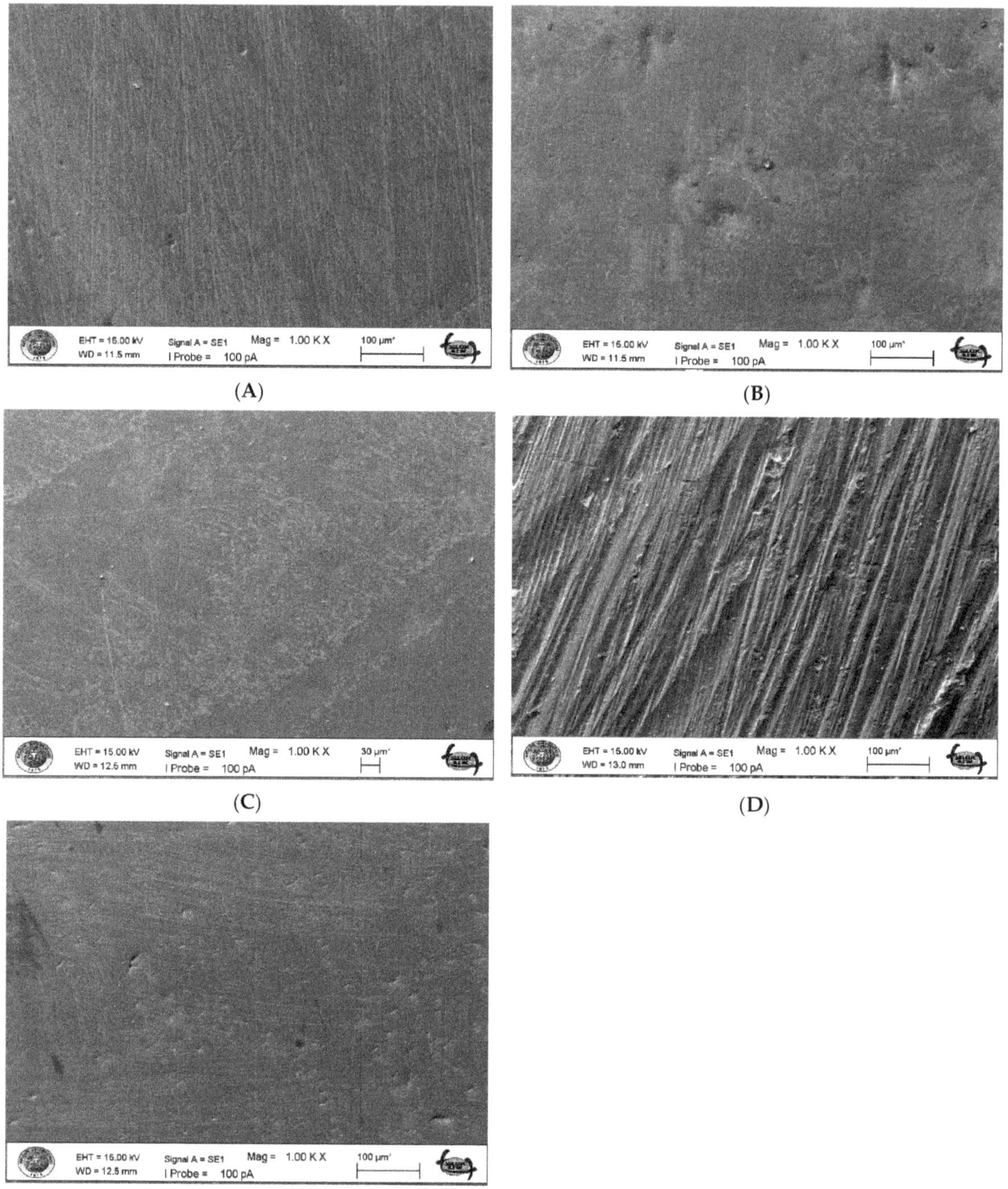

Figure 1. SEM images from CEREC Tessera (original magnification $\times 1000$). (**A**) Control. (**B**) Mechanical polishing group. (**C**) Glazing group. (**D**) Grinding group. (**E**) Repolishing group.

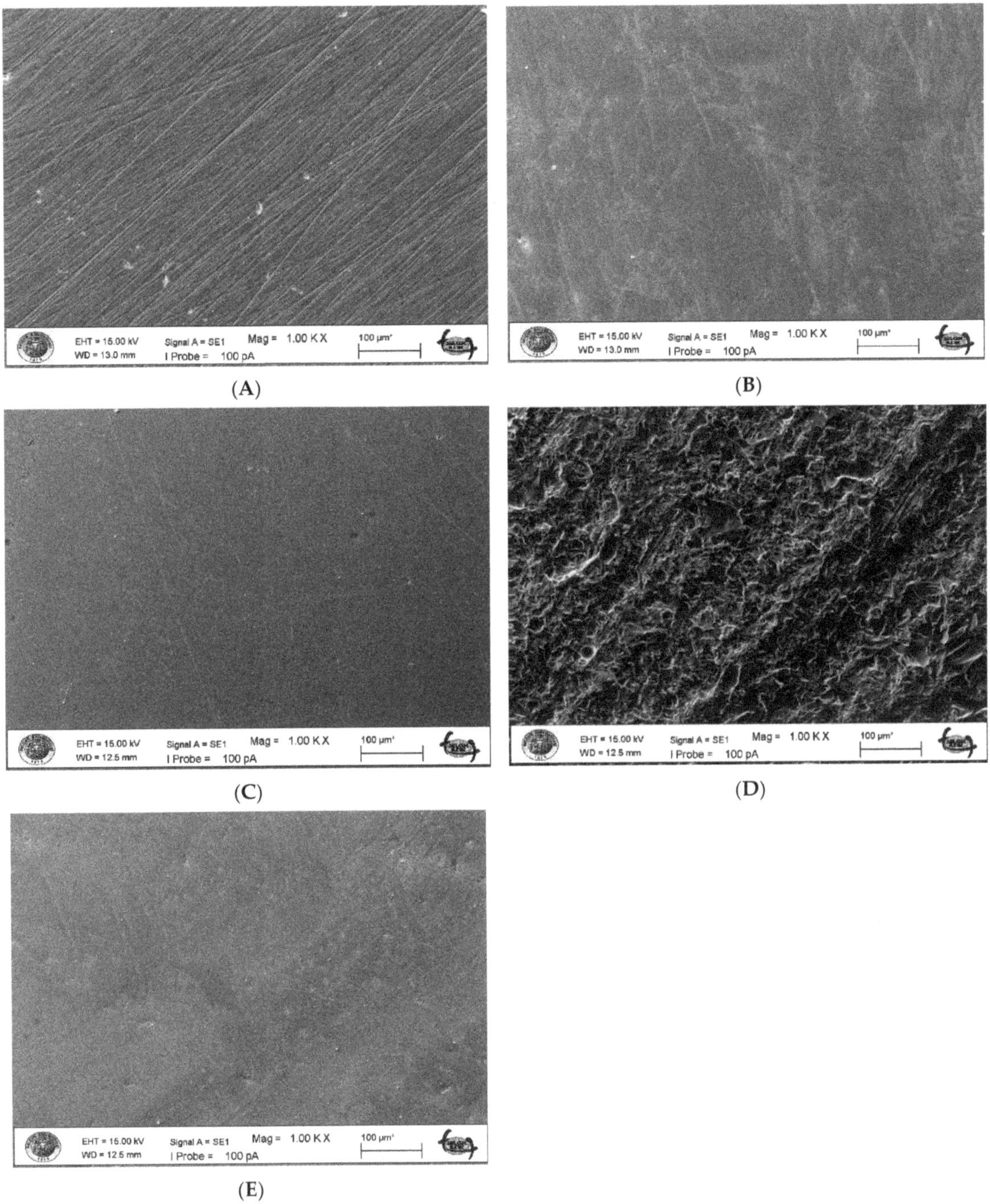

Figure 2. SEM images from GC Initial LiSi (original magnification ×1000). (**A**) Control. (**B**) Mechanical polishing group. (**C**) Glazing group. (**D**) Grinding group. (**E**) Repolishing group.

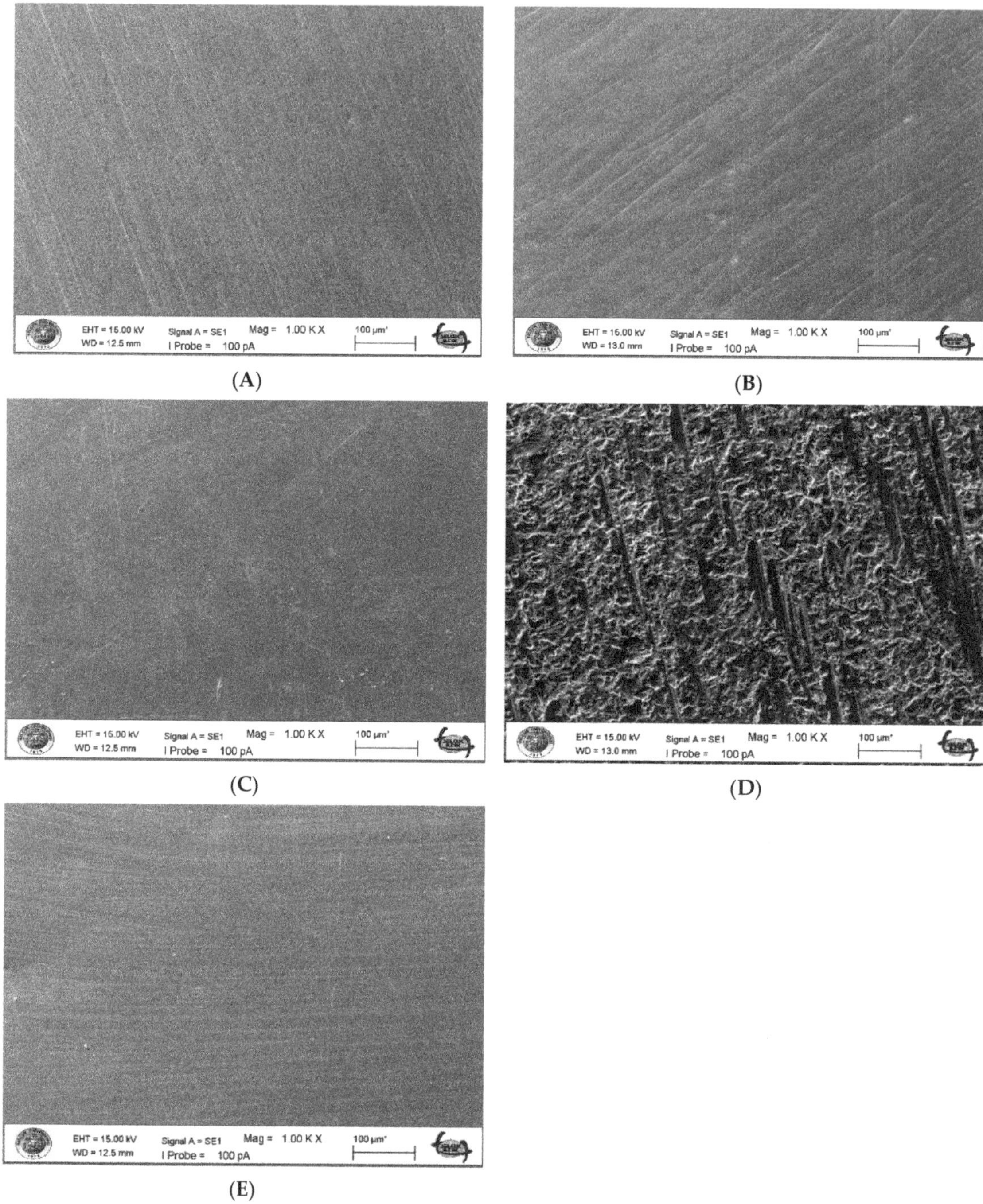

Figure 3. SEM images from IPS e.max CAD (original magnification ×1000). (**A**) Control. (**B**) Mechanical polishing group. (**C**) Glazing group. (**D**) Grinding group. (**E**) Repolishing group.

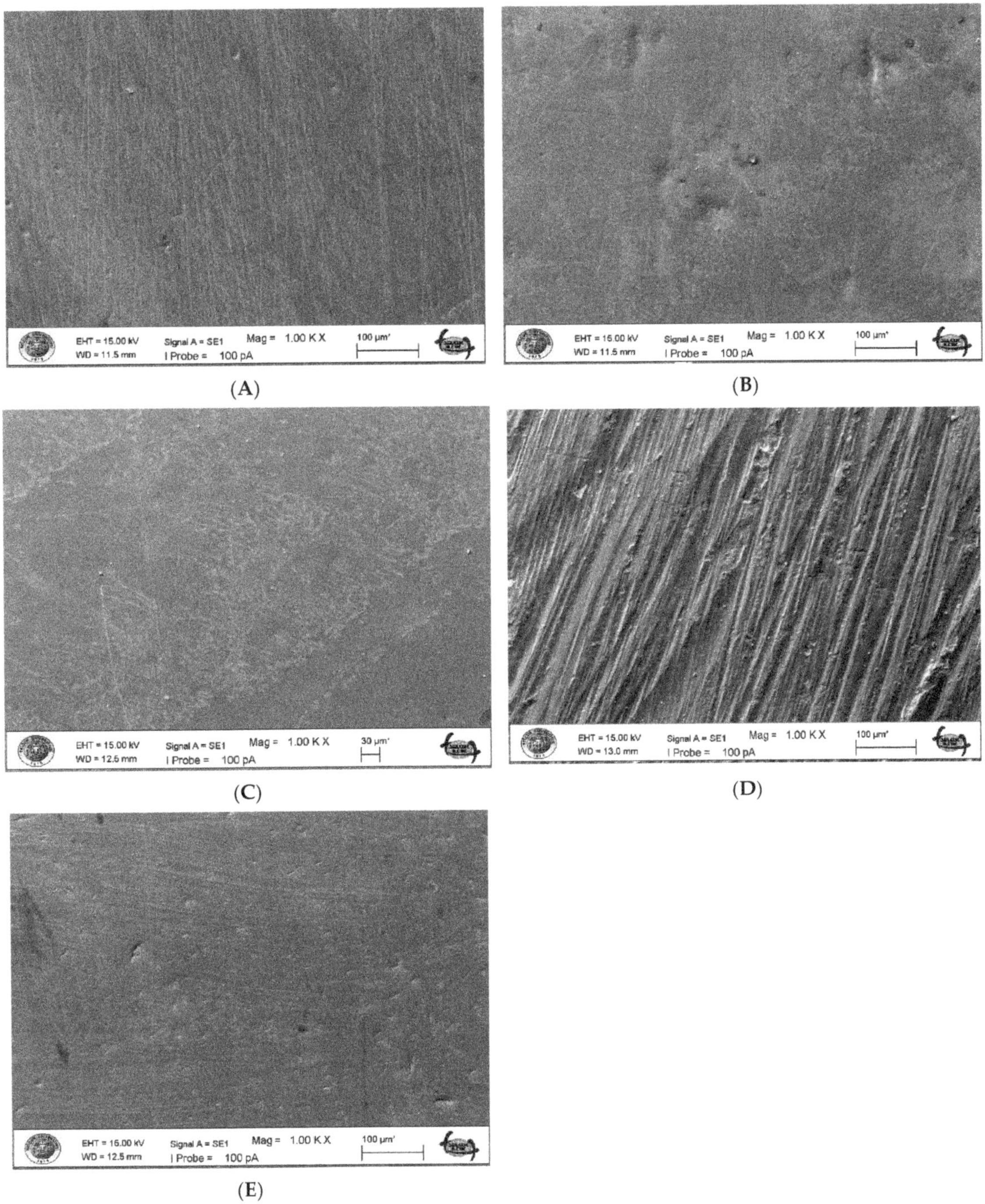

Figure 4. SEM images from KATANA UTML (original magnification ×1000). (**A**) Control. (**B**) Mechanical polishing group. (**C**) Glazing group. (**D**) Grinding group. (**E**) Repolishing group.

4. Discussion

The primary aim of this study was to evaluate the impact of various surface finishing and grinding procedures on the surface gloss and roughness of three types of monolithic lithium disilicate ceramics and one monolithic ultra-translucent zirconia ceramic. This investigation is particularly important because ceramic restorations often undergo intraoral adjustments during clinical procedures, which can compromise their surface integrity. Ensuring that these restorations maintain optimal surface properties—such as smoothness and gloss—is essential for achieving aesthetic satisfaction, minimizing plaque accumulation, and prolonging the lifespan of the restoration. However, there remains a lack of consensus in the literature regarding the most effective method to restore or enhance surface quality following such adjustments. This study contributes valuable insights by comparing the performance of mechanical polishing, glazing, and repolishing protocols across different ceramic materials. Based on the study's outcome, glazing and mechanical polishing had a significant effect on the roughness and gloss values of the ceramic materials ($p < 0.050$), thereby rejecting the first null hypothesis. According to the results from the glazing, grinding, and repolishing groups, the second null hypothesis is partially rejected. After grinding the glaze layer, the mechanical polishing process was significantly able to eliminate the adverse effects of the adjustments. Since mechanical polishing and glazing have varied effects on the smoothness and appearance of dental ceramic surfaces, it was interesting to evaluate in what distinct ways the finishing processes affected surface gloss and roughness [43–45]. Roughness and gloss assessments allow dental ceramics to be analyzed superficially and compared in terms of surface characteristics after surface finishing. Surface roughness and gloss are two essential components that contribute to a restoration's aesthetic appearance [46,47].

Despite advancements in CAD-CAM equipment, chairside adjustments—such as grinding, polishing, and glazing—are frequently required during prosthetic rehabilitation to refine the emergence profile and occlusal or proximal relationships of restorations [48]. Occasionally, additional surface modifications may be necessary even after the restoration has been glazed and permanently cemented to address minor interferences. For long-term clinical success, the surfaces of all ceramic restorations must be adequately smoothed [37,49]. Well-finished surfaces minimize technical and aesthetic complications by enhancing material hardness [50,51], gloss [46], translucency, and color stability [47,52]. A smooth surface also significantly improves patient comfort. Studies have shown that surface roughness (Ra) values exceeding the critical threshold of 0.2 µm are associated with increased risks of dental caries, plaque accumulation, and periodontal inflammation [53]. As a result, numerous investigations have examined the impact of various finishing and polishing techniques on the surface roughness of dental restorative materials [54–56]. Multiple studies consistently report that mechanical polishing not only matches but often surpasses glazing [42,57–59] in producing smooth ceramic surfaces. Kilinc and Turgut, for example, found that manual polishing techniques yielded outcomes comparable to those achieved with glazing [60]. According to Akar et al., using polishing kits and pastes for clinical polishing of ceramics can serve as a secure and efficient substitute for glazing procedures, particularly concerning surface roughness [61]. Mosallam et al. recommended polishing as an alternative to glazing for IPS e.max Press restorations [62]. In a study investigating the effect of polishing and glazing on surface roughness for two distinct hybrid ceramics and a lithium disilicate glass ceramic (EC), the polished surfaces demonstrated lower and clinically acceptable surface roughness values compared to the glazed surfaces across all materials [63]. Numerous studies have shown that mechanical polishing significantly reduces the surface roughness of zirconia, and that the application of polishing results in acceptable intraoral roughness values [64–66]. Similar to the previously mentioned studies, our research found that mechanical polishing led to lower surface roughness values than glazing for all lithium disilicate ceramic materials. Furthermore, the average roughness values of all polished ceramics were within the acceptable threshold for intraoral applications (critical value: 0.2 μm), with the following results: CT—0.09 μm, LS Block—0.08 μm, EC—0.08 μm, and KAT—0.12 μm. As a result, the study concluded that mechanical polishing can be a viable alternative to glazing. Zirconia, with its homogeneous polycrystalline structure and high hardness, presents challenges for conventional polishing systems as they may not achieve a satisfactory polishing effect [67–69]. Numerous studies have shown that zirconia-specific polishing systems outperform universal polishing systems when used on zirconia restorations. These specialized polishing sets are equipped with abrasives, such as diamonds, SiC, and Al_2O_3, that are highly effective in dealing with the elevated hardness of zirconia [70–73]. According to Sasahara et al., the variations in ceramic microstructures make it highly challenging to determine the best polishing technique for each ceramic [23]. A study by Al-Shammery et al. confirmed that different materials require different polishing techniques [74]. In our study, the mechanical polishing and glazing groups exhibited comparable average surface roughness values for the monolithic zirconia ceramic samples. This finding aligns with previous research by several investigators, who also reported similar surface roughness values for both polishing and glazing of monolithic zirconia materials [75,76]. Nonetheless, the outcomes for our lithium disilicate samples were distinct from those obtained for the zirconia samples. These disparities could potentially be ascribed to the different polishing sets utilized or variations in the microstructure of the materials, as indicated in the previously mentioned research [69,70]. Several studies in the literature have examined the effectiveness of mechanical polishing versus glazing after ceramic surfaces have been adjusted with a diamond bur. One study [34] reported that monolithic zirconia specimens, when repolished or overglazed after grinding, exhibited comparable surface roughness values within clinically acceptable limits, supporting the use of chairside mechanical polishing as a viable method to restore smoothness after adjustments [34]. Similarly, research on a newer generation of translucent zirconia [77] found no significant difference in surface roughness between specimens that underwent mechanical polishing and those that were glazed following diamond-bur grinding [77]. Another study [78] comparing monolithic zirconia and feldspathic ceramics demonstrated that samples polished after grinding showed roughness values similar to their glazed counterparts [78]. In a separate investigation on lithium disilicate ceramics (IPS e.max Press) [79], immediate mechanical polishing after glaze removal with a fine-grit diamond bur produced surface roughness levels comparable to those achieved through glazing [79]. Lawson et al. [80] also reported that, for both zirconia and lithium disilicate ceramics, mechanical polishing and glazing following grinding yielded similar roughness values, while the ground-only group exhibited the highest roughness 80]. In agreement with these findings, our study demonstrated that all ceramic materials tested—both lithium disilicate and monolithic zirconia—achieved clinically acceptable surface roughness values after glazing and after grinding followed by mechanical polishing. These results support the effectiveness of mechanical polishing as a chairside alternative to glazing for restoring surface quality.

Surface gloss is one of the desirable properties for restorative materials to mimic the appearance of enamel [81]. The American Dental Association considers a gloss of 40 to 60 GU to be appropriate for dental restorations [40]. Cook and Thomas reported that a poorly finished restoration is generally considered to be below 60 GU, while an acceptable finish is between 60 and 70 GU, and a finish above 80 GU is considered excellent [82]. A gloss value of more than 70 GU means that the human eye cannot distinguish between high and very high gloss [83]. In other words, a material that reaches 70 GU does not appear to be brighter than a material that reaches 90 GU. In contrast to roughness, a clinically accepted threshold for gloss in terms of GU has not yet been established. Nevertheless, some data are available for enamel surface gloss. When the visual luster of different composites was compared to and approximated natural enamel, the gloss of the latter ranged from 40 to 47 GU. In this study, after mechanical polishing, glazing, and repolishing processes, gloss values higher than 80 GU with an excellent finish were obtained in all materials [83].

Chavali et al. [72] conducted a study to evaluate the effects of different polishing systems on the surface roughness and gloss of conventional zirconia. Glazed specimens were used as the control group and were mechanically polished after being ground with a fine-grit diamond bur. The polishing process led to gloss values that were clinically acceptable and either comparable to or better than the glazed control specimens [72,84,85]. Algahtani investigated the impact of various surface finishing techniques on the surface roughness and gloss of different ceramic materials. The gloss values obtained in the glaze and mechanical polishing after grinding groups were within the clinically acceptable values for EC ceramic, as we found in our study [86]. The gloss values achieved by glazing, mechanical polishing, and repolishing for all the ceramic groups in our study were within acceptable intraoral limits, indicating that these procedures can be successfully applied in dental restorations for achieving clinically satisfactory outcomes. In a separate study [87], evaluating the gloss retention and surface roughness of contemporary aesthetic CAD-CAM dental restorative materials, the average gloss value of monolithic translucent zirconia was found to be higher than that of IPS e.max CAD (EC) following polishing. This difference was attributed to zirconia's high refractive index and whiteness, which enhance light reflection 87]. In a similar study, Lee et al. [88] reported that the gloss values of polished monolithic zirconia ceramics were higher than those of the lithium disilicate ceramic groups [88]. In line with previous research, our study also showed that the gloss attained through mechanical polishing for monolithic zirconia was significantly higher than that achieved by EC. The different responses of lithium disilicate and zirconia ceramics to surface treatments can be attributed to their distinct microstructures and compositions. Lithium disilicate ceramics (e.g., EC, LS) contain a glassy matrix and are less hard, allowing polishing to create smoother, glossier surfaces [3]. In contrast, zirconia (e.g., KAT) is a fully crystalline, harder material with no glassy phase, making it more resistant to polishing and requiring specialized protocols to achieve similar gloss. These intrinsic differences explain the variation in surface outcomes after identical treatments [47].

Heintze et al. [46] conducted a study to investigate the relationship between surface roughness and gloss in various dental materials. The study revealed that surface roughness is a contributing factor to gloss, but it is not the sole determinant. In other words, high surface roughness does not always mean low gloss, and vice versa [46]. Monaco et al. [40] investigated the impact of prophylactic polishing pastes on leucite-reinforced glass ceramics, lithium disilicate glass ceramics, and zirconia, focusing on roughness and gloss [40]. They observed a negative relationship between surface roughness and gloss. Similar findings have been reported in other studies concerning the mechanical polishing of feldspathic and hybrid CAD-CAM ceramics; Monaco et al. [40] found that the relationship between 2D roughness and gloss was statistically significant and negatively correlated: roughness increased as surface gloss decreased. The correlation between 2D roughness and translucency was weak for e.max. Further, as a novel study we also found a negative correlation between gloss and roughness in our own study [89,90]. If the restoration was subjected to furnace glazing, the procedure would require a considerable delay of cementation or, more likely, a second appointment. This could save operator time but cannot be considered an effective chairside procedure. [85]. However, there is no "gold standard" finishing and polishing material and/or technique patterned in the literature. In order to improve the comparison of data concerning the efficacy of finishing and polishing systems, it would be useful to standardize methodologies among studies [91].

The difference in gloss values observed between mechanically polished and glazed ceramics can be attributed to both the mechanism of surface modification and inherent material properties. Mechanical polishing involves gradual abrasion using finer-grit abrasives, resulting in a uniform and microscopically smoother surface. This process effectively removes surface irregularities and flattens the microstructure, enhancing specular light reflection, which directly correlates with higher gloss levels [90]. In contrast, glazing relies on applying and firing a thin glassy layer over the ceramic. While it improves esthetics and seals porosities, the glaze layer may exhibit microcracks, uneven thickness, or surface waviness—especially after clinical adjustments—which can diffuse reflected light and reduce gloss [92,93]. Moreover, the ceramic material itself plays a crucial role. Lithium disilicate ceramics (e.g., EC, LS) consist of a fine crystalline phase embedded in a glassy matrix, allowing for more effective polishing due to their relatively homogeneous and softer microstructure). In contrast, zirconia ceramics (e.g., KAT) are fully crystalline, harder, and denser, making them more resistant to mechanical abrasion and more difficult to polish to the same degree of smoothness [37]. These differences impact the surface topography after finishing, and consequently, the gloss outcome.

This study has some limitations. The main limitation of this study is that it was conducted in vitro. While linear roughness parameters such as Ra have been widely used to characterize surfaces, it is also true that these alone are insufficient to fully understand most of the features present in the topography of a material. Therefore, 3D profilometry could be used in future investigations. The specimens were not milled using CAD-CAM but prepared with a low-speed sectioning device. In contrast to our study, the majority of surfaces on crowns or bridges are anatomically curved. For forthcoming investigations, a specialized apparatus capable of enabling standardized pressure during polishing could be employed. This study was performed purely in vitro. While the roughness values (<0.2 μm) and gloss (>60 GU) met clinically acceptable thresholds, the absence of biological testing (e.g., bacterial adhesion, wear resistance) limits direct clinical applicability [92,93]. Future work should consider these factors. The findings of this research are applicable solely to the specific zirconia and lithium disilicate brands utilized in the study and the testing conditions employed. The performance of other ceramic brands might vary due to variations in grain size, sintering temperature, or phase stability.

5. Conclusions

Both mechanical polishing and glaze application significantly affected the surface roughness and gloss of the materials. Surface roughness decreased substantially after surface finishing, reaching clinically acceptable levels (<0.2 μm), while gloss values increased notably, exceeding the clinically acceptable threshold (>60 GU). Among the materials tested, KAT achieved the highest gloss values in the mechanical polishing and repolishing groups. The highest roughness values were observed in KAT for the mechanical polishing groups and LS Block for the repolishing groups.

The mechanical polishing performed after the diamond-bur adjustment of the glaze layer effectively eliminated the negative effects of grinding. A ceramic surface roughened by grinding following clinical adjustments can be restored to its optimal condition through mechanical polishing rather than reglazing.

Clinical Considerations

Manual polishing systems enable chairside restorations in a single session, delivering results comparable to or even better than glazing. This approach allows clinicians to avoid heat treatment and streamline the workflow, which is especially beneficial with the increasing popularity of monolithic restorations. By choosing the appropriate polishing system for the specific ceramic material, clinicians can achieve outcomes as effective as glazing and dependable in clinical practice.

Author Contributions: Conceptualization, N.D. and E.Y.; methodology, N.D. and C.C.T.; validation, N.D., E.Y., and C.C.T.; format analysis, N.D., E.Y., and C.C.T.; investigation, C.C.T.; writing—original draft preparation, N.D. and C.C.T.; writing—review and editing, N.D. and E.Y.; supervision, N.D. and E.Y. All authors have read and agreed to the published version of the manuscript.

Funding: This study was supported by Selcuk University Scientific Research Projects, Konya, Turkey (project number 22132007).

Institutional Review Board Statement: Not applicable.

Informed Consent Statement: Not applicable.

Data Availability Statement: The datasets used and/or analyzed during the current study are available from the corresponding author upon reasonable request.

Conflicts of Interest: The authors declare no conflict of interest.

References

1. Alessandretti, R.; Borba, M.; Benetti, P.; Corazza, P.H.; Ribeiro, R.; Della Bona, A. Reliability and mode of failure of bonded monolithic and multilayer ceramics. *Dent. Mater.* **2017**, *33*, 191–197. [CrossRef] [PubMed]
2. Sfondrini, M.F.; Gandini, P.; Malfatto, M.; Di Corato, F.; Trovati, F.; Scribante, A. Computerized Casts for Orthodontic Purpose Using Powder-Free Intraoral Scanners: Accuracy, Execution Time, and Patient Feedback. *BioMed Res. Int.* **2018**, *2018*, 4103232. [CrossRef] [PubMed]
3. Kelly, J.R.; Benetti, P. Ceramic materials in dentistry: Historical evolution and current practice. *Aust. Dent. J.* **2011**, *56* (Suppl. S1), 84–96. [CrossRef]
4. Tinschert, J.; Natt, G.; Mautsch, W.; Augthun, M.; Spiekermann, H. Fracture resistance of lithium disilicate-, alumina-, and zirconia-based three-unit fixed partial dentures: A laboratory study. *Int. J. Prosthodont.* **2001**, *14*, 231–238.
5. Alaniz, J.; Perez-Gutierrez, F.; Aguilar, G.; Garay, J. Optical properties of transparent nanocrystalline yttria stabilized zirconia. *Opt. Mater.* **2009**, *32*, 62–68. [CrossRef]
6. Johansson, C.; Kmet, G.; Rivera, J.; Larsson, C.; Vult Von Steyern, P. Fracture strength of monolithic all-ceramic crowns made of high translucent yttrium oxide-stabilized zirconium dioxide compared to porcelain-veneered crowns and lithium disilicate crowns. *Acta Odontol. Scand.* **2014**, *72*, 145–153. [CrossRef]
7. Zhang, Y. Making yttria-stabilized tetragonal zirconia translucent. *Dent. Mater.* **2014**, *30*, 1195–1203. [CrossRef]
8. Sarac, D.; Sarac, Y.S.; Yuzbasioglu, E.; Bal, S. The effects of porcelain polishing systems on the color and surface texture of feldspathic porcelain. *J. Prosthet. Dent.* **2006**, *96*, 122–128. [CrossRef]
9. Yilmaz, C.; Korkmaz, T.; Demirköprülü, H.; Ergün, G.; Ozkan, Y. Color stability of glazed and polished dental porcelains. *J. Prosthodont.* **2008**, *17*, 20–24. [CrossRef]
10. Palla, E.S.; Kontonasaki, E.; Kantiranis, N.; Papadopoulou, L.; Zorba, T.; Paraskevopoulos, K.M.; Koidis, P. Color stability of lithium disilicate ceramics after aging and immersion in common beverages. *J. Prosthet. Dent.* **2018**, *119*, 632–642. [CrossRef]
11. Boaventura, J.M.; Nishida, R.; Elossais, A.A.; Lima, D.M.; Reis, J.M.; Campos, E.A.; de Andrade, M.F. Effect finishing and polishing procedures on the surface roughness of IPS Empress 2 ceramic. *Acta Odontol. Scand.* **2013**, *71*, 438–443. [CrossRef] [PubMed]
12. Camacho, G.B.; Vinha, D.; Panzeri, H.; Nonaka, T.; Gonçalves, M. Surface roughness of a dental ceramic after polishing with different vehicles and diamond pastes. *Braz. Dent. J.* **2006**, *17*, 191–194. [CrossRef] [PubMed]
13. Flury, S.; Lussi, A.; Zimmerli, B. Performance of different polishing techniques for direct CAD/CAM ceramic restorations. *Oper. Dent.* **2010**, *35*, 470–481. [CrossRef] [PubMed]
14. Hmaidouch, R.; Weigl, P. Tooth wear against ceramic crowns in posterior region: A systematic literature review. *Int. J. Oral Sci.* **2013**, *5*, 183–190. [CrossRef]
15. Tuncdemir, A.R.; Dilber, E.; Kara, H.B.; Ozturk, A.N. The effects of porcelain polishing techniques on the color and surface texture of different porcelain systems. *Mater. Sci. Appl.* **2012**, *3*, 294–300. [CrossRef]

16. Kim, H.K.; Kim, S.H.; Lee, J.B.; Han, J.S.; Yeo, I.S. Effect of polishing and glazing on the color and spectral distribution of monolithic zirconia. *J. Adv. Prosthodont.* **2013**, *5*, 296–304. [CrossRef]
17. Brodine, B.A.; Korioth, T.V.; Morrow, B.; Shafter, M.A.; Hollis, W.C.; Cagna, D.R. Surface Roughness of Milled Lithium Disilicate With and Without Reinforcement After Finishing and Polishing: An In Vitro Study. *J. Prosthodont.* **2021**, *30*, 245–251. [CrossRef]
18. Çakmak, G.; Subaşı, M.G.; Sert, M.; Yilmaz, B. Effect of surface treatments on wear and surface properties of different CAD-CAM materials and their enamel antagonists. *J. Prosthet. Dent.* **2023**, *129*, 495–506. [CrossRef]
19. Vieira, A.C.; Oliveira, M.C.; Lima, E.M.; Rambob, I.; Leite, M. Evaluation of the surface roughness in dental ceramics submitted to different finishing and polishing methods. *J. Indian Prosthodont. Soc.* **2013**, *13*, 290–295. [CrossRef]
20. Kim, H.K.; Kim, S.H.; Lee, J.B.; Ha, S.R. Effects of surface treatments on the translucency, opalescence, and surface texture of dental monolithic zirconia ceramics. *J. Prosthet. Dent.* **2016**, *115*, 773–779. [CrossRef]
21. Kim, I.J.; Lee, Y.K.; Lim, B.S.; Kim, C.W. Effect of surface topography on the color of dental porcelain. *J. Mater. Sci. Mater. Med.* **2003**, *14*, 405–409. [CrossRef] [PubMed]
22. Shetty, P.; Purayil, T.P.; Ginjupalli, K.; Pentapati, K.C. Effect of polishing technique and immersion in beverages on color stability of nanoceramic composites. *J. Oral Biol. Craniofac. Res.* **2021**, *11*, 53–56. [CrossRef] [PubMed]
23. Sasahara, R.M.; Ribeiro Fda, C.; Cesar, P.F.; Yoshimura, H.N. Influence of the finishing technique on surface roughness of dental porcelains with different microstructures. *Oper. Dent.* **2006**, *31*, 577–583. [CrossRef]
24. Cenci, M.S.; Venturini, D.; Pereira-Cenci, T.; Piva, E.; Demarco, F.F. The effect of polishing techniques and time on the surface characteristics and sealing ability of resin composite restorations after one-year storage. *Oper. Dent.* **2008**, *33*, 169–176. [CrossRef]
25. Kawai, K.; Urano, M.; Ebisu, S. Effect of surface roughness of porcelain on adhesion of bacteria and their synthesizing glucans. *J. Prosthet. Dent.* **2000**, *83*, 664–667. [CrossRef]
26. Aykent, F.; Yondem, I.; Ozyesil, A.G.; Gunal, S.K.; Avunduk, M.C.; Ozkan, S. Effect of different finishing techniques for restorative materials on surface roughness and bacterial adhesion. *J. Prosthet. Dent.* **2010**, *103*, 221–227. [CrossRef]
27. Coşkun, E.; Aslan, Y.U.; Özkan, Y.K. Evaluation of two different CAD-CAM inlay-onlays in a split-mouth study: 2-year clinical follow-up. *J. Esthet. Restor. Dent.* **2020**, *32*, 244–250. [CrossRef]
28. Karayazgan, B.; Atay, A.; Saracli, M.A.; Gunay, Y. Evaluation of Candida albicans formation on feldspathic porcelain subjected to four surface treatment methods. *Dent. Mater. J.* **2010**, *29*, 147–153. [CrossRef]
29. Lee, Y.K.; Lim, B.S.; Kim, C.W. Effect of surface conditions on the color of dental resin composites. *J. Biomed. Mater.* **2002**, *63*, 657–663. [CrossRef]
30. The Glossary of Prosthodontic Terms: Ninth Edition. *J. Prosthet. Dent.* **2017**, *117*, e1–e105. [CrossRef]
31. Powers, J.M.; Wataha, J.C. *Dental Materials: Properties and Manipulation*, 9th ed.; Elsevier Health Sciences: St. Louis, MO, USA, 2012.
32. Kakaboura, A.; Fragouli, M.; Rahiotis, C.; Silikas, N. Evaluation of surface characteristics of dental composites using profilometry, scanning electron, atomic force microscopy and gloss-meter. *J. Mater. Sci. Mater. Med.* **2007**, *18*, 155–163. [CrossRef] [PubMed]
33. Steiner, R.; Beier, U.S.; Heiss-Kisielewsky, I.; Engelmeier, R.; Dumfahrt, H.; Dhima, M. Adjusting dental ceramics: An in vitro evaluation of the ability of various ceramic polishing kits to mimic glazed dental ceramic surface. *J. Prosthet. Dent.* **2015**, *113*, 616–622. [CrossRef] [PubMed]
34. Mohammadi-Bassir, M.; Babasafari, M.; Rezvani, M.B.; Jamshidian, M. Effect of coarse grinding, overglazing, and 2 polishing systems on the flexural strength, surface roughness, and phase transformation of yttrium-stabilized tetragonal zirconia. *J. Prosthet. Dent.* **2017**, *118*, 658–665. [CrossRef] [PubMed]
35. Al Hamad, K.Q.; Abu Al-Addous, A.M.; Al-Wahadni, A.M.; Baba, N.Z.; Goodacre, B.J. Surface Roughness of Monolithic and Layered Zirconia Restorations at Different Stages of Finishing and Polishing: An In Vitro Study. *J. Prosthodont.* **2019**, *28*, 818–825. [CrossRef]
36. Jin, M.; Zhao, J.; Zheng, Y. Effects of Grinding and Polishing on Surface Characteristics of Monolithic Zirconia Fabricated by Different Manufacturing Processes: Wet Deposition and Dry Milling. *J. Prosthodont.* **2022**, *31*, 714–721. [CrossRef]
37. Preis, V.; Behr, M.; Handel, G.; Schneider-Feyrer, S.; Hahnel, S.; Rosentritt, M. Wear performance of dental ceramics after grinding and polishing treatments. *J. Mech. Behav. Biomed. Mater.* **2012**, *10*, 13–22. [CrossRef]
38. Matzinger, M.; Hahnel, S.; Preis, V.; Rosentritt, M. Polishing effects and wear performance of chairside CAD/CAM materials. *Clin. Oral Investig.* **2019**, *23*, 725–737. [CrossRef]
39. Limpuangthip, N.; Poosanthanasarn, E.; Salimee, P. Surface roughness and hardness of CAD/CAM ceramic materials after polishing with a multipurpose polishing kit: An in vitro study. *Eur. J. Dent.* **2022**, *17*, 1075–1083. [CrossRef]
40. Monaco, C.; Arena, A.; Scheda, L.; Di Fiore, A.; Zucchelli, G. In vitro 2D and 3D roughness and spectrophotometric and gloss analyses of ceramic materials after polishing with different prophylactic pastes. *J. Prosthet. Dent.* **2020**, *124*, 787.e1–787.e8. [CrossRef]

41. Vichi, A.; Fabian Fonzar, R.; Goracci, C.; Carrabba, M.; Ferrari, M. Effect of Finishing and Polishing on Roughness and Gloss of Lithium Disilicate and Lithium Silicate Zirconia Reinforced Glass Ceramic for CAD/CAM Systems. *Oper. Dent.* **2018**, *43*, 90–100. [CrossRef]
42. Lawson, N.C.; Burgess, J.O. Gloss and Stain Resistance of Ceramic-Polymer CAD/CAM Restorative Blocks. *J. Esthet. Restor. Dent.* **2016**, *28* (Suppl. 1), S40–S45. [CrossRef] [PubMed]
43. Brunot-Gohin, C.; Duval, J.L.; Azogui, E.E.; Jannetta, R.; Pezron, I.; Laurent-Maquin, D.; Gangloff, S.; Egles, C. Soft tissue adhesion of polished versus glazed lithium disilicate ceramic for dental applications. *Dent. Mater.* **2013**, *29*, e205–e212. [CrossRef] [PubMed]
44. Odatsu, T.; Jimbo, R.; Wennerberg, A.; Watanabe, I.; Sawase, T. Effect of polishing and finishing procedures on the surface integrity of restorative ceramics. *Am. J. Dent.* **2013**, *26*, 51–55.
45. Silva, T.M.; Salvia, A.C.; Carvalho, R.F.; Pagani, C.; Rocha, D.M.; Silva, E.G. Polishing for glass ceramics: Which protocol? *J. Prosthodont. Res.* **2014**, *58*, 160–170. [CrossRef]
46. Heintze, S.D.; Forjanic, M.; Rousson, V. Surface roughness and gloss of dental materials as a function of force and polishing time in vitro. *Dent. Mater.* **2006**, *22*, 146–165. [CrossRef]
47. Awad, D.; Stawarczyk, B.; Liebermann, A.; Ilie, N. Translucency of esthetic dental restorative CAD/CAM materials and composite resins with respect to thickness and surface roughness. *J. Prosthet. Dent.* **2015**, *113*, 534–540. [CrossRef]
48. Ludovichetti, F.S.; Trindade, F.Z.; Adabo, G.L.; Pezzato, L.; Fonseca, R.G. Effect of grinding and polishing on the roughness and fracture resistance of cemented CAD-CAM monolithic materials submitted to mechanical aging. *J. Prosthet. Dent.* **2019**, *121*, 866.e1–866.e8. [CrossRef]
49. Fasbinder, D.J. Clinical performance of chairside CAD/CAM restorations. *J. Am. Dent. Assoc.* **2006**, *137*, 22S–31S. [CrossRef]
50. de Jager, N.; Feilzer, A.J.; Davidson, C.L. The influence of surface roughness on porcelain strength. *Dent. Mater.* **2000**, *16*, 381–388. [CrossRef]
51. Lohbauer, U.; Müller, F.A.; Petschelt, A. Influence of surface roughness on mechanical strength of resin composite versus glass ceramic materials. *Dent. Mater.* **2008**, *24*, 250–256. [CrossRef]
52. Motro, P.F.; Kursoglu, P.; Kazazoglu, E. Effects of different surface treatments on stainability of ceramics. *J. Prosthet. Dent.* **2012**, *108*, 231–237. [CrossRef] [PubMed]
53. Bollen, C.M.; Lambrechts, P.; Quirynen, M. Comparison of surface roughness of oral hard materials to the threshold surface roughness for bacterial plaque retention: A review of the literature. *Dent. Mater.* **1997**, *13*, 258–269. [CrossRef] [PubMed]
54. Kou, W.; Molin, M.; Sjögren, G. Surface roughness of five different dental ceramic core materials after grinding and polishing. *J. Oral Rehabil.* **2006**, *33*, 117–124. [CrossRef] [PubMed]
55. Elmaria, A.; Goldstein, G.; Vijayaraghavan, T.; Legeros, R.Z.; Hittelman, E.L. An evaluation of wear when enamel is opposed by various ceramic materials and gold. *J. Prosthet. Dent.* **2006**, *96*, 345–353. [CrossRef]
56. Saraç, D.; Turk, T.; Elekdag-Turk, S.; Saraç, Y.S. Comparison of 3 polishing techniques for 2 all-ceramic materials. *Int. J. Prosthodont.* **2007**, *20*, 465–468.
57. Oliveira-Junior, O.B.; Buso, L.; Fujiy, F.H.; Lombardo, G.H.; Campos, F.; Sarmento, H.R.; Souza, R. Influence of polishing procedures on the surface roughness of dental ceramics made by different techniques. *Gen. Dent.* **2013**, *61*, e4–e8.
58. Schneider, J.; Dias Frota, B.M.; Passos, V.F.; Santiago, S.L.; Freitas Pontes, K.M. Effects of 2 polishing techniques and reglazing on the surface roughness of dental porcelain. *Gen. Dent.* **2013**, *61*, e6–e9.
59. Fasbinder, D.J.; Neiva, G.F. Surface Evaluation of Polishing Techniques for New Resilient CAD/CAM Restorative Materials. *J. Esthet. Restor. Dent.* **2016**, *28*, 56–66. [CrossRef]
60. Kilinc, H.; Turgut, S. Optical behaviors of esthetic CAD-CAM restorations after different surface finishing and polishing procedures and UV aging: An in vitro study. *J. Prosthet. Dent.* **2018**, *120*, 107–113. [CrossRef]
61. Akar, G.C.; Pekkan, G.; Çal, E.; Eskitaşçıoğlu, G.; Özcan, M. Effects of surface-finishing protocols on the roughness, color change, and translucency of different ceramic systems. *J. Prosthet. Dent.* **2014**, *112*, 314–321. [CrossRef]
62. Mosallam, R.; Taymour, M.; Katamish, H.; Kheirallah, L. Clinical assessment of color stability and patient satisfaction for polished versus glazed lithium disilicate glass ceramic restorations: Randomized controlled clinical trial. *Int. J. Health Sci.* **2022**, *6*, 2819–2830. [CrossRef]
63. Akan, E.; Colgecen, O.; Meşe, I.T.; Bağiş, B. Effects of Different Finishing Procedures on Surface Roughness of Hybrid CAD/CAM Materials. *J. Dent. Indones.* **2021**, *28*, 185–191. [CrossRef]
64. Alves, L.M.M.; da Silva Rodrigues, C.; Ramos, G.F.; Campos, T.M.B.; de Melo, R.M. Wear behavior of silica-infiltrated monolithic zirconia: Effects on the mechanical properties and surface characterization. *Ceram. Int.* **2022**, *48*, 6649–6656. [CrossRef]
65. Pott, P.C.; Hoffmann, J.P.; Stiesch, M.; Eisenburger, M. Polish of interface areas between zirconia, silicate-ceramic, and composite with diamond-containing systems. *J. Adv. Prosthodont.* **2018**, *10*, 315–320. [CrossRef]

66. Park, C.; Vang, M.S.; Park, S.W.; Lim, H.P. Effect of various polishing systems on the surface roughness and phase transformation of zirconia and the durability of the polishing systems. *J. Prosthet. Dent.* **2017**, *117*, 430–437. [CrossRef]
67. Amer, R.; Kürklü, D.; Johnston, W. Effect of simulated mastication on the surface roughness of three ceramic systems. *J. Prosthet. Dent.* **2015**, *114*, 260–265. [CrossRef]
68. Miyazaki, T.; Nakamura, T.; Matsumura, H.; Ban, S.; Kobayashi, T. Current status of zirconia restoration. *J. Prosthodont. Res.* **2013**, *57*, 236–261. [CrossRef]
69. Happe, A.; Röling, N.; Schäfer, A.; Rothamel, D. Effects of different polishing protocols on the surface roughness of Y-TZP surfaces used for custom-made implant abutments: A controlled morphologic SEM and profilometric pilot study. *J. Prosthet. Dent.* **2015**, *113*, 440–447. [CrossRef]
70. Goo, C.L.; Yap, A.; Tan, K.; Fawzy, A.S. Effect of Polishing Systems on Surface Roughness and Topography of Monolithic Zirconia. *Oper. Dent.* **2016**, *41*, 417–423. [CrossRef]
71. Huh, Y.H.; Park, C.J.; Cho, L.R. Evaluation of various polishing systems and the phase transformation of monolithic zirconia. *J. Prosthet. Dent.* **2016**, *116*, 440–449. [CrossRef]
72. Chavali, R.; Lin, C.P.; Lawson, N.C. Evaluation of Different Polishing Systems and Speeds for Dental Zirconia. *J. Prosthodont.* **2017**, *26*, 410–418. [CrossRef] [PubMed]
73. Caglar, I.; Ates, S.M.; Yesil Duymus, Z. The effect of various polishing systems on surface roughness and phase transformation of monolithic zirconia. *J. Adv. Prosthodont.* **2018**, *10*, 132–137. [CrossRef] [PubMed]
74. Al-Shammery, H.A.; Bubb, N.L.; Youngson, C.C.; Fasbinder, D.J.; Wood, D.J. The use of confocal microscopy to assess surface roughness of two milled CAD-CAM ceramics following two polishing techniques. *Dent. Mater.* **2007**, *23*, 736–741. [CrossRef] [PubMed]
75. Sabrah, A.H.; Cook, N.B.; Luangruangrong, P.; Hara, A.T.; Bottino, M.C. Full-contour Y-TZP ceramic surface roughness effect on synthetic hydroxyapatite wear. *Dent. Mater.* **2013**, *29*, 666–673. [CrossRef]
76. Hafezeqoran, A.; Sabanik, P.; Koodaryan, R.; Ghalili, K.M. Effect of sintering speed, aging processes, and different surface treatments on the optical and surface properties of monolithic zirconia restorations. *J. Prosthet. Dent.* **2022**, *130*, 917–926. [CrossRef]
77. Zucuni, C.P.; Pereira, G.K.R.; Valandro, L.F. Grinding, polishing and glazing of the occlusal surface do not affect the load-bearing capacity under fatigue and survival rates of bonded monolithic fully-stabilized zirconia simplified restorations. *J. Mech. Behav. Biomed. Mater.* **2020**, *103*, 103528. [CrossRef]
78. Incesu, E.; Yanikoglu, N. Evaluation of the effect of different polishing systems on the surface roughness of dental ceramics. *J. Prosthet. Dent.* **2020**, *124*, 100–109. [CrossRef]
79. Auškalnis, A.; Žekonis, G.; Sūdžiūtė, G.; Povilaitytė, G.; Milčius, D. Lithium disilicate ceramic roughness evaluation after different finishing methods and comparison before and after surface reduction and intraoral polishing imitation. *Eur. Int. J. Sci. Technol.* **2017**, *6*, 44–52.
80. Lawson, N.C.; Janyavula, S.; Syklawer, S.; McLaren, E.A.; Burgess, J.O. Wear of enamel opposing zirconia and lithium disilicate after adjustment, polishing and glazing. *J. Dent.* **2014**, *42*, 1586–1591. [CrossRef]
81. Yazici, A.R.; Tuncer, D.; Antonson, S.; Onen, A.; Kilinc, E. Effects of delayed finishing/polishing on surface roughness, hardness and gloss of tooth-coloured restorative materials. *Eur. J. Dent.* **2010**, *4*, 50–56. [CrossRef]
82. Cook, M.; Thomas, K. Evaluation of gloss meters for measurement of moulded plastics. *Polym. Test.* **1990**, *9*, 233–244. [CrossRef]
83. Jin, J.; Takahashi, R.; Hickel, R.; Kunzelmann, K.H. Surface properties of universal and flowable nanohybrid composites after simulated tooth brushing. *Am. J. Dent.* **2014**, *27*, 149–154. [PubMed]
84. Yilmaz, K.; Ozkan, P. Profilometer evaluation of the effect of various polishing methods on the surface roughness in dental ceramics of different structures subjected to repeated firings. *Quintessence Int.* **2010**, *41*, e125–e131.
85. Carrabba, M.; Vichi, A.; Vultaggio, G.; Pallari, S.; Paravina, R.; Ferrari, M. Effect of Finishing and Polishing on the Surface Roughness and Gloss of Feldspathic Ceramic for Chairside CAD/CAM Systems. *Oper. Dent.* **2017**, *42*, 175–184. [CrossRef]
86. Algahtani, F. Evaluation of Surface Characteristics for Three Milled CAD/CAM Monolithic Ceramic Restorations. Master's Thesis, Nova Southeastern University, Fort Lauderdale, FL, USA, 2018.
87. Vagkopoulou, T.; Koutayas, S.O.; Koidis, P.; Strub, J.R. Zirconia in dentistry: Part 1. Discovering the nature of an upcoming bioceramic. *Eur. J. Esthet. Dent.* **2009**, *4*, 130–151.
88. Lee, J.-H.; Kim, S.-H.; Han, J.-S.; Yeo, I.-S.L.; Yoon, H.-I.; Lee, J. Effects of ultrasonic scaling on the optical properties and surface characteristics of highly translucent CAD/CAM ceramic restorative materials: An in vitro study. *Ceram. Int.* **2019**, *45*, 14594–14601. [CrossRef]
89. Alhassan, M.; Maawadh, A.; Labban, N.; Alnafaiy, S.M.; Alotaibi, H.N.; BinMahfooz, A.M. Effect of different surface treatments on the surface roughness and gloss of resin-modified CAD/CAM ceramics. *Appl. Sci.* **2022**, *12*, 11972. [CrossRef]
90. Yu, P.; Luo, H.; Yap, A.U.; Tian, F.C.; Wang, X.Y. Effects of polishing press-on force on surface roughness and gloss of CAD-CAM composites. *J. Oral Sci.* **2023**, *65*, 131–135. [CrossRef]

91. Vinagre, A.; Barros, C.; Gonçalves, J.; Messias, A.; Oliveira, F.; Ramos, J. Surface Roughness Evaluation of Resin Composites after Finishing and Polishing Using 3D-Profilometry. *Int. J. Dent.* **2023**, *2023*, 4078788. [CrossRef]
92. Rosentritt, M.; Hmaidouch, R.; Behr, M. Influence of exposure to drinks on the color stability of shaded zirconia ceramics and glazes. *Dent. Mater. J.* **2009**, *28*, 546–552.
93. Al-Hiyasat, A.S.; Darmani, H.; Elbetieha, A. The effects of surface roughness and polishing techniques on plaque accumulation and wear behavior of ceramic restorations. *J. Prosthet. Dent.* **2010**, *104*, 211–217.

applied sciences

MDPI

Article

Tuning BMI.NTf$_2$ Ionic Liquid Concentration in Dental Adhesives Towards a Rational Design of Antibacterial Materials

Isadora Martini Garcia [1], Andressa Simionato [2], Virgínia Serra Souza [3], Jackson Damiani Scholten [3,*], Mary Anne Sampaio Melo [1,*] and Fabrício Mezzomo Collares [2,*]

1 Division of Cariology and Operative Dentistry, Department of Comprehensive Dentistry, University of Maryland School of Dentistry, 650 W Baltimore Street, Baltimore, MD 21201, USA; igarcia1@umaryland.edu
2 Department of Dental Materials, School of Dentistry, Federal University of Rio Grande do Sul, Ramiro Barcelos Street, 2492, Rio Branco, Porto Alegre 90035-004, RS, Brazil; matjje_simionato@hotmail.com
3 Laboratory of Molecular Catalysis, Institute of Chemistry, Federal University of Rio Grande do Sul, Bento Gonçalves Avenue, 9500, Agronomia, Porto Alegre 91501-970, RS, Brazil; vivi_qui@hotmail.com
* Correspondence: jackson.scholten@ufrgs.br (J.D.S.); mmelo@umaryland.edu (M.A.S.M.); fabricio.collares@ufrgs.br (F.M.C.)

Abstract: 1-Butyl-3-methylimidazolium bis(trifluoromethylsulfonyl)imide (BMI.NTf$_2$) is a hydrophobic ionic liquid with potential antibacterial properties for dental materials. This study aimed to (1) incorporate different mass fractions of BMI.NTf$_2$ into a dental adhesive and (2) assess its impact on physical and chemical properties. Adhesive resins were prepared with 1 ($G_{1\%}$), 2.5 ($G_{2.5\%}$), and 5 wt.% ($G_{5\%}$) BMI.NTf$_2$, with a control group (G_{CTRL}) lacking the ionic liquid. Evaluations included polymerization kinetics, degree of conversion (DC), softening in solvent (ΔKHN%), and ultimate tensile strength (UTS). Groups with BMI.NTf$_2$ showed accelerated polymerization kinetics, with $G_{5\%}$ achieving a higher DC and ΔKHN% compared to G_{CTRL} ($p < 0.05$). Lower concentrations (1% and 2.5%) did not affect ΔKHN%, and no significant differences were found in UTS across groups ($p > 0.05$). Notably, 2.5 wt.% of BMI.NTf$_2$ increased the DC without affecting other properties, indicating optimal polymerization rates and handling characteristics. These results support the development of BMI.NTf$_2$-based antibacterial adhesives that may assist in preventing secondary caries in restorative dentistry.

Keywords: dental caries; dental materials; dentin-bonding agents; ionic liquids; polymers; in vitro techniques

1. Introduction

The prevention of secondary caries around bonded restorations triggered by bacterial growth and infiltration into the bonding interface is a challenge. A method is urgently required to help preserve the bonding quality and performance over time [1,2]. Therefore, developing antibacterial, biocompatible, and strong dental adhesives with mechanical and physical properties that match the rate of bacterial growth inhibition is a valuable pursuit [1,2]. Researchers are exploring various additives to improve dental adhesives, focusing on strength and antimicrobial protection. Silver nanoparticles can prevent bacterial growth [3], while quaternary ammonium compounds help break down bacterial cell membranes, reducing plaque buildup [4]. To enhance mechanical properties, nano-fillers like silica are added, making polymers more resistant [5]. By reinforcing the seal against the oral environment, these enhanced adhesives could help prevent secondary caries and extend the life of dental restorations [6,7].

Ionic liquids are organic salts formed by aliphatic chains connected to a high-molecular-weight cation associated with a low-molecular-weight anion [8]. Organic molecules, such as pyridine and imidazole, are commonly used to synthesize pyridinium and imidazolium-based ionic liquids, respectively [9,10]. Among these, imidazole is well known for its biocompatibility and antifungal effect. Ionic liquids can present a broad-spectrum antimicrobial property, affecting gram-positive and gram-negative bacteria, mycobacteria, and fungi [10]. In the pharmaceutical industry, these salts are associated with polymers for drug delivery systems to participate in antibacterial polymer coating synthesis and other processes [9].

In dentistry, imidazolium ionic liquids have already been used to coat titanium implants, testing their adherence to the implant and antimicrobial and anti-corrosion properties [11]. In another study, an imidazolium ionic liquid was used with silver nanoparticles to disinfect root canals against *Enterococcus faecalis*. This material demonstrated greater fibroblast viability than 2.5% sodium hypochlorite and 0.2% chlorhexidine solutions [12].

More recently, the ionic liquid 1-n-butyl-3-methylimidazolium tetrafluoroborate ($BMI.BF_4$) was used to functionalize titanium dioxide quantum dots embedded in an experimental adhesive resin. Its incorporation associated with titanium dioxide quantum dots resulted in immediate and long-term antibacterial activity without showing cytotoxic effects on pulp cells [12]. Another ionic liquid, 1-n-butyl-3-methylimidazolium bis(trifluoromethanesulfonyl)imide ($BMI.NTf_2$) [13], shows the same cation but an anion (bis(trifluoromethanesulfonyl)imide, NTf_2) with higher hydrophobicity compared to the previously used tetrafluoroborate (BF_4), which could bring advantages to dental polymeric materials.

The increased hydrophobicity can enhance the durability of dental polymers by reducing their susceptibility to water absorption. Materials that absorb less water are less likely to undergo hydrolytic degradation, which can weaken their structural integrity and shorten their useful life [14]—consequently, $BMI.NTf_2$ may help extend the longevity of dental restorations. The hydrophobic nature of NTf_2 may reduce the adhesion of bacteria and the absorption of staining agents, which are common issues in dental applications [15]. This property not only helps maintain the aesthetic appearance of dental restorations but also promotes better oral hygiene by reducing the potential for bacterial growth on the surface of the materials.

To initiate studies with $BMI.NTf_2$, this ionic liquid was tested in an experimental orthodontic resin, demonstrating an antimicrobial effect against *Streptococcus mutans* and no cytotoxicity against human keratinocytes when tested up to 5 wt.% [13]. In the present study, $BMI.NTf_2$ was incorporated into an experimental adhesive resin and tested at 1, 2.5, and 5 wt.%. This study aimed to analyze the physical and chemical properties of the adhesives with $BMI.NTf_2$. In this study, we designed $BMI.NTf_2$ containing adhesives with different concentrations (control = no addition of $BMI.NTf_2$, 1%, 2.5%, 5%), and we investigated the concentration-dependent changes in their physico-chemical and mechanical properties in vitro. The null hypothesis of this study is that the addition of the ionic liquid does not change the evaluated properties.

2. Materials and Methods

This is an in vitro and controlled study. The analyzed factor was the different concentrations (control group = no addition of $BMI.NTf_2$, 1 wt.%, 2 wt.%, or 5 wt.%) of ionic liquid added to the adhesive.

2.1. Formulation of Adhesive Resin Samples

The samples used in this study were composed of polymerized or unpolymerized adhesive resins formulated by blending 66.66 wt.% bisphenol A glycerolate dimethacrylate (BisGMA) (Sigma-Aldrich, St. Louis, MO, USA) and 33.33 wt.% 2-hydroxyethyl methacrylate (HEMA) (Sigma-Aldrich, St. Louis, MO, USA). Camphorquinone (Sigma-Aldrich, St. Louis, MO, USA) and ethyl 4-dimethylamino benzoate (Sigma-Aldrich, St. Louis, MO, USA) were added as a photoinitiator system in 1 mol%. Butylhydroxy toluene (Sigma-Aldrich, St. Louis, MO, USA) was added as a polymerization inhibitor at 0.01 wt.%. The ionic liquid 1-*n*-butyl-3-methylimidazolium bis(trifluoromethanesulfonyl)imide ($BMI.NTf_2$) was formulated according to a previous study [13] and incorporated at 1 ($G_{1\%}$), 2.5 ($G_{2.5\%}$), and 5 ($G_{5\%}$) wt.% in the adhesive resin. A control group (G_{CTRL}) was formulated without $BMI.NTf_2$. The adhesives were hand-mixed for 5 min, sonicated for 180 s, and hand-mixed again for 5 min [12]. The adhesives were stored in tubes covered with aluminum foil.

An illustration of the ionic liquid $BMI.NTf_2$ incorporated into the adhesive is shown schematically in Figure 1. All specimens were light-cured using a light-emitting diode (LED, Radii Cal, SDI, Bayswater, Victoria, Australia) at 1200 mW/cm^2 and kept in distilled water for 24 h at 37 °C before testing, except for specimens of polymerization kinetics and degree of conversion (DC), which were prepared during the tests.

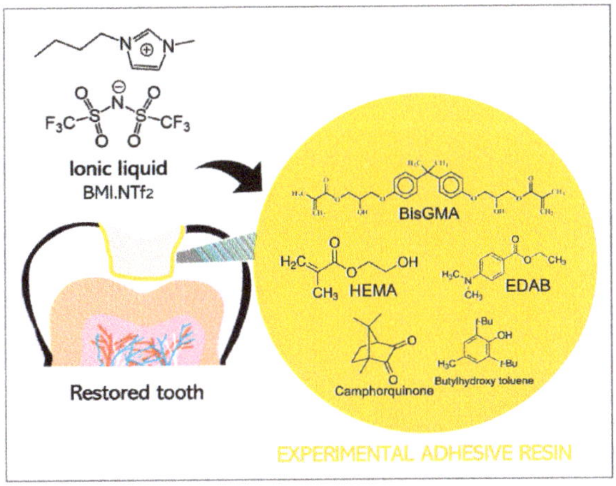

Figure 1. The scheme evidences the structure of the ionic liquid added into the experimental adhesive resin for dental restoration.

2.2. Polymerization Kinetics and Degree of Conversion (DC)

The polymerization kinetics and degree of conversion (DC) were evaluated by Fourier Transform Infrared (FTIR) spectroscopy (Bruker Optics, Ettinger, Germany) with a spectrometer equipped with an attenuated total reflectance (ATR) device consisting of a horizontal diamond crystal. Three samples per adhesive group (n = 3) were dispensed onto the ATR using an auxiliary polyvinylsiloxane matrix with a 4 mm diameter and 1 mm thickness to standardize the samples' thickness. The LED unit tip was standardized and positioned as close as possible to the top of each sample. The absorbance spectra were obtained during 40 s of adhesive photoactivation. Data were evaluated using the Opus 6.5 software (Bruker Optics), in the range of 4000–800 cm^{-1} with 2 scans per second, at a speed of 160 kHz and resolution of 4 cm^{-1}. The DC was calculated based on the height of the following absorption peaks: 1640 cm^{-1} (aliphatic C=C bond) and 1610 cm^{-1} (aromatic C=C bond), which was used as an internal standard (Equation (1)). The DC result was expressed as percentages. The DC calculated the polymerization rate (Rp) as a function of the light-activation time [12].

$$DC(\%) = 1 \times \frac{1640/1610\ (polymer)}{1640/1610\ (monomer)} \times 100 \quad (1)$$

2.3. Softening in Solvent

Five adhesive samples from each group ($n = 5$) were prepared with 5 mm diameter and 1 mm thickness after light-curing for 20 s on each side. After the polymerization, the samples were stored in distilled water for 24 h at 37 °C. Then, the adhesive samples were bonded with double-face tape on a glass table and soaked in self-cure acrylic resin (Clássico Produtos Odontológicos, São Paulo, Brazil). Each acrylic resin set contained five samples per group, which were polished using sandpapers (600, 1200, 2000-grit, 1 min each paper) and distilled water, followed by felt disks with 0.5 µm alumina suspension (3 min) (Fortel, São Paulo, SP, Brazil). After 24 h, the samples were subjected to a microhardness test in which five indentations (10 g for 5 s) were performed per sample at 40× magnification (HMV 2, Shimadzu, Tokyo, Japan) to obtain the initial Knoop hardness number (KHN1). The samples were immersed in a solvent solution (70% ethanol and 30% water) for two hours, washed with distilled water, and tested again to obtain the final Knoop hardness number (KHN2). The Knoop hardness values were recorded as the five indentations per sample average. Softening in solvent (ΔKHN) was calculated by the percentage difference between KHN1 and KHN2 for each group [16].

2.4. Ultimate Tensile Strength

An hourglass-shaped metal mold (8.0 mm long × 2.0 mm wide × 1.0 mm thick and 1 mm^2 in constriction area) was used to prepare five samples per group ($n = 5$). The samples were light-cured for 20 s on each side. After 24 h, the samples were kept in distilled water at 37 °C, and the samples were measured in the constriction area using a digital caliper. Then, the samples were fixed with cyanoacrylate resin into jigs. The samples were submitted to tensile strength in a universal testing machine (Series EZ-SX, Shimadzu, Kyoto, Japan) at 1 mm/min until the fracture of the samples. The force values (N) were divided by the constriction area of each sample and reported as MPa [17].

2.5. Statistical Analysis

The physical and chemical properties of the adhesives were statistically analyzed using SigmaPlot software (version 12.0, Systat Software, San Jose, CA, USA). The Shapiro–Wilk test was used to analyze the data distribution. DC, UTS, KHN1, and ΔKHN were analyzed via one-way ANOVA and Tukey's post-hoc test. Differences between KHN1 and KHN2 within each group were assessed using paired *t* tests. All tests were analyzed with a significance level of 0.05.

3. Results

The results from the polymerization kinetics analysis are indicated in Figure 2. Figure 2A shows the results of DC versus time, evidencing the differences in the conversion process among the experimental adhesives. The groups with the ionic liquid started converting carbon–carbon double bonds (C=C) into single carbon–carbon single bonds (C-C) before the G_{CTRL}. In Figure 3A, it is possible to observe the mean and standard deviation values of DC for each group. The values ranged from 65.16 (±0.83)% for $G_{1\%}$ to 69.75 (±0.09)% for $G_{5\%}$ ($p < 0.05$). There was no statistical difference from the G_{CTRL} to $G_{2.5\%}$ ($p > 0.05$). However, the addition of 5 wt.% of ionic liquid increased the DC compared to G_{CTRL} and $G_{1\%}$ ($p < 0.05$), without statistical difference for $G_{2.5\%}$ ($p > 0.05$).

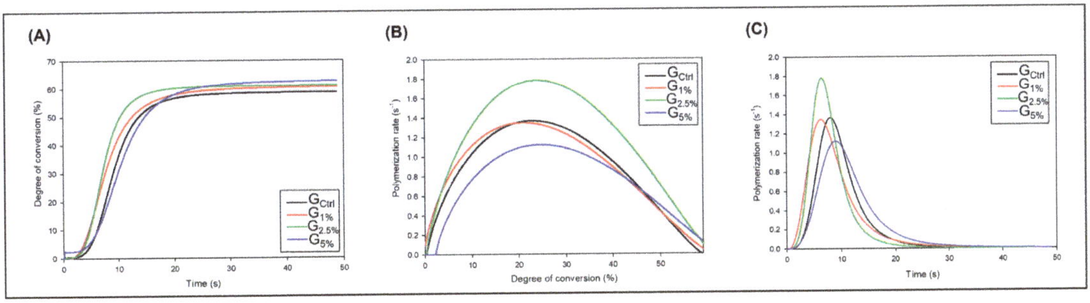

Figure 2. Degree of conversion as a function of time (image (**A**)); polymerization rate as a function of time (image (**B**)); polymerization rate as a function of the degree of conversion (image (**C**)) of the experimental dental adhesives.

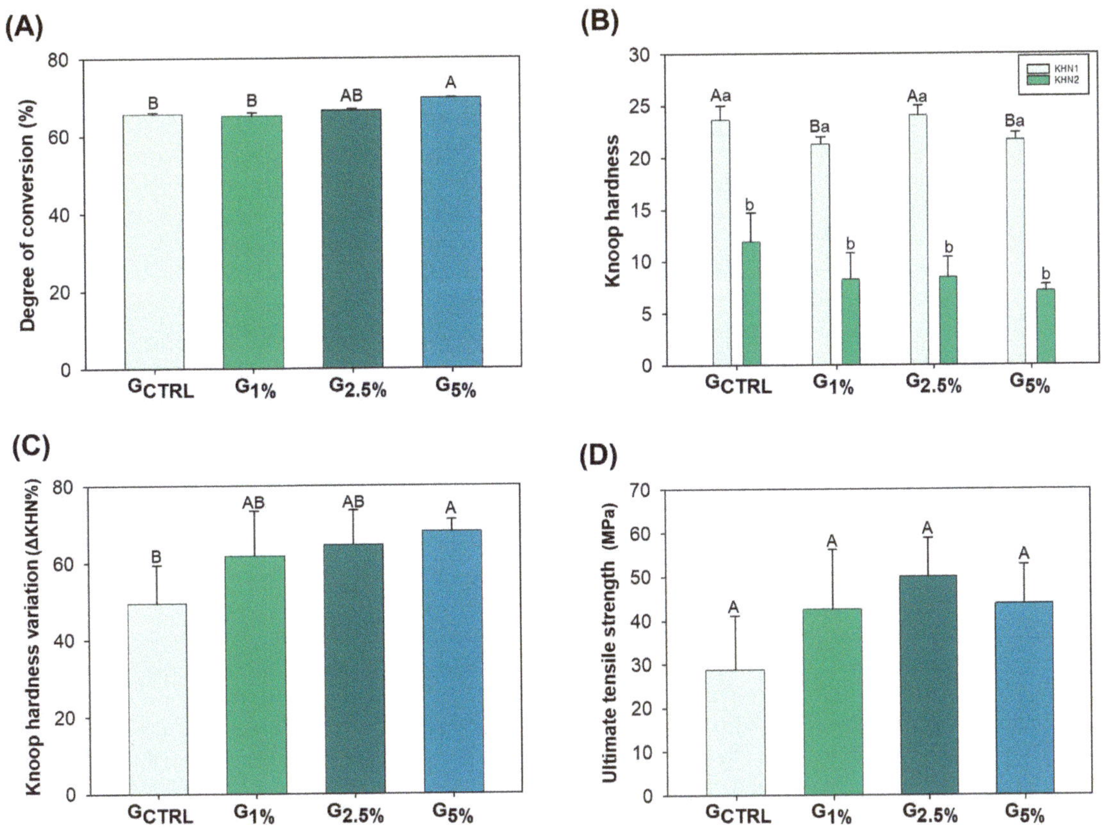

Figure 3. Graphs evidencing the results of degree of conversion (image (**A**)), Knoop hardness (image (**B**)), Knoop hardness variation (image (**C**)), and ultimate tensile strength (image (**D**)). The values are expressed as mean and standard deviation values. Different capital letters indicate statistically significant differences among groups in the same test ($p < 0.05$). Different lowercase letters indicate statistically significant differences within the same group before and after the alcoholic solution immersion ($p < 0.05$).

Still, in Figure 2B, we observed that the ionic liquid groups reached higher maximum polymerization rates than G_{CTRL}. In addition, Figure 2B,C evidence that groups with the ionic liquid started the self-acceleration process before G_{CTRL}.

Figure 3 also shows the experimental adhesive resin's initial and final Knoop hardness (Figure 3B) and Knoop hardness variation (ΔKHN%, Figure 3C). The groups showed different initial Knoop hardness ($p < 0.05$), but all of them decreased the hardness after immersion in the alcoholic solution ($p < 0.05$). The ΔKHN% ranged from 49.47 (±9.94)% for G_{CTRL} to 68.04 (±3.08)% for $G_{5\%}$ ($p < 0.05$). From G_{CTRL} to $G_{2.5\%}$, there were no differences in the softening in solvent ($p > 0.05$), with higher softening in solvent values for $G_{5\%}$ ($p < 0.05$). However, there were no statistical differences among the ionic liquid groups ($p > 0.05$).

Figure 3D shows the ultimate tensile strength (UTS) mean and standard deviation values. The values ranged from 28.71 (±12.37) MPa for G_{CTRL} to 49.99 (±8.88) MPa for $G_{2.5\%}$. There was no statistically significant difference among groups for this mechanical test ($p > 0.05$).

4. Discussion

Incorporating antimicrobial agents into resins aims to reduce biofilm at the tooth–restorative material interface [1,2,7,18]. BMI.NTf_2 was previously incorporated into an orthodontic resin and demonstrated an antibacterial effect against biofilms of *S. mutans* and planktonic *S. mutans* [13]. However, the physicochemical properties were impaired by 10 wt.% of BMI.NTf_2 [13]. This ionic liquid was added to an experimental adhesive resin in the present study, and its physicochemical properties were analyzed. There was no statistical difference in the DC among G_{TRL}, $G_{1\%}$, and $G_{2.5\%}$. The incorporation of 5 wt.% of BMI.NTf_2 increased the DC compared to G_{CTRL} and $G_{1\%}$ ($p < 0.05$), while the softening in solvent was higher with 5 wt.% addition.

Ionic liquids are exploited as solvents [10], and their properties are responsible for increasing the stability of the drug formulation and strengthening the association between drugs and surfactants or polymers. Furthermore, they facilitate drug transport to the target site of action and increase the solubility of moderately water-soluble drugs [10]. The chemical structure of BMI.NTf_2 gives it antimicrobial activity: the cationic structure is attracted by the negative charge at the bacterial wall and membrane compounds by electrostatic forces [9]. Moreover, its alkyl chain and anion, NTf_2, present hydrophobicity, assisting in disorganizing the bacterial wall and membranes [9].

The increase in the concentration of BMI.NTf_2 demonstrated a higher DC. Ionic liquids are characterized by molecular properties such as charge distribution, dipole moment, polarizability, hydrogen acceptance/donation, and electron pair acceptance/donation [10]. The carbon double bonds present in the monomers can interact with the presence of ionic liquids through hydrogen bonds or interaction of the electron pair of the double bond with the electronic cloud of ionic liquid [10]. This interaction can increase the conversion of carbon double bonds for groups with a higher concentration of BMI.NTf_2. In addition to the DC being altered, the polymerization kinetics can change depending on the compound added by modifying the mobility of the polymer chains [13,17].

The polymerization kinetics of the dental adhesive resins incorporating the ionic liquid BMI.NTf_2 provided insightful data that helped elucidate the underlying mechanisms of the observed results. Notably, the polymerization reaction in the samples containing BMI.NTf_2 demonstrated a marked acceleration compared to the control group (G_{CTRL}). The increased polymerization rate for the BMI.NTf_2 groups may be attributed to a reduction in the viscosity of the adhesive resin [13]. The handling properties of the material changed according to ionic liquid concentration. Despite not being tested in the present study, the adhesive with 5 wt.% of ionic liquid seemed to have a lower viscosity than the control group. It is possible that the increased DC% observed for this group was due to a greater mobility of the polymer chains during the curing process [13]. The addition of BMI.NTf$_2$ possibly interfered with the mobility of the chains and the density of crosslinks, leading to plasticizing effects [14,19,20]. Polymers with lower crosslink density are prone to soften more when in contact with alcoholic solutions [19]. Similar results were observed in a previous study with orthodontic adhesive resins with the addition of BMI.NTf$_2$ [13]. This effect was also investigated by thermogravimetric analysis (TGA), and the higher the ionic liquid concentration, the higher the formation of novel derivative (DTG) of the TGA curve. This result was attributed to forming regions with different crosslink densities, with areas more linear than others, when the ionic liquid was incorporated in greater quantities [13].

The immersion of dental adhesive resins in solvent is a critical test to assess their durability and resistance to the oral environment, particularly to the effects of moisture. In the study under consideration, all experimental groups exhibited a reduction in hardness upon solvent immersion. Notably, the group with 5 wt.% of BMI.NTf$_2$ ($G_{5\%}$) demonstrated a more significant decrease in hardness compared to the control group (GCTRL). This finding contrasts with previous research conducted on an orthodontic resin formulation, which showed different behavior under similar conditions [13].

The divergent results between the two studies [13] can largely be attributed to the differences in the base resin compositions used in each. The orthodontic resin did not contain hydroxyethyl methacrylate (HEMA), a commonly used monomer in dental adhesives that is known for its hydrophilic properties. Instead, the orthodontic resin included triethylene glycol dimethacrylate (TEGDMA), which is less hydrophilic than HEMA. This reduced hydrophilicity likely contributed to the orthodontic resin's enhanced resistance to softening when exposed to solvents [13].

Additionally, the orthodontic resin incorporated silanized colloidal silica, a filler known to improve the physicochemical properties of polymers [5,14]. The presence of this filler helps to increase the resin's mechanical strength and stability, making it less susceptible to softening and degradation upon solvent immersion. This enhancement is particularly important in orthodontic applications where the material must withstand prolonged exposure to a moist and mechanically challenging environment [21].

In contrast, the current study involving BMI.NTf$_2$ in dental adhesives explored concentrations of 1% and 2.5% ($G_{1\%}$ and $G_{2.5\%}$), which did not significantly influence the solvent's softening behavior. This suggests that the crosslinking density within these groups, including the control (GCTRL), is likely similar. The addition of BMI.NTf$_2$ at these concentrations does not alter the resin's network structure significantly enough to affect its solvent resistance [22].

The comparison of these two distinct resin formulations highlights the importance of base resin composition and the selection of appropriate additives and fillers in the achieving desired material properties [23]. The difference in behavior underscores the need for tailored resin formulations depending on the specific requirements of the dental application, be it orthodontic or adhesive applications. For future formulations, understanding the interaction between the resin matrix, fillers, and any ionic liquids like BMI.NTf$_2$ will be crucial in developing materials that combine optimal mechanical properties and resist environmental challenges.

Furthermore, an assessment of the cohesive strength of the polymers was conducted in addition to the evaluation of softening in solvent. In congruence with a prior study [13], no significant statistical disparities were observed among the various groups. Despite the adverse impact of incorporating 5 wt.% BMI.NTf$_2$ on the adhesive's softening behavior, this concentration exhibited no discernible alteration in the adhesive's ultimate tensile strength (UTS). Nonetheless, given the outcomes of the softening in solvent tests and the understanding of the potential effects of high concentrations of ionic liquids on polymer structure formation, the utilization of 2.5 wt.% BMI.NTf_2 emerged as the most suitable choice for the experimental adhesive resin.

As a limitation of this study, the mechanical property was not tested directly on dentin. Therefore, the next steps encompass a set of antimicrobial analyses and the microtensile bond strength to dentin. Regulatory considerations for ionic liquid-incorporated dental resins remain evolving due to their unique antibacterial properties and potential interactions with oral tissues. The classification of such materials depends on their mechanism of action and whether the antibacterial effect is purely contact based or involves pharmacological activity [24–27]. In addition, over time, other ionic liquids may be tested to develop increasingly cost-effective materials with a lower environmental impact—particularly regarding the solvents used in chemical processes—and exhibit enhanced biological properties.

5. Conclusions

This study examined the influence of varying percentages of the ionic liquid, BMI.NTf_2, in a novel dental adhesive formulation. Considering clinically pertinent attributes for dental adhesives, the formulation featuring 2.5 wt.% BMI.NTf_2 loading has been identified as the optimal composition. The physical and chemical properties of dental adhesives were analyzed when BMI.NTf_2 was added from 1 to 5 wt.%. It was concluded that BMI.NTf_2 at 2.5 wt.% increases adhesives' degree of conversion without changing other properties. Consequently, this approach holds significant promise in developing a strong bonding interface tooth composite to promote bacterial inhibition and curtailing secondary caries development around bonded restorations.

Author Contributions: Conceptualization, I.M.G., V.S.S., J.D.S. and F.M.C.; formal analysis; I.M.G., A.S. and V.S.S.; project administration, J.D.S. and F.M.C.; resources, J.D.S. and F.M.C.; validation, J.D.S. and F.M.C.; visualization, I.M.G. and M.A.S.M.; writing—original draft, I.M.G., A.S. and V.S.S.; writing—review and editing, M.A.S.M., J.D.S. and F.M.C. All authors have read and agreed to the published version of the manuscript.

Funding: This study was supported by the National Institute of Science and Technology in 3D Printing and Advanced Materials Applied to Human and Veterinary Health—INCT _3D-Saúde, CNPq/Brazil (Grant #406436/2022-3) and CNPq/MCTI/FNDCT N° 18/2021 (408075/2021-0). This study was financed in part by the Coordenação de Aperfeiçoamento de Pessoal de Nível Superior—Brasil (CAPES)—Finance Code 001.

Institutional Review Board Statement: Not applicable.

Informed Consent Statement: Not applicable.

Data Availability Statement: The raw data supporting the conclusions of this article will be made available by the authors on request.

Conflicts of Interest: The authors declare no conflicts of interest.

References

1. Bourbia, M.; Ma, D.; Cvitkovitch, D.G.; Santerre, J.P.; Finer, Y. Cariogenic bacteria degrade dental resin composites and adhesives. *J. Dent. Res.* **2013**, *92*, 989–994. [CrossRef] [PubMed]
2. Melo, M.A.S.; Garcia, I.M.; Mokeem, L.; Weir, M.D.; Xu, H.H.K.; Montoya, C.; Orrego, S. Developing Bioactive Dental Resins for Restorative Dentistry. *J. Dent. Res.* **2023**, *102*, 220345231182357.
3. Mallineni, S.K.; Sakhamuri, S.; Kotha, S.L.; AlAsmari, A.R.G.M.; AlJefri, G.H.; Almotawah, F.N.; Mallineni, S.; Sajja, R. Silver nanoparticles in dental applications: A descriptive review. *Bioengineering* **2023**, *10*, 327. [CrossRef] [PubMed]

4. Makvandi, P.; Jamaledin, R.; Jabbari, M.; Nikfarjam, N.; Borzacchiello, A. Antibacterial quaternary ammonium compounds in dental materials: A systematic review. *Dent. Mater.* **2018**, *34*, 851–867.
5. Ferracane, J.L. Resin composite—State of the art. *Dent. Mater.* **2011**, *27*, 29–38.
6. Breschi, L.; Mazzoni, A.; Ruggeri, A.; Cadenaro, M.; Di Lenarda, R.; De Stefano Dorigo, E. Dental adhesion review: Aging and stability of the bonded interface. *Dent. Mater.* **2008**, *24*, 90–101.
7. Bedran-Russo, A.; Leme-Kraus, A.A.; Vidal, C.M.P.; Teixeira, E.C. An Overview of Dental Adhesive Systems and the Dynamic Tooth-Adhesive Interface. *Dent. Clin. N. Am.* **2017**, *61*, 713–731. [CrossRef]
8. Łuczak, J.; Paszkiewicz, M.; Krukowska, A.; Malankowska, A.; Zaleska-Medynska, A. Ionic liquids for nano-and microstructures preparation. Part 1: Properties and multifunctional role. *Adv. Colloid Interface Sci.* **2016**, *230*, 13–28.
9. Pendleton, J.N.; Gilmore, B.F. The antimicrobial potential of ionic liquids: A source of chemical diversity for infection and biofilm control. *Int. J. Antimicrob. Agents* **2015**, *46*, 131–139.
10. Weingärtner, H. Understanding ionic liquids at the molecular level: Facts, problems, and controversies. *Angew. Chem. Int. Ed. Engl.* **2008**, *47*, 654–670.
11. Kitagawa, H.; Izutani, N.; Kitagawa, R.; Maezono, H.; Yamaguchi, M.; Imazato, S. Evolution of resistance to cationic biocides in *Streptococcus mutans* and *Enterococcus faecalis*. *J. Dent.* **2016**, *47*, 18–22. [CrossRef] [PubMed]
12. Garcia, I.M.; Souza, V.S.; Hellriegel, C.; Scholten, J.D.; Collares, F.M. Ionic liquid–stabilized titania quantum dots applied in adhesive resin. *J. Dent. Res.* **2019**, *98*, 682–688. [CrossRef] [PubMed]
13. Garcia, I.M.; Ferreira, C.J.; de Souza, V.S.; Leitune, V.C.B.; Samuel, S.M.W.; de Souza Balbinot, G.; de Souza da Motta, A.; Visioli, F.; Scholten, J.D.; Collares, F.M. Ionic liquid as antibacterial agent for an experimental orthodontic adhesive. *Dent. Mater.* **2019**, *35*, 1155–1165. [CrossRef] [PubMed]
14. Ferracane, J.L. Hygroscopic and hydrolytic effects in dental polymer networks. *Dent. Mater.* **2006**, *22*, 211–222. [CrossRef]
15. Tu, Y.; Ren, H.; He, Y.; Ying, J.; Chen, Y. Interaction between microorganisms and dental material surfaces: General concepts and research progress. *J. Oral Microbiol.* **2023**, *15*, 2196897. [CrossRef]
16. Bendary, I.M.; Garcia, I.M.; Collares, F.M.; Takimi, A.; Samuel, S.M.W.; Leitune, V.C.B. Wollastonite as filler of an experimental dental adhesive. *J. Dent.* **2020**, *102*, 103472. [CrossRef]
17. Cramer, N.B.; Stansbury, J.W.; Bowman, C.N. Recent Advances and Developments in Composite Dental Restorative Materials. *J. Dent. Res.* **2011**, *90*, 402–416. [CrossRef]
18. Fugolin, A.P.P.; Pfeifer, C.S. New resins for dental composites. *J. Dent. Res.* **2017**, *96*, 1085–1091. [CrossRef]
19. Schneider, L.F.J.; Moraes, R.R.; Cavalcante, L.M.; Sinhoreti, M.A.C.; Correr-Sobrinho, L.; Consani, S. Cross-link density evaluation through softening tests: Effect of ethanol concentration. *Dent. Mater.* **2008**, *24*, 199–203. [CrossRef]
20. Filho, J.D.N.; Poskus, L.T.; Guimarães, J.G.A.; Barcellos, A.A.L.; Silva, E.M. Degree of conversion and plasticization of dimethacrylate-based polymeric matrices: Influence of light-curing mode. *J. Oral Sci.* **2008**, *50*, 315–321. [CrossRef]
21. Selvaraj, M.; Mohaideen, K.; Sennimalai, K.; Gothankar, G.S.; Arora, G. Effect of oral environment on contemporary orthodontic materials and its clinical implications. *J. Orthod. Sci.* **2023**, *12*, 1. [PubMed]
22. Hossain, M.I.; Shams, A.B.; Das Gupta, S.; Blanchard, G.J.; Mobasheri, A.; Hoque Apu, E. The Potential Role of Ionic Liquid as a Multifunctional Dental Biomaterial. *Biomedicines* **2023**, *11*, 3093. [CrossRef] [PubMed]
23. Alluhaidan, T.; Qaw, M.; Garcia, I.M.; Montoya, C.; Orrego, S.; Melo, M.A. Seeking Endurance: Designing Smart Dental Composites for Tooth Restoration. *Designs* **2024**, *8*, 92. [CrossRef]
24. Fernandes, M.M.; Carvalho, E.O.; Correia, D.M.; Esperança, J.M.S.S.; Padrão, J.; Ivanova, K.; Hoyo, J.; Tzanov, T.; Lanceros-Mendez, S. Ionic Liquids as Biocompatible Antibacterial Agents: A Case Study on Structure-Related Bioactivity on *Escherichia coli*. *ACS Appl. Bio Mater.* **2022**, *5*, 5181–5189. [CrossRef]
25. Hassanpour, M.; Torabi, S.M.; Afshar, D.; Kowsari, M.H.; Meratan, A.A.; Nikfarjam, N. Tracing the Antibacterial Performance of Bis-Imidazolium-based Ionic Liquid Derivatives. *ACS Appl. Bio Mater.* **2024**, *7*, 1558–1568. [CrossRef]
26. Ben, C.; He, D.; Wu, Q.; Zhao, S.; Liu, D.; Li, S.; Guo, F.; Li, C.; Jin, L.; Wang, Q.; et al. Regulation of nanotopography of ionic liquid gel particles through the introduction of a second network and its impact on antibacterial properties. *J. Colloid Interface Sci.* **2025**, *686*, 864–877. [CrossRef]
27. Bedair, H.M.; Hamed, M.; Mansour, F.R. New emerging materials with potential antibacterial activities. *Appl. Microbiol. Biotechnol.* **2024**, *108*, 515. [CrossRef]

applied sciences

MDPI

Article

Comparative Evaluation of Temporomandibular Condylar Changes Using Texture Analysis of CT and MRI Images

Celso Massahiro Ogawa [1], Everton Flaiban [1], Ana Lúcia Franco Ricardo [1], Diana Lorena Garcia Lopes [1], Lays Assolini Pinheiro de Oliveira [1], Bruna Maciel de Almeida [2], Adriana de Oliveira Lira [1], Kaan Orhan [3], Sérgio Lúcio Pereira de Castro Lopes [2] and Andre Luiz Ferreira Costa [1,*]

[1] Postgraduate Program in Dentistry, Cruzeiro do Sul University (UNICSUL), São Paulo 1506-000, SP, Brazil; celsomassahiro@gmail.com (C.M.O.); evertonflaiban@hotmail.com (E.F.); anaricardo19@gmail.com (A.L.F.R.); dilomagar@hotmail.com (D.L.G.L.); lays_08@hotmail.com (L.A.P.d.O.); aliraort@uol.com.br (A.d.O.L.)

[2] Department of Diagnosis and Surgery, São José dos Campos School of Dentistry, São Paulo State University (UNESP), São José dos Campos 2245-000, SP, Brazil; brunamacieldealmeida@gmail.com (B.M.d.A.); sergioluciolopes@gmail.com (S.L.P.d.C.L.)

[3] Department of Dentomaxillofacial Radiology, Faculty of Dentistry, Ankara University, Ankara 06560, Turkey; call53@yahoo.com

* Correspondence: alfcosta@gmail.com

Abstract: This study aims to compare computed tomography (CT) with magnetic resonance imaging (MRI) of the temporomandibular joint (TMJ) by using texture analysis (TA) to detect condylar bone marrow changes associated with the flattening and erosion of cortical bone. A total of 47 patients from the Dentomaxillofacial Radiology Division at São Paulo State University were evaluated. Images from 250 CT and 250 MRI images were assessed by experienced radiologists employing OnDemand3D software. Texture parameters were extracted with MaZda software (version 4.6), and we focused on regions of interest within the condyles. Statistical analysis revealed significant differences in texture parameters between the affected and control groups. CT images showed higher correlation values in cases of flattening, whereas MRI images demonstrated substantial changes in texture parameters for both flattening and erosion. These findings suggest that the texture analysis of CT and MRI images can effectively detect early and advanced degenerative changes in the TMJ, thus providing valuable insights into the underlying pathophysiology and aiding in early intervention and treatment planning.

Keywords: computer-assisted diagnosis; condyle; degenerative changes; diagnostic imaging; radiomics

1. Introduction

The morphology of the condyle of the temporomandibular joint (TMJ) changes according to age, gender, facial type, functional load, occlusal force, and type of malocclusion, and between the left and right sides [1]. Parafunctional factors such as bruxism and clenching overload the joints, leading to remodeling [1,2] and articular disc derangement [3].

The trabecular bone organization is characterized by porosity, trabecular thickness, and anisotropy, which can be altered depending on the movements resulting from chewing [4]. The remodeling of the condylar cartilage of the mandible occurs in response to mechanical deformations, in which chondrogenesis and endochondral ossification are regulated to obtain a better balance between mechanical stress and the load capacity of the joint [5]. Among the degenerative signs affecting the condyle, one can cite flattening, formation of osteophytes, presence of subchondral sclerosis, and erosion of cortical bone [6,7], with flattening being a condition that reflects an initial process and cortical erosion occurring in a more advanced stage. The destruction of the condyle can cause malformations such as retrognathism, anterior open bite, and facial asymmetry [7]. Addressing this condition in its early stages is crucial for several reasons:

- Prevention of progressive deformity: Early intervention can halt or slow the progression of facial asymmetry and malocclusion, potentially avoiding more complex surgical corrections in the future [8];
- Preservation of growth potential: In younger patients, timely treatment may allow for more normal facial growth and development [9];
- Functional improvement: Early management can help maintain or restore proper jaw function, including mastication and speech [10];
- Psychosocial benefits: Preventing severe facial deformities can have significant positive impacts on a patient's self-esteem and social interactions, particularly in adolescents [11];
- Simplified treatment: Early detection and treatment may allow for less invasive procedures and potentially better outcomes compared to addressing advanced deformities [12].

Computed tomography (CT) has been used to evaluate TMJ since the early 1980s as it offers superior image quality for assessing bone structures. Therefore, CT is a highly recommended examination in the evaluation of condyles, particularly in the diagnosis of ankyloses, arthritis, and osteoarthritis [13].

Magnetic resonance imaging (MRI) is considered the most accurate method for showing structural alterations, particularly in the TMJ soft tissues, as it can identify the articular disc [9]. MRI is essential to detect changes in the condylar bone marrow, such as avascular necrosis and edema [14].

Radiomics is a field of medical imaging dedicated to quantitative analysis of original medical images [15]. Features extracted from the images (e.g., shape, texture, and pixel intensity) and their analysis are used to obtain detailed information about the morphology and heterogeneity of a lesion or tissue [15,16]. When combined with other clinical data, this information can be valuable for the diagnosis, treatment, and prognosis of a disease [16].

Although MRI is the gold standard for detecting bone marrow changes, identifying these changes through a visual inspection of images remains challenging due to the limitations of the human eye in distinguishing subtle differences in grayscale intensities [17]. Therefore, incorporating radiomics into the methodology enhances the MRI contrast, which allows for a more detailed and quantitative analysis of imaging features. This significantly improves the detection and evaluation of tissue and lesion heterogeneity [15].

Texture analysis (TA) is a statistical image analysis technique based on the use of radiomics, in which the distribution of pixel signals is quantitatively assessed by comparing them to neighboring pixels in a non-invasive way. TA has been developed by measuring the distribution of grayscale levels in the region of interest (ROI) delineated in the image, thus distinguishing lesions from healthy tissues [18–22]. Therefore, data from TA in combination with clinical information can indicate and validate diagnostic hypotheses [23].

One of the most frequent methods for extracting texture parameters from grayscale images is the co-occurrence matrix (GLCM) [24], which can detect subtle changes in images [25–27]. In recent years, computerized analyses of morphology and texture have been used to aid in the diagnosis of various pathologies [21–24]. Automated patterns applied to medical image analysis for lesion recognition have high accuracy and are recognized as imaging biomarkers [28].

The objective of this study was to compare CT and MRI images of TMJs affected by the flattening and erosion of the cortical bone using TA to detect condylar bone marrow changes in these joints. By applying TA to compare CT and MRI images of TMJs affected by flattening and erosion of the cortical bone, we aim to enhance the detection of subtle condylar bone marrow changes that are often challenging to identify through visual inspection alone. This approach has the potential to improve early diagnosis of TMJ degeneration, enabling more timely interventions. This research also seeks to establish quantitative imaging biomarkers specific to TMJ degeneration, which could help standardize assessment criteria across the field. By focusing on these specific conditions, this study may provide new insights into the progression of TMJ degeneration, aiding clinicians in distinguishing between various stages of the condition. Furthermore, the findings from this study could inform the development of more targeted treatment strategies and contribute to the advancement of computer-aided diagnostic tools in TMJ imaging, potentially enhancing the accuracy, efficiency, and early detection of condyle changes in clinical practice.

2. Materials and Methods

This is a retrospective study. All procedures in this study were conducted in full accordance with the ethical principles set by the Helsinki Declaration of 1975, as revised in 2013. All patients had provided written consent after being informed about the use of CT and MRI images.

This study was approved by the institutional review board of the School of Dentistry of the University of São Paulo (USP) according to protocol number 56631222.9.0000.0075.

All the patients enrolled in the study had been admitted for CT and MRI for the evaluation of TMJ complaints. The database held by the Dentomaxillofacial Radiology Division of the São José dos Campos School of Dentistry, UNESP, was reviewed between January 2019 and April 2021.

2.1. Image Acquisition

Non-contrast enhanced CT examinations were performed by using a 4-channel multidetector CT scanner (Alexion, Toshiba/Canon, Otawara, Japan) with contiguous 1 mm thick slices at 1 mm intervals, operated with 100 kV, 100 mA, 1 s/rotation, 512 × 512 matrix, a gap measuring 0.8 mm, a voxel size of 0.37 mm × 0.37 mm, and a field of view (FOV) of 180 mm × 180 mm.

MRI scans were acquired on a 1.5 Tesla scanner (Sigma, General Electric, Milwaukee, WI, USA) with a dedicated TMJ surface coil measuring 0.6 m in diameter. Sagittal T1 images were obtained in the closed-mouth position (TE 8.5 ms and TR 850 ms), with an FOV of 150 mm × 150 mm, 2 mm thickness, a 1.0 mm intersection gap, and a raw data matrix measuring 512 × 512 mm.

The digital imaging and communications in medicine (DICOM) format was used to export all image data acquired from CT and MRI scanners.

2.2. Image Analysis

Patients with both CT and MRI images acquired within a month were included after being retrieved from the computer database for assessment. A total of 500 examinations, consisting of 250 CT images and 250 MRI images, were analyzed by using OnDemand3D software (version 1.0.9.3223, CyberMed Inc., Seul, Republic of Korea). Two dentomaxillofacial radiologists, with more than 15 years of experience, selected and analyzed the images based on a consensus on bone changes, namely erosion and flattening.

Initially, they considered including cases among those in the sample related to other alterations, such as the presence of osteophytes and subchondral cysts. However, the decision was made to focus exclusively on cases with flattening and erosion of the condylar cortex. This selection was based on the rationale that flattening represents an initial stage of degenerative changes, whereas erosion indicates a more advanced and severe stage. Additionally, the number of cases with other alterations in our sample was small, which could potentially have introduced a bias in the results and reduced the statistical power of our analysis. By concentrating on these two specific alterations, we aimed to capture the progression of TMJ degeneration more clearly to provide a comprehensive understanding of the early and late manifestations of the condition. This approach allowed for a more precise evaluation of the efficacy of TA in identifying varying degrees of degenerative changes, thus enhancing the clinical relevance of our findings. Therefore, the final sample consisted of 47 patients of both genders, which was divided into groups of TMJs with flattening and erosion. TMJs without any alteration constituted the control group.

The inclusion criteria were patients from both genders older than 16 years who presented with bilaterally visible TMJs, whereas exclusion criteria were patients with images showing severe artifacts or a history of systemic diseases, maxillofacial trauma, recent jaw surgery, or congenital bone/cartilage disease.

After applying the inclusion and exclusion criteria, 47 patients aged between 16 and 72 years old were included in the study.

2.3. *Extraction and Analysis of Texture Features*

TA analysis was performed by a different fellowship-trained dentomaxillofacial radiologist with five years of CT and MRI experience who was also unaware of the final diagnosis. The radiologist manually selected the first sagittal slice in the most central region in all cases, where the condyle was more visible. Two additional sequential parallel sections, one more medial and another more distal, were also analyzed. Each DICOM slice was processed and converted into bitmap format by using OnDemand3D software (CyberMed Inc., Seoul, Republic of Korea). The same radiologist chose the region of interest (ROI) by drawing lines that intersected the outer and inner edges of the condyles in the sagittal view as well as the medial and lateral borders in the sagittal perspective. Next, to enhance precision in locating the center of the condyles, a line was drawn in the middle of these aforementioned lines to guide the outline of the ROI with a diameter of 6.5 mm at the center of the condyle (Figure 1). TA analysis of CT and MRI images was based on parameters (i.e., features) extracted by using MaZda software, version 4.6 (Technical University of Lodz, Poland), on a 15-inch MacBook Pro notebook (Apple, Los Altos, CA, USA) with an Intel® CoreTMi5 (Intel, Santa Clara, CA, USA), 2.4 GHz, 4 GB RAM, 1067 MHz, DDR3 processor (Samsung, Suwon, Republic of Korea) and Microsoft Windows version 10. The same diameter of the ROI was used in the three sections to create volumetric data, that is, values of the volume of interest (VOI) for texture analysis [29]. The texture parameters from each of the three sections were extracted, and the mean value was calculated for each condyle.

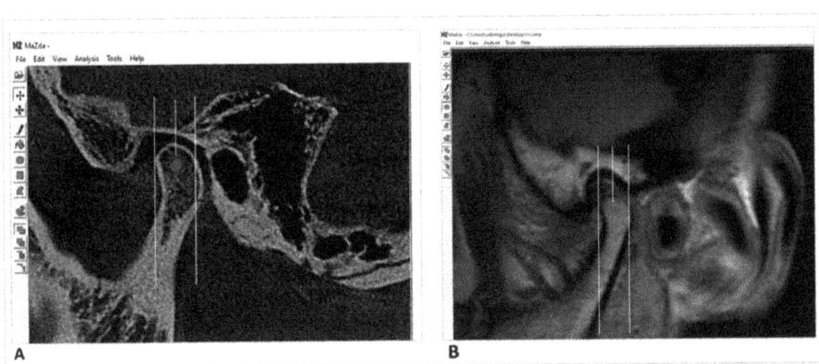

Figure 1. Representative sagittal images showing the central section of the condyle and the manual selection of the ROI to extract texture and image parameters from CT (**A**) and MRI images (**B**).

GLCM is a statistical method for the calculation of the properties of spatial relationships between pixels [29]. Texture parameters were computed from the GLCM, corresponding to distances of 1, 2, and 3 pixels in the four directions of the image (i.e., horizontal, diagonal, vertical, and anti-diagonal, corresponding to 0°, 45°, 90°, and 135°, respectively).

To minimize the factors at play and select seven parameters with a stronger connection with bone tissue, we used a recent study as a basis to select seven texture parameters [29]. The Supplementary Table S1 shows the texture features computed by using MaZda software.

To provide a comprehensive overview of our methodological approach, Figure 2 presents a visual representation of the entire pipeline, from image acquisition to texture analysis. This flowchart illustrates the key steps in our process, including image acquisition, analysis and selection, preparation for texture analysis, feature extraction, and data analysis.

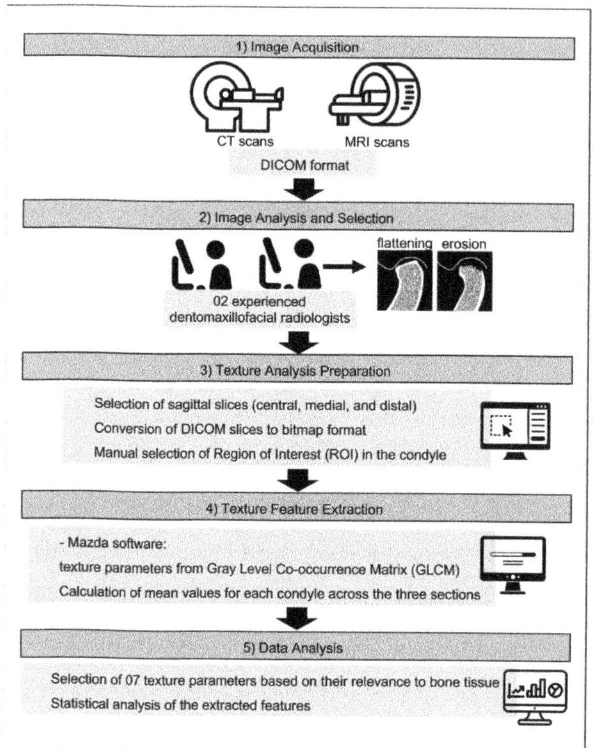

Figure 2. Flowchart of the methodological pipeline for the texture analysis of temporomandibular joints (TMJs) using CT and MRI images.

2.4. Statistical Analysis

Statistical analyses were performed by using R software, version 3.6.0 (R Foundation for Statistical Computing, Vienna, Austria). Spearman's correlation coefficient was used to assess the correlation between distances of the same texture parameter. Groups with and without disease were compared by using the Mann–Whitney test. All statistical analyses were performed at a significance level of 5%.

3. Results

This study included 47 patients of both genders (74% females and 26% males), aged between 16 and 72 years old (mean age of 32.5 years). Texture parameters were measured for each patient by using both CT and MRI images of the condylar bone marrow. Table 1 shows the distribution of the alterations (i.e., flattening and erosion) in the sample. Concerning the pathologies of flattening and erosion, the analysis of the right and left sides was performed as the same patients did not necessarily have the condition on both sides.

Texture parameters were obtained for each patient by using CT and MRI images of both the right and left sides.

Table 1. Number of patients diagnosed for each pathology.

Pathology	Side	Number of Diagnosed Patients	Observation
Flattening	Right	22	Assessment by side
Flattening	Left	20	Assessment by side
Erosion	Right	6	Assessment by side
Erosion	Left	7	Assessment by side

Seven parameters (angular second moment [AngScMom], contrast, correlation [Correlat], entropy, inverse difference moment [InvDfMom], sum of entropy [SumEntrp], and sum of squares [SumOfSqs]) were extracted for 12 positions. Before calculating the average of the 12 positions of each parameter, Spearman's correlation coefficient between them was calculated. As a high correlation was observed between the positions in six of the seven parameters, we decided to use the average between them. Because no strong association was observed between the positions for the correlation parameter, all 12 parameters were analyzed separately. Figure 2 shows the correlation matrix calculated for CT and MRI images. The two distances were organized according to four directions in the following positions: S10 (d1 = 1; ∡ = 0°), S01 (d1 = 1; ∡ = 45°), S11 (d1 = 1; ∡ = 90°), S1m1 (d1 = 1; ∡ = 135°), S20 (d2 = 2; ∡ = 0°), S02 (d2 = 2; ∡ = 45°), S22 (d2 = 2; ∡ = 90°), S2m2 (d2 = 2; ∡ = 135°), S30 (d3 = 3; ∡ = 0°), S03 (d3 = 3; ∡ = 45°), S33 (d3 = 3; ∡ = 90°), S3m3 (d3 = 3; ∡ = 135°).

Figures 3 and 4 show a comparison of the groups with and without pathology regarding the texture parameters of CT and MRI images for both sides. The groups were statistically different at a 5% significance level for the parameters marked with an asterisk (*). The parameters contrast and SumOfSqs were divided by 10 to be included in the graphs without distorting the scale for the other parameters.

Statistically significant differences in texture parameters between the groups with and without TMJ pathologies (flattening and erosion) for CT and MRI images are shown in Table 2.

Texture parameters included angular second moment [AngScMom], contrast, correlation [Correlat], entropy, inverse difference moment [InvDfMom], sum of entropy [SumEntrp], sum of squares [SumOfSqs].

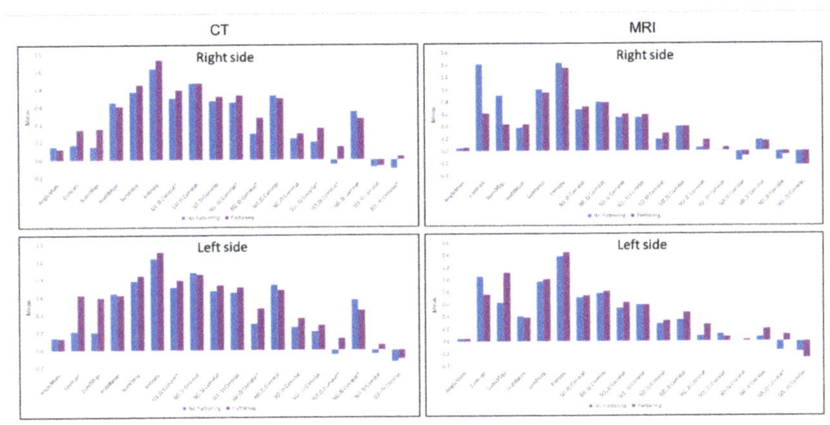

Figure 3. Comparison of patients with and without flattening on the right and left sides for CT and MRI images and texture parameters (angular second moment [AngScMom], contrast, correlation [Correlat], entropy, inverse difference moment [InvDfMom], sum of entropy [SumEntrp], sum of squares [SumOfSqs]). * Significant p-values.

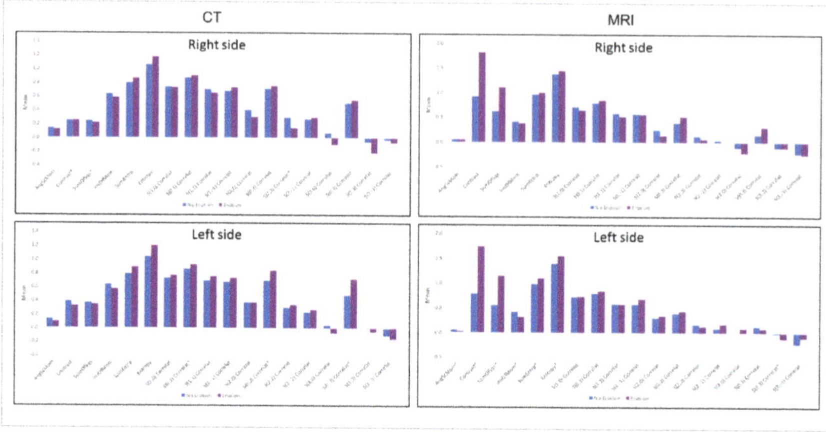

Figure 4. Comparison of patients with and without erosion on the right and left sides for CT and MRI images and texture parameters (angular second moment [AngScMom], contrast, correlation [Correlat], entropy, inverse difference moment [InvDfMom], sum of entropy [SumEntrp], sum of squares [SumOfSqs]). * Significant *p*-values.

Table 2. Statistically significant differences in texture parameters between groups with and without TMJ pathologies (flattening and erosion) for CT and MRI images.

Group	Texture Parameter	Position	*p*-Value
Flattening on the right side: CT	Higher Correlation	S(1,0)	0.005
	Higher Correlation	S(1,−1)	0.007
	Higher Correlation	S(2,0)	0.001
	Higher Correlation	S(2,−2)	0.003
	Higher Correlation	S(3,0)	0.004
	Higher Correlation	S(2,−2)	0.010
Flattening on the left side: CT	Higher Correlation	S(1,0)	0.025
	Higher Correlation	S(2,0)	0.012
	Higher Correlation	S(3,0)	0.004
	Lower Correlation	S(0,3)	0.028
Flattening on the left side: MRI	Higher Correlation	S(3,3)	0.017
Erosion on the right side: CT	Higher Contrast	All	0.018
	Higher SumOfSqs	All	0.045
	Lower Correlation	S(2,2)	0.048
Erosion on the left side: CT	Higher Correlation	S(0,1)	0.003
	Higher Correlation	S(0,2)	0.001
	Higher Correlation	S(0,3)	0.001
Erosion on the left side: MRI	Lower AngScMom	All	0.020
	Higher Contrast	All	0.031
	Higher SumOfSqs	All	0.027
	Lower InvDfMom	All	0.025
	Higher SumEntrp	All	0.027
	Higher Entropy	All	0.023

4. Discussion

This study yielded compelling results by shedding light on the potential of TA in detecting early signs of TMJ degeneration. Texture parameters were meticulously measured for each patient by using both CT and MRI modalities with a focus on the condylar medulla.

In the cases of condylar flattening, which is a precursor to more advanced degenerative changes, TA revealed significant differences between affected and unaffected groups.

Interestingly, the group with flattening showed higher correlation values, particularly in the positions S(1,0), S(1,−1), S(2,0), S(2,−2) and S(3,0), as observed in the CT images. These findings were consistent for both the right and left condyles, thus underscoring the sensitivity of TA in detecting early degenerative changes.

MRI-based TA also yielded notable results, as the group with flattening on the left condyle showed higher correlation values in S(3,3). As the degenerative process progresses, condylar erosion becomes a prominent feature. In this study, TA revealed distinct patterns associated with erosive changes. CT images of the right condyle in the group with erosion showed higher contrast values, a higher sum of squares, and lower correlation values in S(2,2).

On the left condyle, the group with erosion showed higher correlation values in the positions S(0,1), S(0,2), and S(0,3), as detected via CT images.

MRI-based TA also contributed with valuable insights, in which the group with erosion on the left condyle showed a lower angular second moment, higher contrast, higher sum of squares, lower inverse difference moment, higher sum of entropy, and higher entropy values.

These findings highlight the sensitivity of TA in detecting both early and advanced degenerative changes in TMJ condyles based on complementary information from CT and MRI images.

The textural patterns observed in this study provide valuable insights into the pathophysiological processes underlying TMJ degeneration. Higher correlation values associated with condylar flattening and erosion suggest higher linear interdependence between pixel intensities, which reflects changes in bone density and organization.

As the degenerative process progresses, the body attempts to adapt by altering the trabecular architecture and increasing bone density in the affected regions [30]. This adaptive response manifests as higher correlation values in TA, indicating a more organized and interdependent distribution of pixel intensities.

Furthermore, the observed changes in the contrast, sum of squares, and entropy parameters in the cases of condylar erosion reflect alterations in the heterogeneity and complexity of the medullary bone structure [31,32]. These findings align with the expected pathophysiological changes associated with advanced degenerative processes, such as bone remodeling, trabecular disruption, and the formation of erosive lesions [33].

This study's findings underscore the complementary nature of CT and MRI in assessing TMJ degeneration through TA. While CT excels in capturing changes related to cortical bone integrity and density, MRI provides valuable insights into alterations within the medullary bone and surrounding soft tissues.

By combining the strengths of both imaging modalities, TA offers a comprehensive evaluation of the degenerative process by encompassing cortical and medullary bone changes, including associated soft tissue alterations. This multimodal approach enhances diagnostic accuracy and facilitates a more holistic understanding of the disease's progression.

The ability to detect early degenerative changes within TMJ condyles through TA holds significant clinical implications. Early intervention is essential in mitigating the progression of TMJ degeneration and preventing irreversible damage to the joint [34,35].

By identifying subtle alterations in the medullary bone structure, TA can serve as a valuable tool for clinicians in enabling them to initiate appropriate treatment strategies at the earliest possible stage. This proactive approach may include conservative measures, such as lifestyle modifications, physical therapy, or pharmacological interventions, aimed at slowing or halting the degenerative process.

Moreover, the quantitative nature of TA parameters opens the door for personalized treatment planning and monitoring. By tracking changes in these parameters over time, clinicians can tailor treatment regimens to individual patient needs, thus optimizing outcomes and minimizing potential complications.

As the field of medical imaging continues to evolve, the integration of artificial intelligence (AI) and machine learning (ML) techniques holds immense potential for further enhancing the diagnostic capabilities of TA [36].

By leveraging large datasets of TA parameters and clinical outcomes, AI algorithms can be developed to recognize intricate patterns and correlations that may be imperceptible to human observers [37]. These algorithms can then assist in the automated detection, classification, and prognosis of TMJ degenerative conditions by streamlining the diagnostic process and reducing the potential for human error.

Additionally, the incorporation of ML techniques can facilitate the development of predictive models to enable clinicians to anticipate the progression of degenerative changes and tailor treatment strategies accordingly. This proactive approach can significantly improve patient outcomes and quality of life.

Our study's methodology aligns with and builds upon recent advancements in TA for TMJ evaluation. Girondi et al. [38] applied TA to MRI to identify changes in TMJ discs affected by effusion, utilizing similar GLCM parameters in MaZda software. Their findings of distinct texture patterns in effusion-affected discs support the potential of TA in detecting subtle TMJ changes. In a related study, Ricardo et al. [39] employed MRI-based TA for the quantitative evaluation of the mandibular condyle in juvenile idiopathic arthritis, demonstrating the technique's utility in assessing bone changes in inflammatory conditions. Furthermore, Nussi et al. [40] extended the application of TA to cone beam computed tomography (CBCT) images of the mandibular condyle, correlating texture features with gender and age. These studies collectively underscore the growing importance of TA in TMJ research and its potential to enhance diagnostic accuracy across various imaging modalities. Our work contributes to this emerging field by focusing specifically on TMJ degeneration, thereby expanding the application of TA in TMJ disorders and reinforcing its value as a quantitative tool in radiological assessment.

Despite the promising results, this study has several limitations that need to be addressed. Firstly, the relatively small sample size limits the robustness and generalizability of our findings; a larger cohort would provide more comprehensive data. Secondly, the retrospective study design may introduce selection bias. Thirdly, while experienced radiologists performed image analysis, there is a potential annotation bias due to the inherent subjectivity in interpreting imaging findings, which could have impacted our results. This limitation underscores the need for future studies to implement measures for quantifying inter-rater reliability. Additionally, the study has primarily focused on imaging findings, and clinical correlation with symptoms, functional outcomes, and patient-reported measures is crucial to validate the clinical use of TA in the evaluation of TMJ degeneration. Future research should address these limitations to further strengthen the applicability of texture analysis in assessing TMJ degeneration.

5. Conclusions

With the aid of TA, CT can identify changes in the condylar medullary bone for more subtle processes, such as flattening, whereas MRI allows the identification of more advanced processes that compromise cortical integrity, such as erosion. Therefore, TA can serve as a supplement to morphological MRI and CT to enhance the identification of minor cartilage changes and as an aid in the initial treatment at an early stage.

Supplementary Materials: The following supporting information can be downloaded at: https://www.mdpi.com/article/10.3390/app14167020/s1, Table S1: The texture features computed by using MaZda software.

Author Contributions: Conceptualization, A.L.F.C., C.M.O. and S.L.P.d.C.L.; investigation, C.M.O., E.F. and A.L.F.R.; formal analysis, D.L.G.L., L.A.P.d.O., B.M.d.A. and C.M.O.; data curation, E.F., A.d.O.L., K.O. and C.M.O.; methodology, A.L.F.C., A.L.F.R. and C.M.O.; project administration, A.d.O.L.; supervision, A.L.F.C. and S.L.P.d.C.L.; writing—original draft, A.L.F.C., C.M.O., S.L.P.d.C.L. and K.O.; writing—review and editing, A.L.F.C., C.M.O., E.F., D.L.G.L., L.A.P.d.O., B.M.d.A., A.d.O.L., K.O. and S.L.P.d.C.L. All authors have read and agreed to the published version of the manuscript.

Funding: This research was supported by Coordenação de Aperfeiçoamento de Pessoal de Nível Superior (Capes), funding number "001".

Institutional Review Board Statement: This study has been approved by the institutional review board (Ethical Committee of the School of Dentistry, University of São Paulo/USP); no. 56631222.9.0000.0075, date of approval: May 2nd 2020.

Informed Consent Statement: Informed consent was obtained from all subjects involved in the study.

Data Availability Statement: The datasets generated and/or analyzed during the current study are available from the corresponding author upon reasonable request.

Conflicts of Interest: The authors declare no conflicts of interest.

References

1. Valladares Neto JEC, B.M.; Guedes, O.A.; Porto, O.C.L.; Pécora, J.D. Prevalence of degenerative disease in temporomandibular disorder patients with disc displacement: A systematic review and meta-analysis. *Dent. Press J. Orthod.* **2010**, *15*, 172–181.
2. Widmalm, S.E.; Westesson, P.L.; Kim, I.K.; Pereira, F.J., Jr.; Lundh, H.; Tasaki, M.M. Temporomandibular joint pathosis related to sex, age, and dentition in autopsy material. *Oral Surg. Oral Med. Oral Pathol.* **1994**, *78*, 416–425. [CrossRef] [PubMed]
3. Honey, O.B.; Scarfe, W.C.; Hilgers, M.J.; Klueber, K.; Silveira, A.M.; Haskell, B.S.; Farman, A.G. Accuracy of cone-beam computed tomography imaging of the temporomandibular joint: Comparisons with panoramic radiology and linear tomography. *Am. J. Orthod. Dentofac. Orthop.* **2007**, *132*, 429–438. [CrossRef] [PubMed]
4. Arsan, B.; Kose, T.E.; Cene, E.; Ozcan, I. Assessment of the trabecular structure of mandibular condyles in patients with temporomandibular disorders using fractal analysis. *Oral Surg. Oral Med. Oral Pathol. Oral Radiol.* **2017**, *123*, 382–391. [CrossRef] [PubMed]
5. Chen, J.; Sobue, T.; Utreja, A.; Kalajzic, Z.; Xu, M.; Kilts, T.; Young, M.; Wadhwa, S. Sex differences in chondrocyte maturation in the mandibular condyle from a decreased occlusal loading model. *Calcif. Tissue Int.* **2011**, *89*, 123–129. [CrossRef] [PubMed]
6. Seo, B.Y.; Huh, K.H.; An, J.S.; Chang, M.S.; Ahn, S.J. Relationship of computed tomography-verified degenerative condylar morphology with temporomandibular joint disk displacement and sex. *Oral Surg. Oral Med. Oral Pathol. Oral Radiol.* **2021**, *132*, 93–103. [CrossRef] [PubMed]
7. Song, H.; Lee, J.Y.; Huh, K.H.; Park, J.W. Long-term Changes of Temporomandibular Joint Osteoarthritis on Computed Tomography. *Sci. Rep.* **2020**, *10*, 6731. [CrossRef] [PubMed]
8. Olate, S.; Ravelo, V.; Alister, J.P.; Netto, H.D.; Haidar, Z.S.; Sacco, R. Early Treatment of Unilateral Condylar Hyperplasia in Adolescents: Preliminary Results. *J. Clin. Med.* **2023**, *12*, 3408. [CrossRef] [PubMed]
9. Vajda, D.; Chen, V.; Shailendrasinh, V.; Borg, J.; Freymiller, E. Severe skeletal deformity following post-traumatic condylar resorption: A case report. *Oral Maxillofac. Surg. Cases* **2021**, *7*, 100227. [CrossRef]
10. Saeed, N.R.; Gerber, B. Management of the secondary growth defect. *J. Oral Biol. Craniofacial Res.* **2022**, *12*, 833–837. [CrossRef]
11. Crerand, C.E.; Sarwer, D.B.; Kazak, A.E.; Clarke, A.; Rumsey, N. Body Image and Quality of Life in Adolescents With Craniofacial Conditions. *Cleft Palate Craniofacial J.* **2017**, *54*, 2–12. [CrossRef] [PubMed]
12. Shoohanizad, E.; Garajei, A.; Enamzadeh, A.; Yari, A. Nonsurgical management of temporomandibular joint autoimmune disorders. *AIMS Public Health* **2019**, *6*, 554–567. [CrossRef] [PubMed]
13. Talmaceanu, D.; Lenghel, L.M.; Bolog, N.; Hedesiu, M.; Buduru, S.; Rotar, H.; Baciut, M.; Baciut, G. Imaging modalities for temporomandibular joint disorders: An update. *Clujul Med.* **2018**, *91*, 280–287. [CrossRef] [PubMed]
14. Emshoff, R.; Brandlmaier, I.; Bertram, S.; Rudisch, A. Relative odds of temporomandibular joint pain as a function of magnetic resonance imaging findings of internal derangement, osteoarthrosis, effusion, and bone marrow edema. *Oral Surg. Oral Med. Oral Pathol. Oral Radiol. Endod.* **2003**, *95*, 437–445. [CrossRef] [PubMed]
15. Gillies, R.J.; Kinahan, P.E.; Hricak, H. Radiomics: Images Are More than Pictures, They Are Data. *Radiology* **2016**, *278*, 563–577. [CrossRef]
16. An, P.; Zhang, J.; Li, M.; Duan, P.; He, Z.; Wang, Z.; Feng, G.; Guo, H.; Li, X.; Qin, P. Clinical Data-CT Radiomics-Based Model for Predicting Prognosis of Patients with Gastrointestinal Pancreatic Neuroendocrine Neoplasms (GP-NENs). *Comput. Math. Methods Med.* **2022**, *2022*, 4186305. [CrossRef] [PubMed]
17. Samei, E.; Badano, A.; Chakraborty, D.; Compton, K.; Cornelius, C.; Corrigan, K.; Flynn, M.J.; Hemminger, B.; Hangiandreou, N.; Johnson, J.; et al. Assessment of display performance for medical imaging systems: Executive summary of AAPM TG18 report. *Med. Phys.* **2005**, *32*, 1205–1225. [CrossRef] [PubMed]
18. Castellano, G.; Bonilha, L.; Li, L.M.; Cendes, F. Texture analysis of medical images. *Clin. Radiol.* **2004**, *59*, 1061–1069. [CrossRef] [PubMed]
19. de Oliveira, M.S.; Betting, L.E.; Mory, S.B.; Cendes, F.; Castellano, G. Texture analysis of magnetic resonance images of patients with juvenile myoclonic epilepsy. *Epilepsy Behav.* **2013**, *27*, 22–28. [CrossRef]
20. de Oliveira, M.S.; D'Abreu, A.; Franca, M.C., Jr.; Lopes-Cendes, I.; Cendes, F.; Castellano, G. MRI-texture analysis of corpus callosum, thalamus, putamen, and caudate in Machado-Joseph disease. *J. Neuroimaging* **2012**, *22*, 46–52. [CrossRef]
21. De Rosa, C.S.; Bergamini, M.L.; Palmieri, M.; Sarmento, D.J.S.; de Carvalho, M.O.; Ricardo, A.L.F.; Hasseus, B.; Jonasson, P.; Braz-Silva, P.H.; Ferreira Costa, A.L. Differentiation of periapical granuloma from radicular cyst using cone beam computed tomography images texture analysis. *Heliyon* **2020**, *6*, e05194. [CrossRef] [PubMed]

22. Raja, J.V.; Khan, M.; Ramachandra, V.K.; Al-Kadi, O. Texture analysis of CT images in the characterization of oral cancers involving buccal mucosa. *Dentomaxillofacial Radiol.* **2012**, *41*, 475–480. [CrossRef] [PubMed]
23. Feng, J.; Li, C. Editorial: Incorporation of texture analysis in diagnosing and characterizing cancer. *Front. Oncol.* **2023**, *13*, 1224644. [CrossRef] [PubMed]
24. Gomes, J.P.P.; Ogawa, C.M.; Silveira, R.V.; Castellano, G.; De Rosa, C.S.; Yasuda, C.L.; Rocha, A.C.; Hasseus, B.; Orhan, K.; Braz-Silva, P.H.; et al. Magnetic resonance imaging texture analysis to differentiate ameloblastoma from odontogenic keratocyst. *Sci. Rep.* **2022**, *12*, 20047. [CrossRef]
25. Oliveira, M.S.; Fernandes, P.T.; Avelar, W.M.; Santos, S.L.; Castellano, G.; Li, L.M. Texture analysis of computed tomography images of acute ischemic stroke patients. *Braz. J. Med. Biol. Res.* **2009**, *42*, 1076–1079. [CrossRef] [PubMed]
26. Santos, T.A.; Maistro, C.E.; Silva, C.B.; Oliveira, M.S.; Franca, M.C., Jr.; Castellano, G. MRI Texture Analysis Reveals Bulbar Abnormalities in Friedreich Ataxia. *AJNR Am. J. Neuroradiol.* **2015**, *36*, 2214–2218. [CrossRef] [PubMed]
27. Goncalves, B.C.; de Araujo, E.C.; Nussi, A.D.; Bechara, N.; Sarmento, D.; Oliveira, M.S.; Santamaria, M.P.; Costa, A.L.F.; Lopes, S. Texture analysis of cone-beam computed tomography images assists the detection of furcal lesion. *J. Periodontol.* **2020**, *91*, 1159–1166. [CrossRef] [PubMed]
28. Varghese, B.A.; Cen, S.Y.; Hwang, D.H.; Duddalwar, V.A. Texture Analysis of Imaging: What Radiologists Need to Know. *AJR Am. J. Roentgenol.* **2019**, *212*, 520–528. [CrossRef] [PubMed]
29. Costa, A.L.F.; de Souza Carreira, B.; Fardim, K.A.C.; Nussi, A.D.; da Silva Lima, V.C.; Miguel, M.M.V.; Jardini, M.A.N.; Santamaria, M.P.; de Castro Lopes, S.L.P. Texture analysis of cone beam computed tomography images reveals dental implant stability. *Int. J. Oral Maxillofac. Surg.* **2021**, *50*, 1609–1616. [CrossRef]
30. Burr, D.B.; Gallant, M.A. Bone remodelling in osteoarthritis. *Nat. Rev. Rheumatol.* **2012**, *8*, 665–673. [CrossRef]
31. Auger, J.D.; Frings, N.; Wu, Y.; Marty, A.G.; Morgan, E.F. Trabecular Architecture and Mechanical Heterogeneity Effects on Vertebral Body Strength. *Curr. Osteoporos. Rep.* **2020**, *18*, 716–726. [CrossRef]
32. Wegrzyn, J.; Roux, J.P.; Arlot, M.E.; Boutroy, S.; Vilayphiou, N.; Guyen, O.; Delmas, P.D.; Chapurlat, R.; Bouxsein, M.L. Role of trabecular microarchitecture and its heterogeneity parameters in the mechanical behavior of ex vivo human L3 vertebrae. *J. Bone Miner. Res.* **2010**, *25*, 2324–2331. [CrossRef] [PubMed]
33. Brandi, M.L. Microarchitecture, the key to bone quality. *Rheumatology* **2009**, *48* (Suppl. S4), iv3–iv8. [CrossRef] [PubMed]
34. Cardoneanu, A.; Macovei, L.A.; Burlui, A.M.; Mihai, I.R.; Bratoiu, I.; Rezus, I.I.; Richter, P.; Tamba, B.I.; Rezus, E. Temporomandibular Joint Osteoarthritis: Pathogenic Mechanisms Involving the Cartilage and Subchondral Bone, and Potential Therapeutic Strategies for Joint Regeneration. *Int. J. Mol. Sci.* **2022**, *24*, 171. [CrossRef] [PubMed]
35. Roberts, W.E.; Stocum, D.L. Part II: Temporomandibular Joint (TMJ)-Regeneration, Degeneration, and Adaptation. *Curr. Osteoporos. Rep.* **2018**, *16*, 369–379. [CrossRef] [PubMed]
36. Nurzynska, K.; Piórkowski, A.; Strzelecki, M.; Kociołek, M.; Banyś, R.P.; Obuchowicz, R. Differentiating age and sex in vertebral body CT scans—Texture analysis versus deep learning approach. *Biocybern. Biomed. Eng.* **2024**, *44*, 20–30. [CrossRef]
37. Obuchowicz, R.; Strzelecki, M.; Piorkowski, A. Clinical Applications of Artificial Intelligence in Medical Imaging and Image Processing-A Review. *Cancers* **2024**, *16*, 1870. [CrossRef] [PubMed]
38. Girondi, C.M.; de Castro Lopes, S.L.P.; Ogawa, C.M.; Braz-Silva, P.H.; Costa, A.L.F. Texture Analysis of Temporomandibular Joint Disc Changes Associated with Effusion Using Magnetic Resonance Images. *Dent. J.* **2024**, *12*, 82. [CrossRef]
39. Ricardo, A.L.F.; da Silva, G.A.; Ogawa, C.M.; Nussi, A.D.; De Rosa, C.S.; Martins, J.S.; de Castro Lopes, S.L.P.; Appenzeller, S.; Braz-Silva, P.H.; Costa, A.L.F. Magnetic resonance imaging texture analysis for quantitative evaluation of the mandibular condyle in juvenile idiopathic arthritis. *Oral Radiol.* **2023**, *39*, 329–340. [CrossRef]
40. Nussi, A.D.; de Castro Lopes, S.L.P.; De Rosa, C.S.; Gomes, J.P.P.; Ogawa, C.M.; Braz-Silva, P.H.; Costa, A.L.F. In vivo study of cone beam computed tomography texture analysis of mandibular condyle and its correlation with gender and age. *Oral Radiol.* **2023**, *39*, 191–197. [CrossRef]

applied sciences

MDPI

Review

Multidisciplinary Applications of AI in Dentistry: Bibliometric Review

Hela Allani [1,*], Ana Teresa Santos [1,2] and Honorato Ribeiro-Vidal [3]

1 Egas Moniz School of Health & Science, 2829-511 Almada, Portugal; atsantos@egasmoniz.edu.pt
2 Centro de Estudos Internacionais (CEI), Instituto Universitário de Lisboa (ISCTE-IUL), 1649-026 Lisbon, Portugal
3 Department of Periodontology, Faculty of Dentistry, Universidade do Porto, 4200-393 Porto, Portugal
* Correspondence: helaallani95@gmail.com

Abstract: This review explores the impact of Artificial Intelligence (AI) in dentistry, reflecting on its potential to reshape traditional practices and meet the increasing demands for high-quality dental care. The aim of this research is to examine how AI has evolved in dentistry over the past two decades, driven by two pivotal questions: "What are the current emerging trends and developments in AI in dentistry?" and "What implications do these trends have for the future of AI in the dental field?". Utilizing the Scopus database, a bibliometric analysis of the literature from 2000 to 2023 was conducted to address these inquiries. The findings reveal a significant increase in AI-related publications, especially between 2018 and 2023, underscoring a rapid expansion in AI applications that enhance diagnostic precision and treatment planning. Techniques such as Deep Learning (DL) and Neural Networks (NN) have transformed dental practices by enhancing diagnostic precision and reducing workload. AI technologies, particularly Convolutional Neural Networks (CNNs) and Artificial Neural Networks (ANNs), have improved the accuracy of radiographic analysis, from detecting dental pathologies to automating cephalometric evaluations, thereby optimizing treatment outcomes. This advocacy is underpinned by the need for AI applications in dentistry to be both efficacious and ethically sound, ensuring that they not only improve clinical outcomes but also adhere to the highest standards of patient care.

Keywords: dentistry; diagnostics; artificial intelligence; deep learning; bibliometrics

1. Introduction

Artificial Intelligence (AI) has significantly reshaped modern healthcare, introducing groundbreaking enhancements in patient care and medical practice [1]. Its integration into diverse medical fields has not only extended human capabilities but also improved efficiency and accuracy in clinical settings [1]. In this technological surge, the field of dentistry has not remained untouched by the AI wave, witnessing transformative changes in various aspects of dental practice [2]. The integration of digital technologies in dentistry is advancing the frontiers of precision medicine at an unprecedented pace [3].

While the field of dentistry has made considerable strides with the adoption of AI, certain challenges persist. Variability in diagnostic precision and the subjectivity inherent in treatment planning are prominent concerns that require attention [4]. AI stands as a robust solution to these issues, promising to strengthen decision-making processes, bring uniformity to clinical practices, and improve the quality of patient care outcomes.

The growing volume of academic literature underscores the significant advancements in the theoretical and practical utilization of AI within dentistry. AI's applications are extensive and profound. This includes not only diagnosing oral pathologies, such as cancerous lesions, periodontal and periapical diseases, and caries, but also the conception of individualized treatment strategies in orthodontics, and the enhancement of precision in oral surgeries through guidance and positioning techniques [5–7].

The goal of this study is to thoroughly review and synthesize a broad spectrum of literature from 2000 to 2023, applying a bibliometric approach to provide a comprehensive overview of AI's applications and impact in dentistry. The focus extends to understanding emerging trends and pinpointing significant contributions and advancements in the field; additionally, to showcase how AI technologies are effectively being utilized to enhance diagnostic accuracy, treatment planning, and prediction of treatment outcomes.

The expected outcome of our work was to provide a comprehensive overview of AI applications within dentistry, offer valuable contributions to the scientific discourse, and inform further research and developments in this transformative field.

2. Materials and Methods

2.1. Data Collection

To collect data for the article, a Boolean search strategy was deployed on Scopus in December 2023. Scopus has become a substantial collection of peer-reviewed literature consisting of books, scientific journals, and conference papers since it was established in 2004 [8]. It spans a wide range of research topics, spanning from scientific and technical fields to medicine and community studies, and even arts and humanities [9]. It operates as a prominently curated abstract and citation database, boasting an expansive reach at both the global and regional levels [10]. Our strategy involves identifying articles with "dentistry" and "artificial intelligence" mentioned in their title, keywords, or abstract, and restricted to publications between 2000 and 2023 (see Figure 1). By closing our search window in 2023, we strategically aimed to capture the most updated collection of records, coinciding with the apex of interest in AI. Additionally, a rigorous filtering process was instituted to eliminate content forms such as books, book chapters, editorials, letters, retracted articles, non-English articles, those not directly pertinent to AI in dentistry, and any duplicates. Subsequently, these articles were classified according to their primary focus areas, which may encompass diagnostics, treatment planning, or the utilization of AI within specific dental specialties like endodontics, conservative dentistry, prosthodontics, oral pathology, orthodontics, and periodontics.

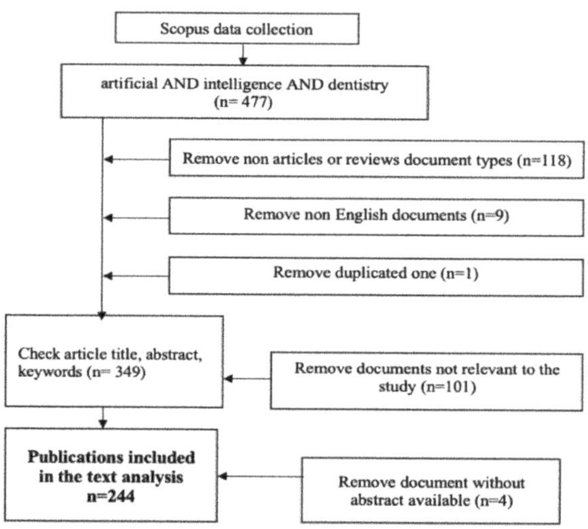

Figure 1. Flowchart of the literature identification and selection for this study.

2.2. Methodology

Bibliometrics is an invaluable method for both qualitative and quantitative analysis of scientific literature, offering an organized framework for assessing study outcomes and their implications and identifying emerging patterns of a specific topic [11]. It enables the exploration of contributions from various countries, institutions, journals, and individual scholars within a particular field. These analyses typically involve the use of specialized software tools and visual assessments, designed to systematically scrutinize the knowledge base and trace the evolutionary trends of a given discipline. In the field of dentistry, bibliometric analyses have proven to be effective in assessing trends and guiding research, as evidenced by the work of Chen et al. [12] and Qasim et al. [13]. It has been widely used, such as in prosthodontics, endodontics, implantology, orthodontics, pediatric dentistry, and periodontology, which concisely delivered valuable information for future advancement [14]. In this study, we applied bibliometric methodologies to conduct an in-depth review of AI applications in dentistry, aiming to identify current trends in this field [7].

This bibliometric analysis follows the BIBLIO framework's guidelines for methodological transparency and quantitative approaches [15], as well as detailed guidance on scientific mapping [16,17] and inclusive bibliometric indicator selection [18]. This allowed us to present our data transparently, promoting replication and comprehension of the review's breadth, while also ensuring that the analysis remained responsible and indicative of the diverse character of this study subject.

3. Results

3.1. The Scientific Discourse

3.1.1. The Development of the Field

The evolution of AI in dentistry from 2000 to 2023 has been marked by a gradual but accelerating interest, culminating in a significant surge in recent years. The early years, particularly from 2000 to 2017, saw a limited number of publications, indicating that AI's application in dentistry was a relatively unexplored area. However, this trend shifted notably in 2019, with an increase in research output. The period from 2020 to 2021 marked a substantial growth phase, reflecting advancements in AI technology and its applicability in dental research and practice [19]. This growth trajectory peaked in 2022 and 2023 is illustrated in Figure 2, with an explosive increase in publications, underscoring a robust and widespread academic and practical interest in AI within the dental field.

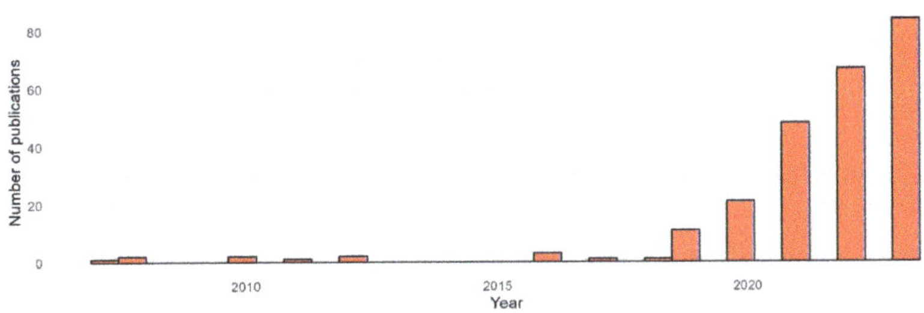

Figure 2. The number of papers published per year between 2000 and 2023.

3.1.2. Publications Outlets

From 2000 to 2023, our analysis uncovered 137 journals that have published 244 articles related to the use of AI in dental specialties; precisely, a significant portion of these sources have published at least one article over the past 4 years. The top 19 journals in terms of the number of published articles are listed in Figure 3. They were responsible for publishing 104 articles, around 42.6% of the whole sample. Throughout the years, the forefront of publishing AI in dentistry has been led by a select few journals. *Diagnostics* emerges as the top publisher with a total of 14 manuscripts, followed closely by the *Journal of Dental Research* with 12 articles. Equally impactful, *Applied Sciences (Switzerland)* and *Journal of Dentistry* have each contributed (n = 8), illustrating their significant roles in advancing the field. Other notable contributors include *Dentomaxillofacial Radiology* and *Oral Radiology*, each adding a substantial number of articles to the growing body of knowledge. This varied landscape of publication venues showcases the multidisciplinary nature of AI research in dentistry, reflecting a widespread academic interest.

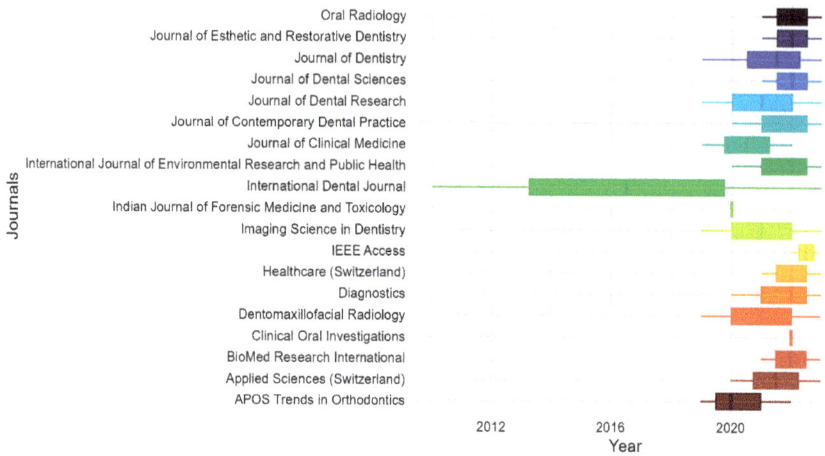

Figure 3. Publication Trends of Top 19 Journals.

3.1.3. Producers' Locations

Regarding the number of countries represented in the authors list, we reviewed all affiliations provided and discovered writers in 54 countries/territories. Figure 4 below shows the distribution of authorships by continent and nation. The darker the color, the larger the number of authors linked with national institutions. The grey color identifies the countries where no authors were found affiliated.

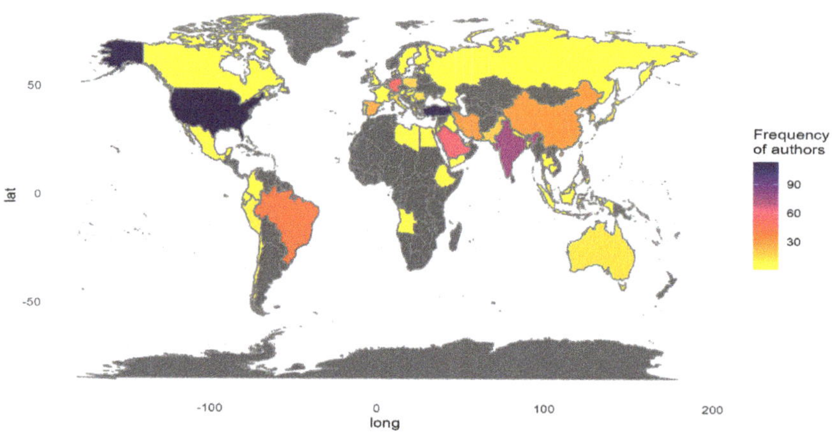

Figure 4. Global distribution of publications (2000–2023).

The United States stands out as the country hosting the highest number of co-authors, with Turkey coming in second place. On the other hand, Africa has the lowest representation among the authors, a trend that mirrors observations in various other fields. For instance, this pattern is evident in geoscience research, as detailed in a comprehensive review [20], and in studies focusing on climate change research within the African continent [21]. The disparity in author representation underscores broader regional imbalances in academic contributions and research outputs across different scientific disciplines.

Upon analyzing publication frequency, India emerges as the leading nation with the highest number of publications (n = 30, 12.30%). The United States follows closely with 27 publications (11.07%), and Turkey ranks third with 24 publications (9.84%). Germany holds the fourth position (n = 19, 7.79%), followed by Saudi Arabia (n = 16, 6.56%). India's prominence in research output has been increasingly recognized since 2022, when it surpassed the United Kingdom and ranked third globally, following only China and the United States.

When examining the contributions of various institutions, the two most prolific are located in Turkey: the University of Ankara with the highest number of publications (n = 16), followed by Eskisehir Osmangazi University (n = 11). The third position is held by Charité-Universitätsmedizin Berlin (n = 8) from Germany. The notable productivity of these institutions underscores their pivotal role in advancing scientific knowledge and the prominence of Turkish and German research outputs in the global academic landscape.

3.2. *Thematic Focus*

3.2.1. Extraction from Keywords

We investigated research publications about the use of AI in dental specialties to identify prevailing themes within this domain. After pre-processing the data, 1061 different keywords were found, but we set a minimum occurrence of two times for each keyword to analyze which ones occurred the most. In total, 58 keywords met this criteria. Both "dentistry" and "artificial intelligence" were removed as these were the words used in the search criteria. These can be seen through a word cloud methodology. Words with darker and larger fonts are more frequent topics.

The most frequently used words, as shown in Figure 5, are "deep learning" and "machine learning" which are both types of AI (Although both systems have the capacity for advanced problem-solving, "deep learning" is a "machine learning" sub-field which employs artificial neural networks with multiple layers to analyze data and make intelligent decisions (see [22])). Each one appears 64 times in the articles selected. Their notable occurrences in the literature are revolutionizing diagnosis and treatment planning, significantly in areas like periodontal disease, orthodontics, and prosthodontics [23]. They are followed by "neural networks", "diagnosis", and "digital dentristry", with frequencies of 21, 18, and 17 times, respectively, which underscore a shift towards more accessible, efficient, and technologically integrated dental care. The integration of robotics, such as for computer-assisted surgery or crown preparation, into dental practices, although less frequent than other topics, still represents a significant trend toward automating and enhancing dental procedures [24]. The existing literature confirms the potential of robotics to improve dental procedure outcomes, but they are understudied due to their limited availability and the technical expertise required for their operation. Thus, progress in dental robotics hinges on collaborations between engineers and dentists [25].

3.2.2. Extraction from Abstracts

In order to gain a broader overview of the context and approaches followed in each article considered, we analyzed the abstracts as short pieces of text, which is seen as a succinct summary of the entire paper. For this purpose, we applied four pivotal steps: text segmentation, purgation of numbers and punctuation, conversion to lowercase, and removal of stop words. Each step aims to guarantee the data quality and accuracy by reducing the noise (irrelevant or redundant information) and the dimensionality of the data, making it more manageable and computationally efficient to process.

The first step developed was the text segmentation, synonymously known as tokenization, pertaining to the fragmentation of the primary text into discrete words based on delineated word boundaries such as white spaces, a process corroborated by Hinterberger et al. [26]. We followed by converting the entire corpus to lowercase and eliminated elements such as numbers, punctuation, and running heads, streamlining the texts to facilitate analytical precision. At the end, words deemed trivial or auxiliary at the terminus of word segments were purged. Recognized as "stop words", these constituents were removed as they have a negligible contribution to the analytical purpose, and their omission does not compromise the integrity of the text analysis outcomes [27]. Finally, the most frequent words, which occurred more than 70 times in the abstracts, were plotted in Figure 6.

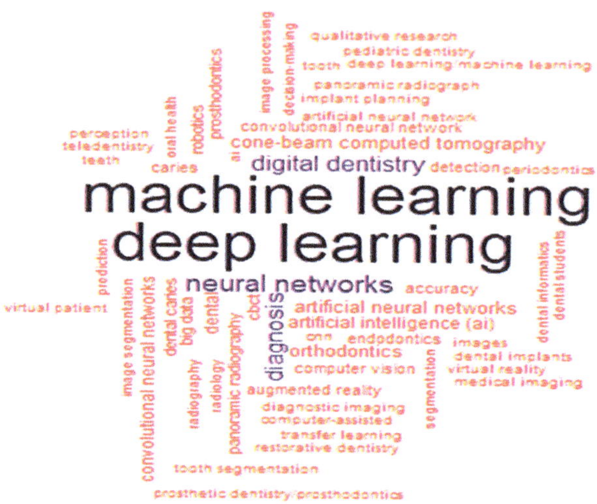

Figure 5. Word cloud visualization of frequently and repeatedly used keywords.

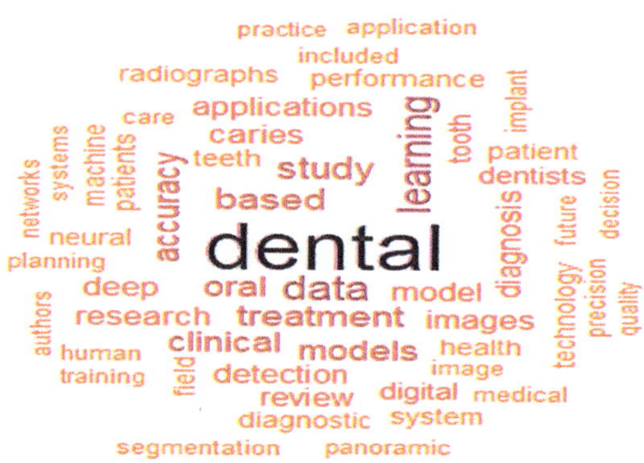

Figure 6. Word cloud visualization of frequently and repeatedly used keywords in articles' abstract.

As expected, the most frequently occurring word was "dental", appearing 556 times, which aligns with the focus of our study. This term is prominent in discussions about the impact of AI on dental implant procedures [28,29], replacing dental personnel [29,30] and providing appropriate dental care [31]. The words "data" and "learning" occurred 236 times in articles exploring AI applications, such as models for assessing and classifying periodontal defects [32] and for caries detection [33]. These findings are consistent with the most frequent keywords identified, pointing out the substantial body of literature focused on the integration of new AI techniques in the field of dentistry.

3.3. *The Evolving Discussion*

3.3.1. Longitudinal Development of Keywords

In order to analyze the longitudinal development of the field, a panel plot was prepared to illustrate the evolution of specific keywords in dentistry as reflected in scientific publications from 2000 to 2023. Figure 7 shows the keywords that experienced the greatest shift in frequency over this period. For most of them, the first appearance occurred in recent years, as did the repetitions.

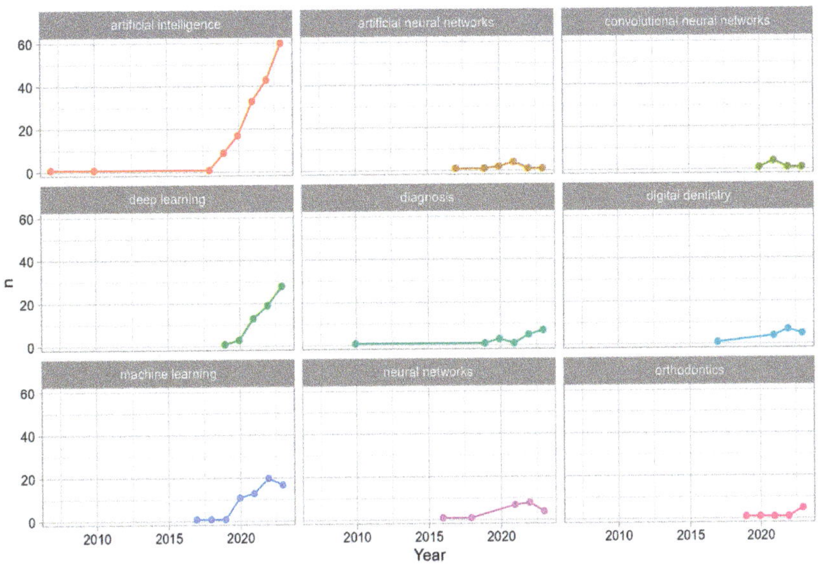

Figure 7. Featuring keyword patterns.

During the early years of the study period (2000–2018), keywords like "artificial intelligence" and "diagnosis" showed a modest consistent presence in dentistry research. More recently, from 2019 to 2023, there has been a notable increase in the frequency of keywords including "Artificial Intelligence", "Deep Learning", "Machine Learning", and "Neural Networks" (see, for example, [34]), indicating a shift toward more sophisticated AI methodologies. This is followed by the increase, although discrete, of keywords related to specific AI techniques, such as "Artificial Neural Networks" and "convolutional neural networks".

Concurrently with the increased usage of technical keywords in recent years, there has also been a marked rise in the frequency of keywords pertinent to the dentistry field, such as "orthodontics", "digital dentistry", and "diagnosis". This trend suggests that the emerging techniques are being mainly applied to these areas within dentistry. The growing prevalence of these keywords underscores the targeted application of advanced methodologies to enhance specific domains within dental research and practice.

3.3.2. Trending Topics in the Abstracts

Considering that abstracts serve as concise representations of complete papers and can provide more information about the context, we conducted a longitudinal analysis to identify the words that exhibited the most significant changes over the studied period. The twelve words with the greatest variation in frequency are illustrated in Figure 8. All those words seem to increase in the last years following the increasing number of articles published.

By far, "model" is the most frequent word with an exponential growth in its usage from 2020 onwards. It has been applied in articles aiming to develop tools to determine automatic tooth numbering, frenulum attachments, gingival overgrowth areas, and gingival inflammation signs on intraoral photographs [35], classifying periodontal defects [32] and assessing the performance of AI models [28].

The second word achieving the highest frequencies is "learning", associated with Deep and Machine learning models, which underscores a shift toward advanced, complex data processing capabilities, particularly in image analysis. These terms surged as the dental field recognized the potential of AI for deep analysis of images and radiographs, using sophisticated techniques like image segmentation for enhanced detection and diagnosis [36]. Simultaneously, "Machine Learning" steadily gained momentum, reflecting its integral role in predictive analytics and individualized treatment planning. The focused emergence of "Dental Implants" as a significant term marks AI's increasing practical application in dental treatments, with AI assisting in precision and accuracy, especially in implantology [28,37,38].

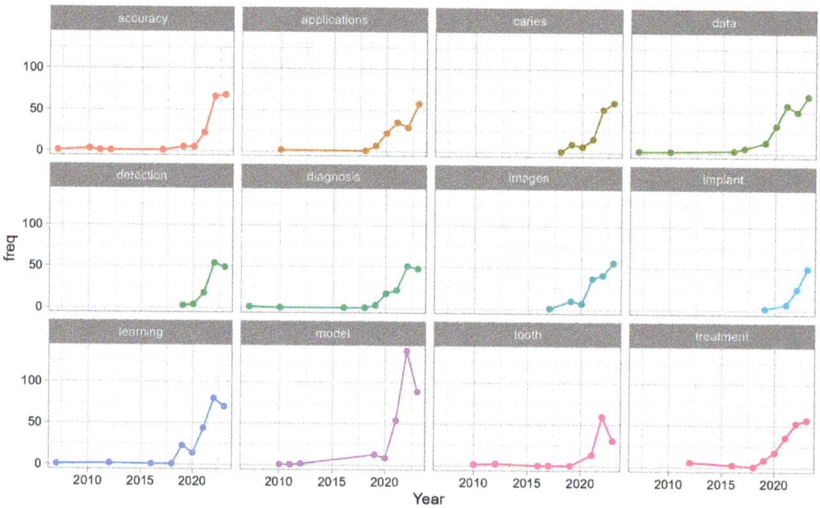

Figure 8. Longitudinal development of specific words in abstracts.

The term "data" emerges as a prominent and fundamental element in the realm of learning models, serving as the cornerstone for the processes of training, testing, and validation. This foundational element underpins the development and refinement of algorithms, providing the required input for models to learn, adapt, and improve. Its growth was accompanied by the term "accuracy" as a performance criterion for classification ensuring the reliability of models. Additionally, terms such as "diagnosis", "detection", and "treatment" have become more prevalent, suggesting the application of these complex techniques (see [37,39]).

3.3.3. Most Relevant Discussion

All the trending topics identified in the abstracts were accompanied by words that contextualize them in countless directions. To explore the subject matters addressed in relation to each topic, we analyzed the co-occurring words within the abstracts, regardless of their proximity to each other. For this purpose, we applied a method that analyzes word occurrence correlations and identifies words commonly associated with previously identified trending topics such as "caries", "learning", and "tooth". The five words with higher correlation to these three are illustrated in Figure 9. Higher correlations indicate more simultaneous occurrences.

It is quite interesting to see some common words being shared between the three topics such as "deep" and "detection", although with different degrees of correlation. In the context of "caries", the term "detection" exhibits the highest correlation, indicating that the interest in identifying this pathology is a frequent topic of discussion. Additionally, the occurrence of the term "machine" suggests that machine learning techniques are being considered for the detection of caries (see [7,30,33]).

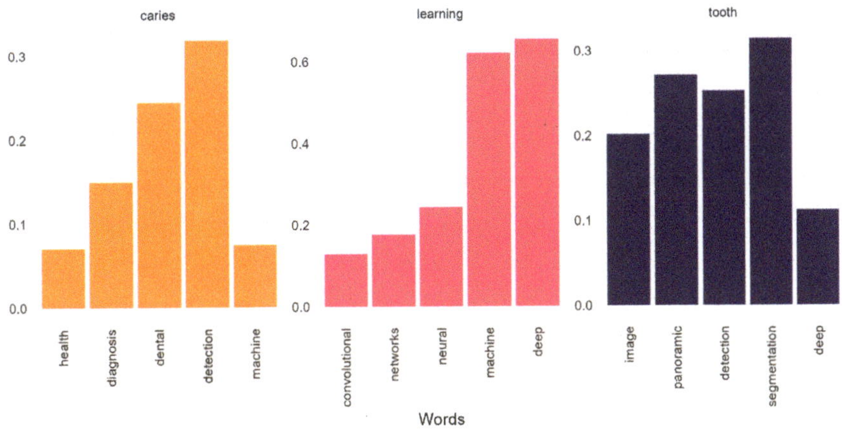

Figure 9. Words co-occurrence correlation.

Regarding "learning", both "deep" and "machine" are the most correlated topics because of the techniques being discussed. However, other methods are also being addressed simultaneously, such as neural networks and convolutional.

About tooth, "segmentation" has the first position as teeth segmentation is a prerequisite for computer-aided dental diagnosis and treatment. It is followed by the word "panoramic" as it is a common diagnostic tool for dentists and oral surgeons for being a quick and non-invasive procedure that enables an accurate assessment of oral health needs.

4. Discussion

The analysis of our study indicated that, between 2000 and 2023, a diverse group of 647 authors from 63 countries and 478 institutions contributed to 244 publications on the application of AI in the dentistry field. These publications emphasize the extensive reach and diverse perspectives in this area of research. Notably, there was a marked escalation in the volume of publications between 2018 and 2023. We observed a significant rise in the number of publications, a trend that aligns with findings in broader literature [7]. This surge can be linked to a variety of crucial factors. Thurzo et al. [40] conducted a comprehensive review, revealing a remarkable and unparalleled increase in research activity in AI dental publications, with an average annual growth of 21.6% over the last decade and a 34.9% increase per year over the last 5 years, particularly in digital diagnostic methods like radiology. Ahmed et al. [41] further supported this trend, highlighting the improvement in AI techniques and their outcomes in dentistry, emphasizing AI's role in accurate patient management, dental diagnosis, prediction, and decision-making. Moreover, another research on dental esthetics indicates a growing interest in research trends and global productivity [42].

Notably, India and the United States have emerged as forefront leaders in this domain. Among these contributions, the University of Ankara, Eskisehir Osmangazi University, and Charité Universitätsmedizin Berlin stand out for their significant impact and leadership in the field. Additionally, the work of highly cited authors like Schwendicke F. and Krois J. has been influential in shaping the current and future directions of AI applications in dentistry [43]. These findings align closely with those reported in a similar study by Xie et al. [7], reinforcing the global relevance and consistency in AI dentistry research trends.

The transformative potential of AI in dentistry, as previously highlighted in our literature review, has been empirically validated by our bibliometric analysis. Between 2018 and 2023, there has been a pronounced surge in publications focusing on advanced AI techniques such as Deep Learning (DL) and Neural Networks (NNs). These methods have transitioned from experimental to core tools in dental AI applications, especially in the areas of diagnosis and treatment planning.

Our findings indicate a significant emphasis on the use of CNNs (Convolutional Neural Networks) and ANNs (Artificial Neural Networks) for critical diagnostic tasks. CNNs, for example, have been increasingly applied to enhance the accuracy of diagnosing periapical lesions and identifying root anatomies from radiographic images, often producing results that surpass the diagnostic capabilities of experienced practitioners [44]. Similarly, ANNs have shown quite high accuracy in predicting post-operative pain and accurately placing cephalometric points on lateral cephalograms and CBCT [44,45]. Studies have highlighted that an ANN not only simplifies the process but also eases the workload for dentists [46]. This correlates strongly with the trends identified in our bibliometric analysis, where these technologies have been employed to analyze a variety of radiographic data including bitewings, periapical and panoramic radiographs, and CBCT scans. Radiographic data are essential for AI use in dentistry, as they serve as a critical resource for training AI models, enhancing accuracy in diagnostics, standardizing interpretations, and facilitating predictive analysis [47].

Notably, the literature underscores AI's capacity for improving image classification and segmentation. Segmentation allows AI systems to isolate specific areas within radiographs, such as distinguishing healthy tissue from pathological areas [48]. Once segmented, these images are classified, enabling detailed diagnostics. For instance, in the literature in periodontics, CNNs are used for segmenting images to identify periodontal cysts and then classifying them as either having cysts or no cysts [49]. Similarly, CNNs are employed to detect approximal dental caries in bitewing radiographic images and classify them according to the severity of the lesion [50]. This aligns with the observed bibliometric trends where AI's role in image segmentation and classification has markedly contributed to enhancing diagnostic precision and optimizing treatment outcomes.

Such advancements reflect a concerted effort within the dental research community to leverage AI not merely as a supplementary tool but as an integral component of modern dental practice, significantly influencing both current methodologies and future directions in dental care.

Future research should explore integrating AI with widely used digital tools, like smartphone applications and daily use software. For instance, combining AI with smartphone apps could make AI-driven diagnostics more accessible and practical in daily practice [51]. Similarly, using AI with software for pediatric dental radiographs could further validate its reliability and ease of use in clinical settings [52]. Addressing these areas will enable the dental research community to more easily test the reliability of AI-based programs in daily clinical practice, ensuring that they are both effective and user-friendly in real-world environments, which is crucial for enhancing dental care.

By synthesizing the empirical data from our bibliometric analysis with the theoretical insights from the literature, it is evident that AI's capabilities in dental diagnostics are both evolving rapidly and proving indispensable. This dual approach not only supports but also enhances our understanding of AI's critical role in advancing dental diagnostics and treatment planning, paving the way for further innovation and application in the field.

However, several limitations should be acknowledged. At the study and outcome levels, there is a potential risk of bias in the selection of studies, possibly leading to an overrepresentation of positive outcomes, especially those involving advanced AI techniques. Methodological differences across studies may also affect result comparability.

At the review level, incomplete retrieval of research is a concern. Despite an extensive search, some studies may have been missed due to language barriers, publication delays, or access issues. Additionally, reporting bias may have skewed the analysis toward studies with significant or favorable results.

5. Conclusions

This bibliometric study highlights the progressive integration of digital technology in oral health from 2000 to 2023, showcasing a significant transformation in dental practices and patient care. The evolution of AI during this period reflects a shift from basic data management to advanced implementations like the use of Deep Learning (DL) and Neural Networks (NNs). This technological advancement has revolutionized diagnostic methods, treatment planning, and outcomes prediction in dentistry, significantly enhancing the efficiency, accuracy, and personalization of treatments across various specialties.

Moreover, this study presents an opportunity for policymakers to understand and leverage these technological trends, types, and applications to improve access, literacy, knowledge, and services in oral health. It emphasizes that technology types and classifications vary over time and across dental areas, underscoring the importance of context-specific applications.

However, it is important to recognize that while AI-developed algorithms have shown promising results, they are still in need of further development and refinement. Challenges like data security, ethical considerations, and maintaining the human element in patient care are crucial. These considerations call for a balanced and cautious approach to the integration of AI in dentistry. The study suggests that continuous evaluation, adaptation, and development are essential for AI to further integrate effectively into the dental field, guiding the future toward an informed, precise, and patient-centered approach in dental healthcare. Additionally, it is important to acknowledge the long learning curve associated with AI, which necessitates ongoing attention and effort as we move forward.

Author Contributions: Conceptualization, H.A. and A.T.S.; methodology, H.A. and A.T.S.; software, H.A. and A.T.S.; validation, H.A., A.T.S. and H.R.-V.; formal analysis, H.A. and A.T.S.; investigation, H.A. and A.T.S.; resources, H.A. and A.T.S.; data curation, H.A.; writing—original draft preparation, H.A.; writing—review and editing, A.T.S. and H.R.-V.; visualization, H.A.; supervision, A.T.S.; project administration, A.T.S. All authors have read and agreed to the published version of the manuscript.

Funding: This research received no external funding.

Institutional Review Board Statement: Not applicable.

Informed Consent Statement: Not applicable.

Data Availability Statement: Not applicable.

Conflicts of Interest: The authors declare no conflicts of interest.

References

1. Davenport, T.; Kalakota, R. The potential for artificial intelligence in healthcare. *Future Healthc. J.* **2019**, *6*, 94–102. [CrossRef] [PubMed]
2. Shan, T.; Tay, F.R.; Gu, L. Application of Artificial Intelligence in Dentistry. *J. Dent. Res.* **2021**, *100*, 232–244. [CrossRef] [PubMed]
3. DaSilva, A.F.; Robinson, M.A.; Shi, W.; McCauley, L.K. The Forefront of Dentistry—Promising Tech-Innovations and New Treatments. *JDR Clin. Transl. Res.* **2022**, *7*, 16S–24S. [CrossRef] [PubMed]
4. Oh, S.L.; Jones, D.; Kim, J.R.; Choi, S.K.; Chung, M.K. Comparison Study of Diagnosis and Treatment Planning for Dental Infections between Dental Students and Practitioners. *Healthcare* **2022**, *10*, 1393. [CrossRef]
5. Hung, K.F.; Ai, Q.Y.H.; Leung, Y.Y.; Yeung, A.W.K. Potential and impact of artificial intelligence algorithms in dento-maxillofacial radiology. *Clin. Oral Investig.* **2022**, *26*, 5535–5555. [CrossRef]
6. Issa, J.; Jaber, M.; Rifai, I.; Mozdziak, P.; Kempisty, B.; Dyszkiewicz-Konwińska, M. Diagnostic Test Accuracy of Artificial Intelligence in Detecting Periapical Periodontitis on Two-Dimensional Radiographs: A Retrospective Study and Literature Review. *Medicina* **2023**, *59*, 768. [CrossRef]
7. Xie, B.; Xu, D.; Zou, X.Q.; Lu, M.J.; Peng, X.L.; Wen, X.J. Artificial intelligence in dentistry: A bibliometric analysis from 2000 to 2023. *J. Dent. Sci.* **2024**, *19*, 1722–1733. [CrossRef] [PubMed]
8. Thelwall, M.; Sud, P. Scopus 1900–2020: Growth in articles, abstracts, countries, fields, and journals. *Quant. Sci. Stud.* **2022**, *3*, 37–50. [CrossRef]
9. Borgohain, D.J. Analysis Based on Scopus Database Analysis Based on Scopus Database Research Output of Dibrugarh University: A Scientometric Analysis Based on Scopus Database. 2020. [Online]. Available online: https://digitalcommons.unl.edu/libphilprac (accessed on 12 March 2024).

10. Baas, J.; Schotten, M.; Plume, A.; Côté, G.; Karimi, R. Scopus as a curated, high-quality bibliometric data source for academic research in quantitative science studies. *Quant. Sci. Stud.* **2020**, *1*, 377–386. [CrossRef]
11. Ninkov, A.; Frank, J.R.; Maggio, L.A. Bibliometrics: Methods for studying academic publishing. *Perspect. Med. Educ.* **2022**, *11*, 173–176. [CrossRef]
12. Chen, Y.; Yeung, A.W.K.; Pow, E.H.N.; Tsoi, J.K.H. Current status and research trends of lithium disilicate in dentistry: A bibliometric analysis. *J. Prosthet. Dent.* **2021**, *126*, 512–522. [CrossRef] [PubMed]
13. Qasim, S.S.B.; Ali, D.; Khan, A.S.; Rehman, S.U.; Iqbal, A.; Baskaradoss, J.K. Evidence-Based Bibliometric Analysis of Research on Silver Diamine Fluoride Use in Dentistry. *BioMed Res. Int.* **2021**, *2021*, 9917408. [CrossRef]
14. Chen, M.-C.; Chen, S.-H.; Cheng, C.-D.; Chung, C.-H.; Mau, L.-P.; Sung, C.-E.; Weng, P.-W.; Tsai, Y.-W.C.; Shieh, Y.-S.; Huang, R.-Y.; et al. Mapping out the bibliometric characteristics of classic articles published in a Taiwanese academic journal in dentistry: A scopus-based analysis. *J. Dent. Sci.* **2023**, *18*, 1493–1509. [CrossRef] [PubMed]
15. Montazeri, A.; Mohammadi, S.; Hesari, P.M.; Ghaemi, M.; Riazi, H.; Sheikhi-Mobarakeh, Z. Preliminary guideline for reporting bibliometric reviews of the biomedical literature (BIBLIO): A minimum requirements. *Syst. Rev.* **2023**, *12*, 239. [CrossRef] [PubMed]
16. Donthu, N.; Kumar, S.; Mukherjee, D.; Pandey, N.; Lim, W.M. How to conduct a bibliometric analysis: An overview and guidelines. *J. Bus. Res.* **2021**, *133*, 285–296. [CrossRef]
17. Gutiérrez-Salcedo, M.; Martínez, M.Á.; Moral-Munoz, J.A.; Herrera-Viedma, E.; Cobo, M.J. Some bibliometric procedures for analyzing and evaluating research fields. *Appl. Intell.* **2018**, *48*, 1275–1287. [CrossRef]
18. Cabezas-Clavijo, A.; Torres-Salinas, D. Bibliometric Reports for Institutions: Best Practices in a Responsible Metrics Scenario. *Front. Res. Metr. Anal.* **2021**, *6*, 696470. [CrossRef]
19. Thurzo, A.; Strunga, M.; Urban, R.; Surovková, J.; Afrashtehfar, K.I. Impact of Artificial Intelligence on Dental Education: A Review and Guide for Curriculum Update. *Educ. Sci.* **2023**, *13*, 150. [CrossRef]
20. North, M.A.; Hastie, W.W.; Hoyer, L. Out of Africa: The underrepresentation of African authors in high-impact geoscience literature. *Earth-Sci. Rev.* **2020**, *208*, 103262. [CrossRef]
21. North, M.A.; Hastie, W.W.; Craig, M.H.; Slotow, R. Tracing primary sources of funding for, and patterns of authorship in, climate change research in Africa. *Environ. Sci. Policy* **2022**, *127*, 196–208. [CrossRef]
22. Janiesch, C.; Zschech, P.; Heinrich, K. Machine learning and deep learning. *Electron. Mark.* **2021**, *31*, 685–695. [CrossRef]
23. Retrouvey, J.M.; Conley, R.S. Decoding Deep Learning applications for diagnosis and treatment planning. *Dent. Press J. Orthod.* **2023**, *27*, e22spe5. [CrossRef] [PubMed]
24. Monterubbianesi, R.; Tosco, V.; Vitiello, F.; Orilisi, G.; Fraccastoro, F.; Putignano, A.; Orsini, G. Augmented, Virtual and Mixed Reality in Dentistry: A Narrative Review on the Existing Platforms and Future Challenges. *Appl. Sci.* **2022**, *12*, 877. [CrossRef]
25. Grischke, J.; Johannsmeier, L.; Eich, L.; Griga, L.; Haddadin, S. Dentronics: Towards robotics and artificial intelligence in dentistry. *Dent. Mater.* **2020**, *36*, 765–778. [CrossRef]
26. Liu, L.; Özsu, M.T. *Encyclopedia of Database Systems*; Springer: Boston, MA, USA, 2009. [CrossRef]
27. Schofield, A.; Magnusson, M.; Mimno, D. Pulling Out the Stops: Rethinking Stopword Removal for Topic Models. In *Proceedings of the 15th Conference of the European Chapter of the Association for Computational Linguistics: Volume 2, Short Papers*; Association for Computational Linguistics: Valencia, Spain, 2017.
28. Revilla-León, M.; Gómez-Polo, M.; Vyas, S.; Barmak, B.A.; Galluci, G.O.; Att, W.; Krishnamurthy, V.R. Artificial intelligence applications in implant dentistry: A systematic review. *J. Prosthet. Dent.* **2023**, *129*, 293–300. [CrossRef]
29. Bonny, T.; Al Nassan, W.; Obaideen, K.; Al Mallahi, M.N.; Mohammad, Y.; El-Damanhoury, H.M. Contemporary Role and Applications of Artificial Intelligence in Dentistry. *F1000Research* **2023**, *12*, 1179. [CrossRef]
30. Tabatabaian, F.; Vora, S.R.; Mirabbasi, S. Applications, functions, and accuracy of artificial intelligence in restorative dentistry: A literature review. *J. Esthet. Restor. Dent.* **2023**, *35*, 842–859. [CrossRef]
31. Sudeep, P.; Gehlot, P.M.; Murali, B.; Mariswamy, A.B. Artificial intelligence in endodontics: A narrative review. *J. Int. Oral Health* **2023**, *15*, 134–141. [CrossRef]
32. Karacaoglu, F.; Kolsuz, M.E.; Bagis, N.; Evli, C.; Orhan, K. Development and validation of intraoral periapical radiography-based machine learning model for periodontal defect diagnosis. *Proc. Inst. Mech. Eng. Part H J. Eng. Med.* **2023**, *237*, 607–618. [CrossRef]
33. Tareq, A.; Faisal, M.I.; Islam, S.; Rafa, N.S.; Chowdhury, T.; Ahmed, S.; Farook, T.H.; Mohammed, N.; Dudley, J. Visual Diagnostics of Dental Caries through Deep Learning of Non-Standardised Photographs Using a Hybrid YOLO Ensemble and Transfer Learning Model. *Int. J. Environ. Res. Public Health* **2023**, *20*, 5351. [CrossRef]
34. Esmaeilyfard, R.; Bonyadifard, H.; Paknahad, M. Dental Caries Detection and Classification in CBCT Images Using Deep Learning. *Int. Dent. J.* **2024**, *74*, 328–334. [CrossRef] [PubMed]
35. Kurt-Bayrakdar, S.; Ugurlu, M.; Yavuz, M.B.; Sali, N.; Bayrakdar, I.S.; Celik, O.; Koese, O.; Beklen, A.; Saylan, B.C.U.; Jagtap, R.; et al. Detection of tooth numbering, frenulum attachment, gingival overgrowth, and gingival inflammation signs on dental photographs using convolutional neural network algorithms: A retrospective study. *Quintessence Int.* **2023**, *54*, 680–693. [CrossRef]
36. Leite, A.F.; Gerven, A.V.; Willems, H.; Beznik, T.; Lahoud, P.; Gaêta-Araujo, H.; Vranckx, M.; Jacobs, R. Artificial intelligence-driven novel tool for tooth detection and segmentation on panoramic radiographs. *Clin. Oral Investig.* **2021**, *25*, 2257–2267. [CrossRef] [PubMed]

37. Bornes, R.S.; Montero, J.; Correia, A.R.M.; das Neves Rosa, N.R. Use of bioinformatic strategies as a predictive tool in implant-supported oral rehabilitation: A scoping review. *J. Prosthet. Dent.* **2023**, *129*, 322.e1–322.e8. [CrossRef]
38. Prados-Privado, M.; Villalón, J.G.; Martínez-Martínez, C.H.; Ivorra, C. Dental Images Recognition Technology and Applications: A Literature Review. *Appl. Sci.* **2020**, *10*, 2856. [CrossRef]
39. Londono, J.; Ghasemi, S.; Shah, A.H.; Fahimipour, A.; Ghadimi, N.; Hashemi, S.; Khurshid, Z.; Dashti, M. Evaluation of deep learning and convolutional neural network algorithms accuracy for detecting and predicting anatomical landmarks on 2D lateral cephalometric images: A systematic review and meta-analysis. *Saudi Dent. J.* **2023**, *35*, 487–497. [CrossRef]
40. Thurzo, A.; Urbanová, W.; Novák, B.; Czako, L.; Siebert, T.; Stano, P.; Mareková, S.; Fountoulaki, G.; Kosnáčová, H.; Varga, I. Where Is the Artificial Intelligence Applied in Dentistry? Systematic Review and Literature Analysis. *Healthcare* **2022**, *10*, 1269. [CrossRef]
41. Ahmed, N.; Abbasi, M.S.; Zuberi, F.; Qamar, W.; Bin Halim, M.S.; Maqsood, A.; Alam, M.K. Artificial Intelligence Techniques: Analysis, Application, and Outcome in Dentistry—A Systematic Review. *BioMed Res. Int.* **2021**, *2021*, 9751564. [CrossRef] [PubMed]
42. Mutlu-Sagesen, H.; Sagesen, A. The evolution of esthetic publications in dentistry, research trends and global productivity: A bibliometric analysis. *Int. J. Prosthodont.* **2024**, *3*, 306–318. [CrossRef]
43. Schwendicke, F.; Samek, W.; Krois, J. Artificial Intelligence in Dentistry: Chances and Challenges. *J. Dent. Res.* **2020**, *99*, 769–774. [CrossRef]
44. Gao, X.; Xin, X.; Li, Z.; Zhang, W. Predicting postoperative pain following root canal treatment by using artificial neural network evaluation. *Sci. Rep.* **2021**, *11*, 17243. [CrossRef] [PubMed]
45. Monill-González, A.; Rovira-Calatayud, L.; d'Oliveira, N.G.; Ustrell-Torrent, J.M. Artificial intelligence in orthodontics: Where are we now? A scoping review. *Orthod. Craniofacial Res.* **2021**, *24*, 6–15. [CrossRef]
46. Bichu, Y.M.; Hansa, I.; Bichu, A.Y.; Premjani, P.; Flores-Mir, C.; Vaid, N.R. Applications of artificial intelligence and machine learning in orthodontics: A scoping review. *Prog. Orthod.* **2021**, *22*, 18. [CrossRef]
47. Al-Sarem, M.; Al-Asali, M.; Alqutaibi, A.Y.; Saeed, F. Enhanced Tooth Region Detection Using Pretrained Deep Learning Models. *Int. J. Environ. Res. Public Health* **2022**, *19*, 15414. [CrossRef] [PubMed]
48. Chen, Y.-W.; Stanley, K.; Att, W. Artificial intelligence in dentistry: Current applications and future perspectives. *Quintessence Int.* **2020**, *51*, 248–257. [CrossRef]
49. Lakshmi, T.K.; Dheeba, J. Classification and Segmentation of Periodontal Cyst for Digital Dental Diagnosis Using Deep Learning. *Comput. Assist. Methods Eng. Sci.* **2022**, *30*, 131–149. [CrossRef]
50. Moran, M.; Faria, M.; Giraldi, G.; Bastos, L.; Oliveira, L.; Conci, A. Classification of Approximal Caries in Bitewing Radiographs Using Convolutional Neural Networks. *Sensors* **2021**, *21*, 5192. [CrossRef] [PubMed]
51. Pascadopoli, M.; Zampetti, P.; Nardi, M.G.; Pellegrini, M.; Scribante, A. Smartphone Applications in Dentistry: A Scoping Review. *Dent. J.* **2023**, *11*, 243. [CrossRef]
52. Kaya, E.; Gunec, H.G.; Gokyay, S.S.; Kutal, S.; Gulum, S.; Ates, H.F. Proposing a CNN Method for Primary and Permanent Tooth Detection and Enumeration on Pediatric Dental Radiographs. *J. Clin. Pediatr. Dent.* **2022**, *46*, 293–298. [CrossRef]

applied sciences

MDPI

Case Report

Modified Lip Repositioning Surgery in the Treatment of Gummy Smile

Cesar Augusto Signori Arruda [1,*], Filipa Passos Sousa [1,2] and Ricardo Castro Alves [1,2]

[1] Egas Moniz School of Health and Science, Campus Universitário Quinta da Granja, Monte de Caparica, 2829-511 Almada, Portugal; filipampsousa@gmail.com (F.P.S.); ralves@egasmoniz.edu.pt (R.C.A.)
[2] Clinical Research Unit (CRU), CiiEM, Egas Moniz—Cooperativa de Ensino Superior, Caparica, 2829-511 Almada, Portugal
* Correspondence: signoriarruda@gmail.com; Tel.: +351-933-129-250

Abstract: The smile is a characteristic that expresses emotions and affects interpersonal relationships, significantly impacting self-esteem and influencing personal and professional life. The growing emphasis on aesthetics has made patients increasingly well-informed and demanding regarding available procedures. Excessive gingival display (EGD) can result from various factors, such as altered passive eruption, vertical maxillary excess, and short or hyperactive upper lip, among others. In this case report, where EGD was caused by upper lip hypermobility, the proposed treatment involved the modified lip repositioning surgical technique (MLRS) using sutures in the modified horizontal mattress technique, aiming to limit muscle and tissue movement and to approximate the mucosal edges. The outcome was an improved aesthetic harmony of the smile, with a more suitable position of the upper lip during spontaneous smiling, as observed in a six-month follow-up.

Keywords: gummy smile; gingival exposure; gingival aesthetics; lip repositioning surgery; LipStat

1. Introduction

The smile plays a significant role in expression and appearance. Nowadays, achieving a 'perfect smile' has become an essential goal for many patients. Therefore, in addition to teeth, the condition of oral tissues, gingival contour, and lip position all affect the final aesthetics of a smile. Creating the ideal smile is a challenge, as treatment requires meticulous planning and a multidisciplinary approach [1]. Excessive gingival display (EGD), commonly known as a 'gummy smile', presents an aesthetic issue and leaves an individual dissatisfied with their smile [2].

One study compared oral health-related quality of life between individuals with and without EGD. Fifty-three patients with EGD and fifty-three control patients were selected in the southern region of Brazil. Through a questionnaire that assessed various aspects, it was observed that the aesthetic satisfaction of patients with EGD was 21.1%, while for control patients it was 78.9% [3].

A smile is defined as pleasant when the upper teeth are fully exposed; however, the degree of gingival exposure considered aesthetically pleasing varies according to the geographic location and culture. Generally, gingival exposure of no more than 2–3 mm is considered pleasant, while exposure exceeding 3 mm is typically regarded as unattractive [4].

Excessive gingival display is a common finding that can occur due to various etiologies. The amount of gingival exposure depends on the position of the smile line, which is defined as the relationship between the upper lip and the visibility of gingival tissues and teeth. There are many factors that contribute to excessive gingival display (EGD), and it is common for this condition to result from the interaction of multiple etiologies [5]. These factors include altered passive eruption, vertical maxillary excess, short upper lip, excessive upper lip mobility, and other conditions that lead to gingival enlargement [4]. To this day, there are still diagnostic and treatment challenges faced by healthcare professionals.

Appropriate treatment techniques should be chosen based on the identification and definitive diagnosis of the causes of EGD [4]. Therefore, more than one procedure can be performed to achieve the desired aesthetic [6].

The most well-known technique for correcting a gummy smile is esthetic crown lengthening. However, when crown proportions are appropriate, other treatment approaches should be considered. Surgical lip repositioning (LipStat) can be used when indicated. It is a minimally invasive procedure with fewer post-operative complications compared to orthognathic surgery, which aims to shorten the depth of the vestibular sulcus, limiting the retraction of the elevators of the upper lip muscles [4].

Historically, in 1973, a technique similar to LipStat was first described in the medical literature by Rubenstein and Kostianovsky [7]. In 1979, a study already advocated this procedure for correcting EGD in the presence of a short upper lip [8]. Subsequently, some authors proposed variations of the technique, including the retention of lip elevator muscles (the levator labii superioris alaeque nasi, the levator labii superioris muscle, the minor zygomatic muscle, and the major zygomatic muscle), resulting in a reduction in EGD [9]. In 2010, another study recommended myotomy of the levator labii superioris muscle after removing the mucosal band in the sulcus base to minimize tension after suturing the edges and prevent recurrence of the lip position at the anterior height [10]. In 2013, a modification was proposed, maintaining the labial frenum. The reasons for this were to maintain a midline reference and reduce post-operative morbidity [11].

In this case report, the modified lip repositioning surgical technique (MLRS) was used, along with internal sutures, to reposition the upper lip and limit its movement during smiling [12]. The aim of this study is to demonstrate the relevance of deep sutures in lip repositioning surgery, providing dentists with an additional safe and predictable treatment option for achieving an ideal smile.

2. Case Presentation

A 47-year-old male patient, despite being a smoker, presented with good systemic and periodontal health. He attended the Egas Moniz School of Health and Science with the main complaint of excessive gingival display (EGD) (Figure 1A). The patient, classified as Angle Class I, had a brachyfacial appearance (Figure 1B), and exhibited clinical crowns without altered passive eruption, along with some incisal wear.

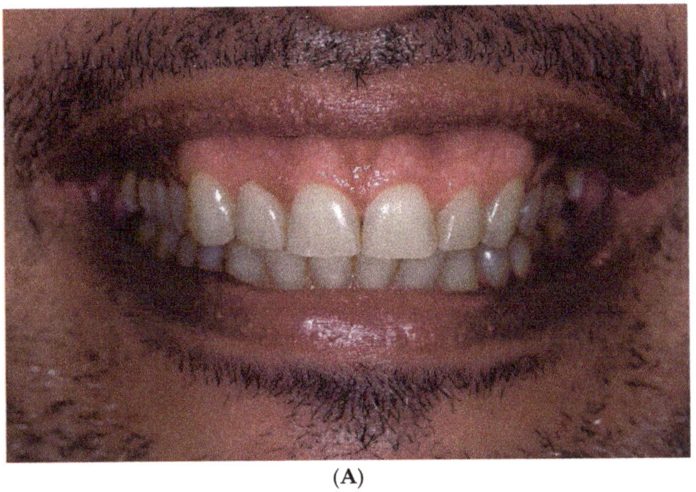

(A)

Figure 1. *Cont.*

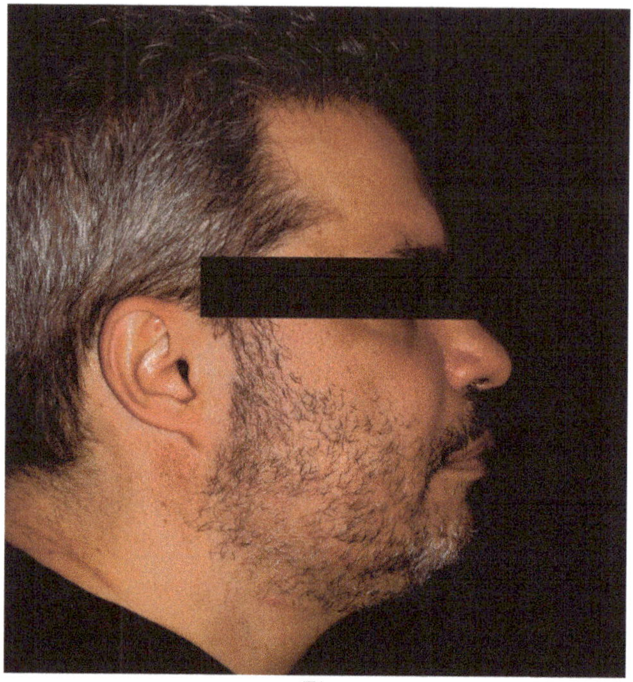

(**B**)

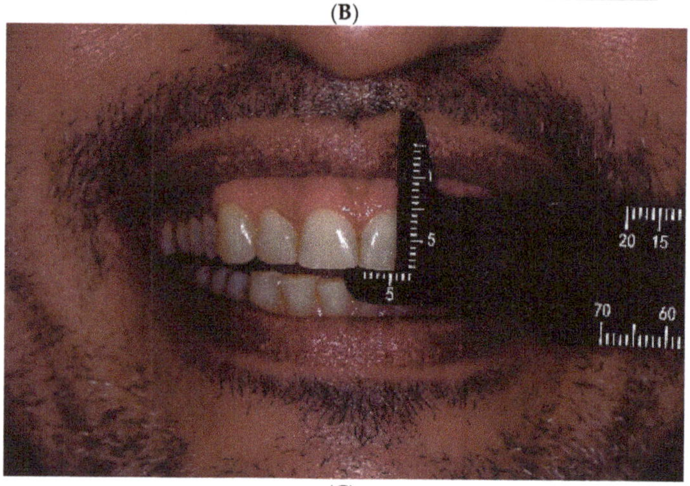

(**C**)

Figure 1. *Cont.*

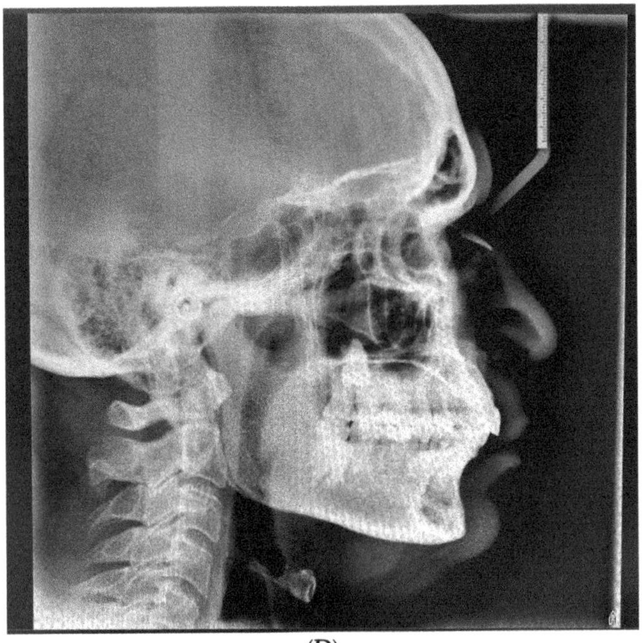

(D)

Figure 1. (**A**) Initial appearance of the smile. (**B**) Side view photograph (brachyfacial appearance). (**C**) Smile with an average 5 mm of EGD. (**D**) Cephalometry where normal size and position of the upper jaw were observed.

A length of 9.5 mm was observed in the central incisors due to incisal edge wear, along with EGD being observed during the smile, extending from the right upper second premolar to the left upper second premolar. The height from the nasal base to the lower edge of the upper lip was 24 mm, which is considered a normal lip height for a male. The patient demonstrated hypermobility of the upper lip elevator muscles during smiling. In a situation considered normal, the upper lip rises 6 to 8 mm from the resting position to the spontaneous smiling position; however, in this case, the upper lip position rose on average 1.5 times more than what is considered normal. The height of exposed gingiva in the central incisor region during spontaneous smiling was approximately 5 mm (Figure 1C). According to the patient's report, there was a genetic predisposition as his father had the same lip condition.

Cephalometric radiograph was obtained to exclude excess vertical growth of the maxilla, which may also lead to excessive gingival display (Figure 1D).

A proposed lip repositioning surgery was performed after extra and intra-oral disinfection using chlorhexidine. The procedure was carried out under local anesthesia of the infraorbital nerve, supplemented with anesthesia in the vestibular sulcus and the keratinized gingival region, bilaterally, using 2% Articaine with 1:100,000 epinephrine. To delineate the areas for incision, a bilateral lip retractor (Espandex) was used to ensure consistent lip expansion on both sides (right and left). The initial contour of the incisions was marked with a sterilized dermatological pencil (Surgical Marker) (Figure 2A). The lower border of the incision was delimited approximately 1 mm above the mucogingival line, and the upper border was delimited 10 mm above the previous one (twice the average gingival exposure height). The two lines were connected at the distal ends (in the regions of the first premolars), and the labial frenulum was preserved in the midline to maintain a reference during closure of the surgical edges.

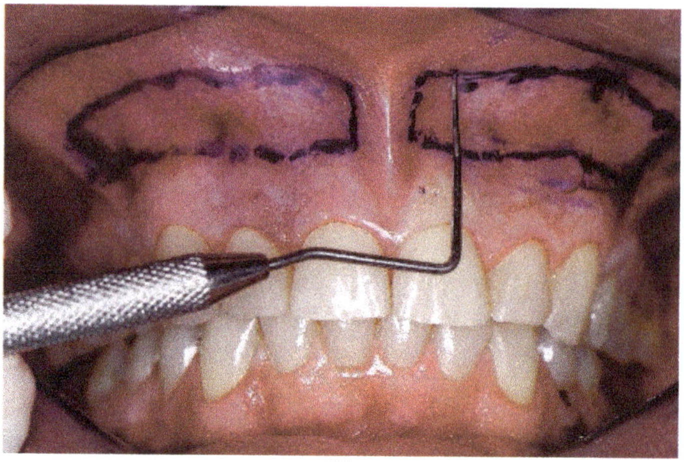

(A)

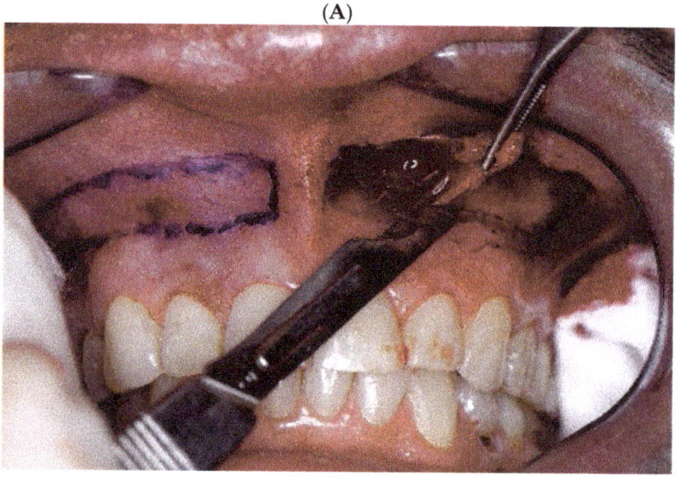

(B)

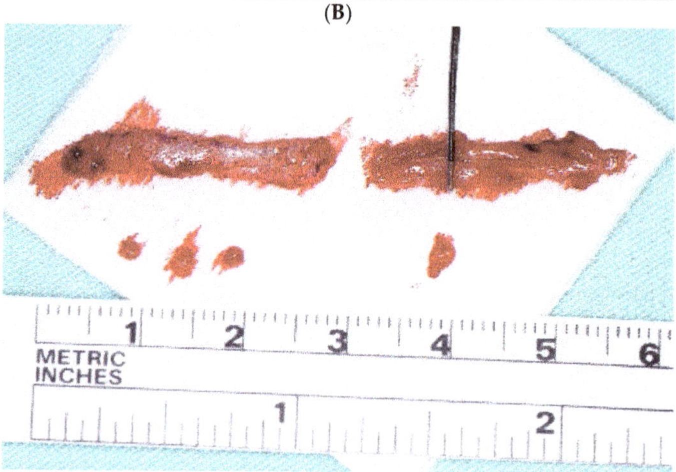

(C)

Figure 2. *Cont.*

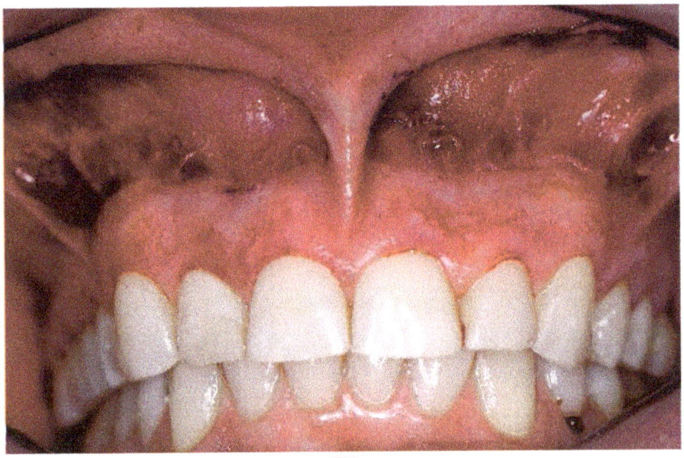

(D)

Figure 2. (**A**) Markings. (**B**) Removal of the mucosal band. (**C**) Strips of mucosa removed. (**D**) Exposure of the connective tissue.

For the superficial mucosal incisions, the same bilateral lip retractor (Espandex) was employed to maintain adequate exposure. N° 15C scalpel blades were used. A partial-thickness dissection was performed, and all epithelium was excised along the rectangular contour, exposing the underlying connective tissue (Figure 2B–D).

After removal of the mucosal strip on both sides, the first stage of deep suturing was initiated using slow-absorbing Polidioxanone (PDS) 5/0 suture (Atramat® Internacional Farmacéutica S.A. de C.V., Cuautitlán Izcalli, Mexico). Modified horizontal mattress sutures were performed to limit movement of the muscles and tissues in the region, as well as to approximate the surgical edges before external sutures (Figure 3A,B).

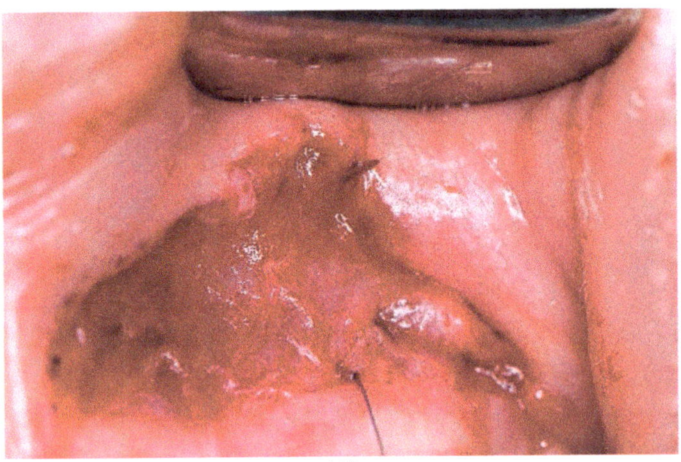

(A)

Figure 3. *Cont.*

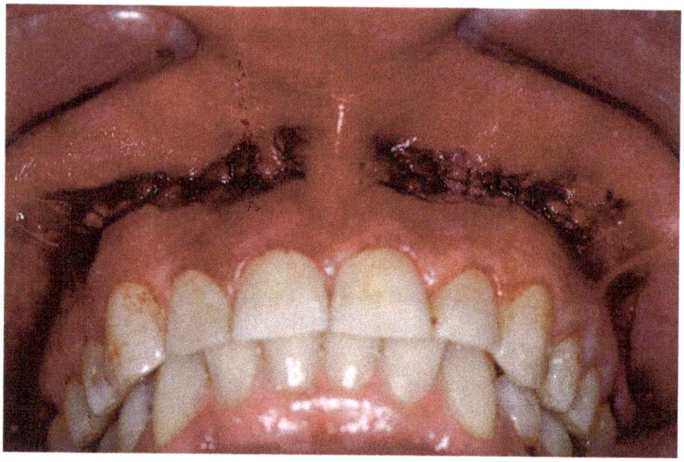

(B)

Figure 3. (**A**) Deep sutures. Needle entry and exit points in the modified horizontal mattress suture. (**B**) Deep sutures (modified horizontal mattress) providing approximation of the upper and lower edges.

The second stage of suturing was performed using the same absorbable thread. The technique used was interrupted simple sutures, ensuring complete coaptation of the surgical edges to guarantee proper alignment of the midline of the lip with the midline of the teeth (Figure 4).

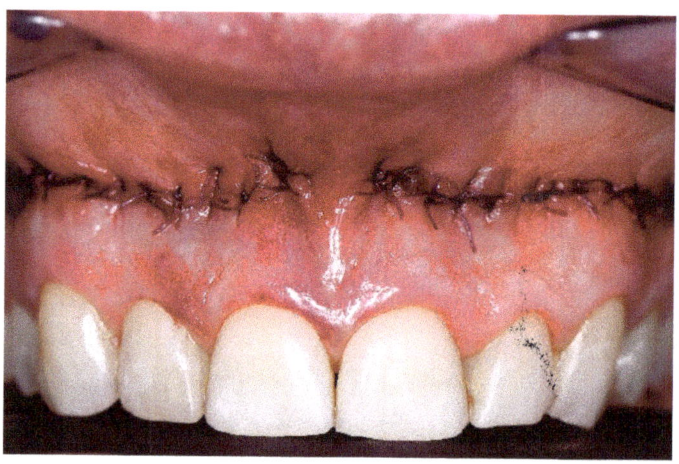

Figure 4. External sutures with complete coaptation of the mucosa.

A corticosteroid (Deflazacort 30 mg) was prescribed, starting 2 h before the procedure and maintained for 2 days; an antibiotic (Amoxicillin 1 g) started 2 h before the procedure and maintained for 7 days; an analgesic (Paracetamol1 g) in case of pain; and a 2% chlorhexidine mouthwash (2 times per day for 15 days). The patient was instructed to rest and apply ice, maintaining a soft and cold diet for 2 days.

The patient was reevaluated after 7 days, reporting minimal discomfort on the first day, with a sensation of tension at the surgical site. The patient also described numbness in the right subnasal region. Healing was considered excellent for the period (Figure 5A,B).

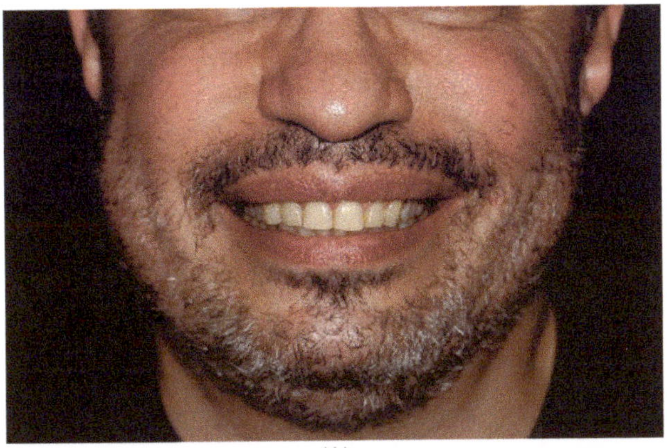

(A)

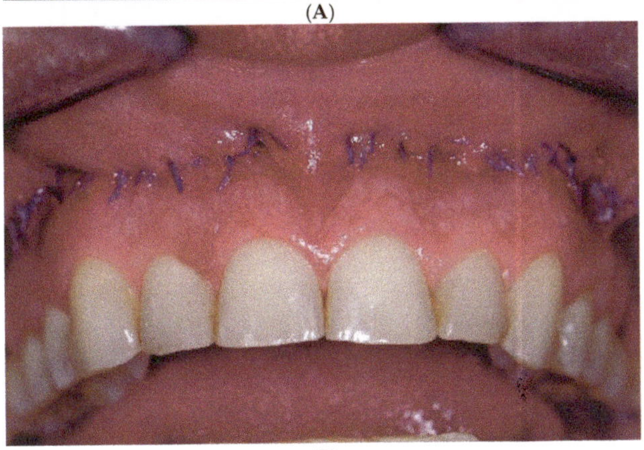

(B)

Figure 5. (**A**) Appearance of the smile 7 days after surgery. (**B**) External sutures after 7 days post-operatively.

After 15 days, the patient was reevaluated, and mucosal healing was complete. The patient did not report any complaints (Figure 6A,B).

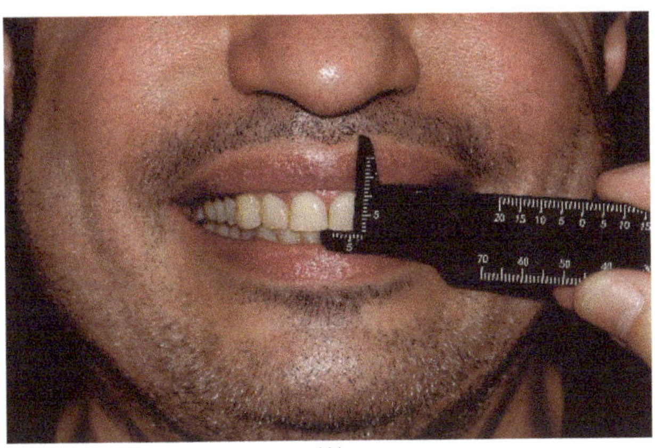

(A)

Figure 6. *Cont.*

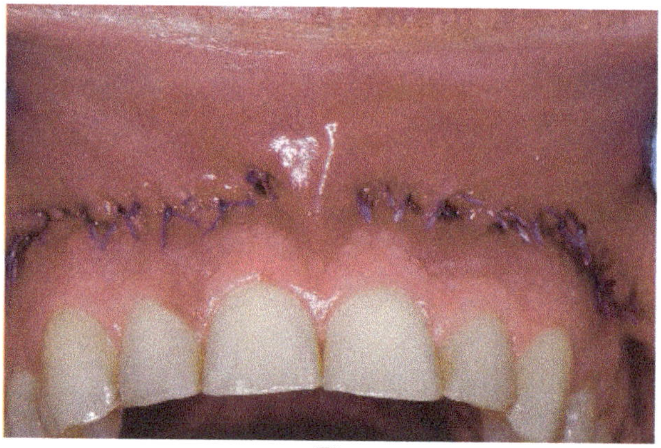

(**B**)

Figure 6. (**A**) 15 days post-operative follow-up. (**B**) External sutures after 15 days post-operatively.

At 30 days post-operatively, a scar line was observed (Figure 7A), confirming other reports in the literature. Gingival exposure decreased to an average of 1.5 mm (Figure 7B).

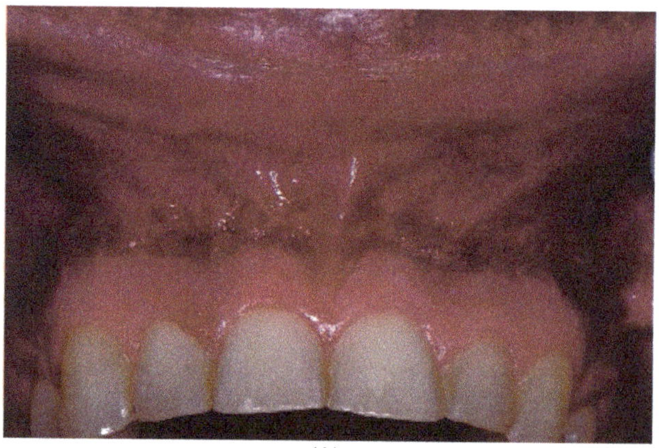

(**A**)

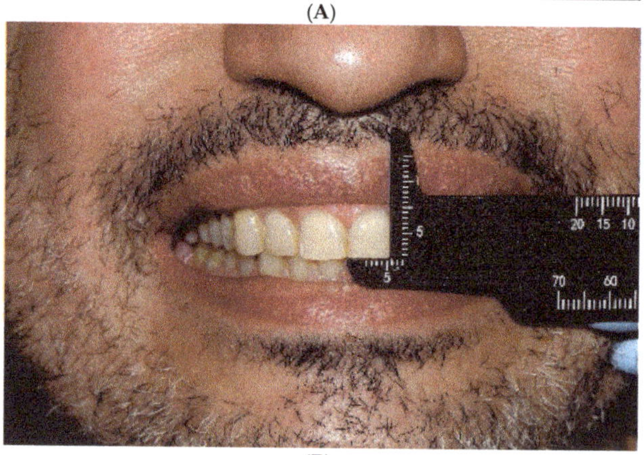

(**B**)

Figure 7. (**A**) Visible scar above the mucogengival line. (**B**) A 30-day of post-operative follow-up with an average gingival exposure of 1.5 mm when smiling.

After 6 months of follow-up, gingival exposure remained reduced, and the mucosa appeared healed. The patient was quite satisfied with the results of the treatment (Figure 8A–C).

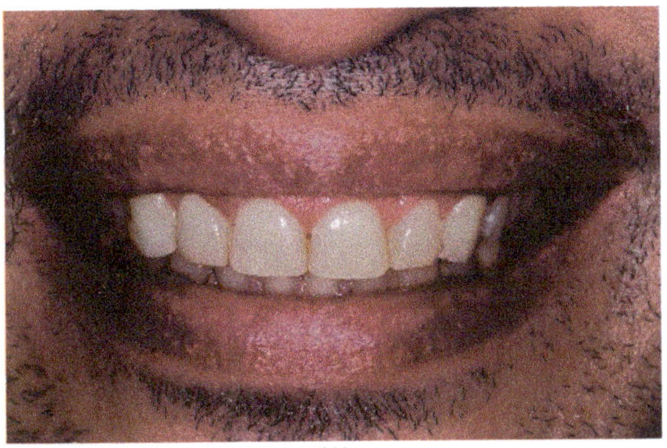

(**A**)

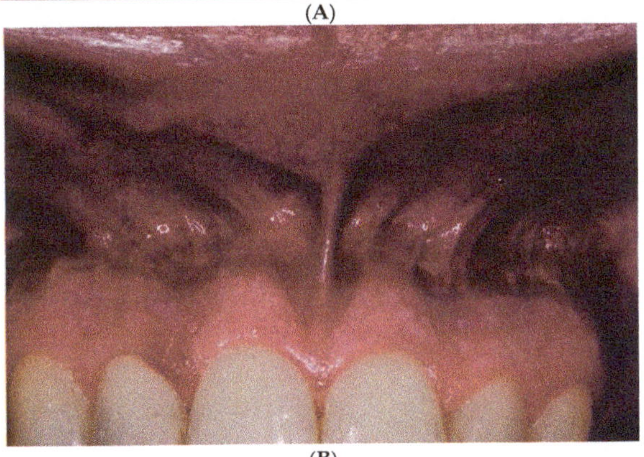

(**B**)

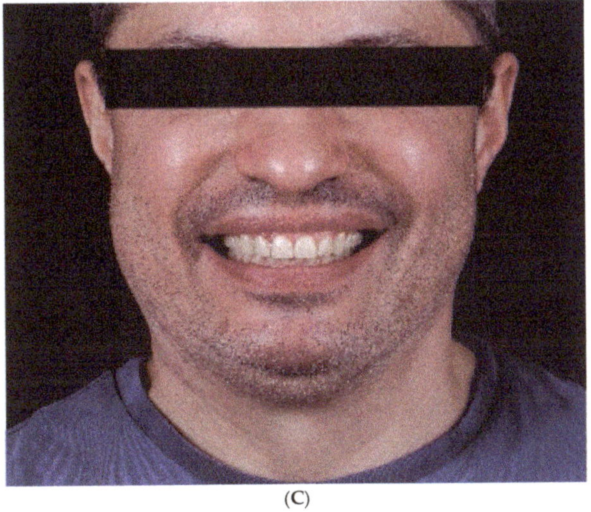

(**C**)

Figure 8. (**A**) At 6 months post-operatively. (**B**) Improvement in healing. (**C**) Aspect of the smile at 6-month post-operative follow-up.

3. Discussion

For many years, aesthetic problems treated by dentists were limited to those involving teeth, without considering the gums. However, it is now well established that these structures must be in balance to appear aesthetically pleasing. More than 3 mm of gingival exposure during smiling is considered excessive gingival display, also known as a gummy smile, which is unattractive [13–16]. When achieving an ideal smile, it is also well established that structures—dental, gingival, skeletal, and muscular—must be in balance to appear aesthetically pleasing [4,13].

The literature classifies gummy smiles according to their different etiologies and reports the possibility of a combination of some of these factors [4,17–19]. The latest classifications confirm that this variety of factors can act alone or in combination. These factors include altered passive eruption, vertical maxillary excess, short upper lip, hyperactive upper lip, among other factors that cause gingival enlargement [4]. In some cases, it is not possible to treat the patient solely through gingival recontouring because the amount of gingival exposure remains significant [20–22].

Many cases of EGD have multiple etiologies and require more than one technique to achieve desirable aesthetic results. Several techniques and variations have been reported, including myotomy or repositioning of the levator labii superioris muscle, Le Fort impaction, maxillary gingivectomies, botulinum toxin injections, and lip stabilization. Treatment is tailored to each type of etiology, and two or more techniques can be combined to resolve the issue [17,23–28].

Surgical lip repositioning (LipStat) for the treatment of EGD in mild to moderate cases is a less invasive procedure, with fewer post-operative complications and provides faster recovery compared to orthognathic surgery [4,18,27,29,30]. It can be said that LipStat is a viable treatment option for improving the gummy smile, provided that a systematic evaluation of the case is performed to choose the appropriate treatment option [29,31].

The contraindications of the technique include cases with severe vertical maxillary excess (>8 mm). These severe skeletal deformities should ideally be treated with orthognathic surgery [4,18]. A reduced width of the inserted gingiva can result in scar exposure during smiling. In such situations, the possibility of scar exposure over the mucogingival line is a limitation for this technique and should be explained to the patient [27].

Reports in the literature have shown some post-operative complications, such as discomfort, bruising, and edema of the upper lip. A less frequent complication may be the formation of a mucocele due to the cutting of the minor salivary glands in the upper lip, which arises in the post-operative period [18]. Other rare complications reported in the literature include paresthesia and transient paralysis [32]. Complications reported regarding the lip repositioning surgery are generally minor and include post-operative edema, mild pain, and tension when smiling or speaking, especially during the first week. Complications such as transient numbness and paresthesia, early recurrence, suture loss, bruising, mucocele development, and double-lip formation are rarer, while mild scarring near the mucogingival junction is often present. When more invasive approaches, such as muscle detachment, are used, complications can increase in both prevalence and duration. Although some authors report significant recurrence rates and severity, several studies show good long-term stability of results; these discrepancies may depend on the technique and possibly the operator. In addition to these complications, inadequate diagnosis or poor treatment planning, where other underlying causes are not adequately considered, can lead to inappropriate use of the lip repositioning surgery, resulting in questionable aesthetic outcomes [27].

The complications of LipStat reported in the literature include discomfort, bruising, post-operative edema, some rare cases of mucocele, paresthesia, and transient paralysis [3,16,18,23,27,31]. Additionally, the risk of recurrence should be thoroughly discussed. Previous reports have shown a higher likelihood of recurrence, especially in cases with limited indications for this technique [21,22,33–35].

A study conducted in 2021 subjected four patients with EGD of 6 to 8 mm to modified lip repositioning surgery, using internal horizontal mattress sutures to immobilize the upper lip elevator muscle. None of the patients experienced complications, and healing occurred without incident. All patients demonstrated favorable results with stability over an average follow-up period of 3.5 years [12].

Accurate case selection is crucial for reducing the risk of recurrence in lip repositioning surgery, and if followed correctly, the results will be sustainable for months [13,36]. The stability of the lip in its new position is crucial for the overall success of the procedure. Therefore, it is recommended to use appropriate suturing techniques for an adequate period to limit the action of the lip elevator muscles for an extended time [37–39]. The stability of the sutures in the post-operative period is crucial. After closing the surgical edges, in cases where orthodontic brackets are present, they can be used as anchorage for suspensory sutures in the sulcus, further limiting the mobility of the upper lip during the post-operative period [35]. The risk of an asymmetric smile can also occur when the surgeon does not pay attention to different levels of gingival exposure in patients who already have a pre-existing asymmetric smile [27]. The use of botulinum toxin can be an alternative in the treatment of gummy smile [6,17,19,23,24,27,39].

A systematic review conducted in 2018 investigated cases of excessive gingival display (EGD) treated with upper lip repositioning (LipStat). On average, they observed a reduction of 3.4 mm in gingival exposure, suggesting that the technique could be successfully used to treat EGD [1]. This reduction in gingival exposure was also observed in the present case (average of 3.5 mm).

Another method used for surgical lip repositioning is the use of a diode laser due to its beneficial characteristics, such as efficient tissue ablation capacity, reduced wound contraction, minimal scar formation, and decreased pain after surgery. Thus, the use of lasers in lip repositioning surgeries aims to minimize pain, bruising, swelling, and discomfort, providing long-term aesthetic benefits [40]. Patients often report that the most challenging aspects are discomfort, pain, hematoma, swelling, and limited lip movement during the initial recovery period. However, laser surgery has proven to be more effective than conventional scalpel surgery, as it can mitigate these effects [41].

Several reports showed improved outcomes, with reduced recurrence, when the surgical lip repositioning technique is combined with myotomy of the levator labii superioris alaeque nasi muscle [18–20,42]. Despite promising results, there are still inconsistencies in the existing evidence. Conducting further structured clinical trials is essential to determine the effectiveness of myotomy compared to the traditional method [42].

In 2021, a study evaluated the long-term clinical results of a modified lip repositioning technique that utilized periosteal sutures in a population of 12 twins with hypermobility of the upper lip. The patients were divided into two groups: the control group received treatment with the original LipStat technique, while the test group was treated with the addition of periosteal sutures. In the control group, there was a slight increase in gingival exposure over 3 years. On the other hand, in the test group, higher satisfaction and more stable results were observed over a 3.5-year follow-up [43].

Another study in 2021 analyzed four patients with 6 to 8 mm of excessive gingival display (EGD) who underwent modified surgical lip repositioning (Modified LipStat) with internal horizontal mattress sutures to immobilize the levator labii superioris muscle. All patients demonstrated stability over a 3.5-year follow-up period [12].

A recent study, involving 20 female patients with hypermobility of the upper lip or short upper lip, compared the standard technique versus the other with dual-layer sutures. Authors observed that after surgery there was a significant reduction in gingival exposure in both groups at 14 days. However, at 3 months, the first group experienced complete relapse, while the second group showed slight improvement, although it also fully relapsed by 6 months [39].

In 2023, a study with 200 patients compared the clinical outcomes and long-term stability following modified surgical lip repositioning with the addition of periosteal sutures (test group, $n = 100$) versus conventional surgical lip repositioning (control group, $n = 100$). The results demonstrated stability and no recurrence with the modified technique up to one year of follow-up [38]. The patient satisfaction level with the results of modified lip repositioning was significantly higher when compared to the satisfaction level of patients undergoing the conventional technique [44].

Several preoperative procedures must be performed, including the administration of analgesics, cleaning of the surgical site, and application of local anesthesia. When appropriate and necessary, prophylactic antibiotic therapy may also be recommended. After the surgery, it is essential to alleviate pain and inflammation to ensure a comfortable recovery period, with specific instructions for the patient [31].

Despite the emergence of studies with larger sample sizes in recent years, the importance of proper patient selection and choosing the best option for internal sutures is still lacking in the current literature.

4. Conclusions

When the diagnosis and classification of excessive gingival display are carried out correctly, modified surgical lip repositioning performed either alone or in conjunction with other techniques, demonstrates itself as an effective and predictable procedure with low post-operative morbidity compared to orthognathic surgery.

According to recent publications, modified lip repositioning surgery is a viable and successful treatment option for patients with EGD. Typically, with MLRS, a 2 to 3 mm reduction in EGD can be expected.

The modified surgical lip repositioning technique, with internal mattress sutures in a modified horizontal mattress pattern, appears to provide more reliable long-term results in patients with excessive gingival display, with a lower risk of recurrence. However, it is important to pay attention to the quality of well-tensioned sutures to ensure effective stabilization of the upper lip.

A limitation of this manuscript was the 6-month follow-up period. Despite the promising results, further longitudinal studies with a larger sample size are needed to determine the efficacy and stability of this treatment modality.

Author Contributions: Conceptualization, R.C.A.; methodology, R.C.A.; validation, F.P.S. and R.C.A.; formal analysis, F.P.S. and R.C.A.; investigation, C.A.S.A.; data curation, C.A.S.A. and F.P.S.; writing—original draft preparation, C.A.S.A.; writing—review and editing, R.C.A.; visualization, F.P.S.; supervision, R.C.A.; project administration, C.A.S.A. All authors have read and agreed to the published version of the manuscript.

Funding: This research received no external funding.

Institutional Review Board Statement: Accordance with the guidelines of the Egas Moniz School of Health and Science, the study in question meets the required ethical standards. The Informed Consent Form was duly signed by the participant involved, ensuring the protection of their identity, as established by the Declaration of Helsinki and Decree-Law No. 80/2018. Therefore, in accordance with current legislation and ethical standards, submission to the Ethics Committee does not apply in this specific case.

Informed Consent Statement: Informed consent was obtained from all subjects involved in the study.

Data Availability Statement: The data presented in this study are available in the article.

Conflicts of Interest: The authors declare no conflicts of interest.

References

1. Tawfik, O.K.; El-Nahass, H.E.; Shipman, P.; Looney, S.W.; Cutler, C.W.; Brunner, M. Lip repositioning for the treatment of excess gingival display: A systematic review. *J. Esthet. Restor. Dent.* **2018**, *30*, 101–112. [CrossRef]
2. Jananni, M.; Sivaramakrishnan, M.; Libby, T.J. Surgical correction of excessive gingival display in class I vertical maxillary excess: Mucosal strip technique. *J. Nat. Sci. Biol. Med.* **2014**, *5*, 494–498. [CrossRef]

3. Antoniazzi, R.P.; Fischer, L.S.; Balbinot, C.E.A.; Antoniazzi, S.P.; Skupien, J.A. Impact of excessive gingival display on oral health-related quality of life in a Southern Brazilian young population. *J. Clin. Periodontol.* **2017**, *44*, 996–1002. [CrossRef] [PubMed]
4. Bhola, M.; Fairbairn, P.J.; Kolhatkar, S.; Chu, S.J.; Morris, T.; de Campos, M. LipStaT: The Lip Stabilization Technique-Indications and Guidelines for Case Selection and Classification of Excessive Gingival Display. *Int. J. Periodontics Restor. Dent.* **2015**, *35*, 549–559. [CrossRef]
5. Gaddale, R.; Desai, S.R.; Mudda, J.A.; Karthikeyan, I. Lip repositioning. *J. Indian Soc. Periodontol.* **2014**, *18*, 254–258. [CrossRef] [PubMed]
6. Dinker, S.; Anitha, A.; Sorake, A.; Kumar, K. Management of gummy smile with Botulinum Toxin Type-A: A case report. *J. Int. Oral Health JIOH* **2014**, *6*, 111–115.
7. Rubenstein, A.M.; Kostianovsky, A.S. Cirugia estetica de la malformacion de la sonrisa. *Pren. Med. Argent.* **1973**, *60*, 952–954.
8. Litton, C.; Fournier, P. Simple surgical correction of the gummy smile. *Plast. Reconstr. Surg.* **1979**, *63*, 372–373. [CrossRef]
9. Rosenblatt, A.; Simon, Z. Lip repositioning for reduction of excessive gingival display: A clinical report. *Int. J. Periodontics Restor. Dent.* **2006**, *26*, 433–437.
10. Ishida, L.H.; Ishida, L.C.; Ishida, J.; Grynglas, J.; Alonso, N.; Ferreira, M.C. Myotomy of the levator labii superioris muscle and lip repositioning: A combined approach for the correction of gummy smile. *Plast. Reconstr. Surg.* **2010**, *126*, 1014–1019. [CrossRef]
11. Silva, C.O.; Ribeiro-Júnior, N.V.; Campos, T.V.; Rodrigues, J.G.; Tatakis, D.N. Excessive gingival display: Treatment by a modified lip repositioning technique. *J. Clin. Periodontol.* **2013**, *40*, 260–265. [CrossRef] [PubMed]
12. Mateo, E.; Collins, J.R.; Rivera, H.; Nart, J. New Surgical Approach for Labial Stabilization: A Long Term Follow-up Case Series. *Int. J. Periodontics Restor. Dent.* **2021**, *41*, 405–410. [CrossRef]
13. Haddadi, P.; Zare, H.; Azadikhah, A. Lip Repositioning, a Solution for Gummy Smile. *Front. Dent.* **2021**, *18*, 15. [CrossRef] [PubMed]
14. Nunes, L.; Teixeira, S.; Guevara, H.A.G.; Ferrão Junior, J.P.; Leandro, L.F.L. Tratamiento de la sonrisa gingival con la toxina botulínica tipo A: Caso clínico. *Rev. Española Cirurgía Oral Y Maxilofac.* **2015**, *37*, 229–232. [CrossRef]
15. Mostafa, D. A successful management of sever gummy smile using gingivectomy and botulinum toxin injection: A case report. *Int. J. Surg. Case Rep.* **2018**, *42*, 169–174. [CrossRef] [PubMed]
16. Faus-Matoses, V.; Faus-Matoses, I.; Jorques-Zafrilla, A.; Faus-Llácer, V.J. Lip repositioning technique. A simple surgical procedure to improve the smile harmony. *J. Clin. Exp. Dent.* **2018**, *10*, e408–e412. [CrossRef] [PubMed]
17. Mantovani, M.B.; Souza, E.C.; Marson, F.C.; Corrêa, G.O.; Progiante, P.S.; Silva, C.O. Use of modified lip repositioning technique associated with esthetic crown lengthening for treatment of excessive gingival display: A case report of multiple etiologies. *J. Indian Soc. Periodontol.* **2016**, *20*, 82–87. [CrossRef] [PubMed]
18. Alammar, A.M.; Heshmeh, O.A. Lip repositioning with a myotomy of the elevator muscles for the management of a gummy smile. *Dent. Med. Probl.* **2018**, *55*, 241–246. [CrossRef] [PubMed]
19. Bastidas, J.A. Surgical Correction of the "Gummy Smile". *Oral Maxillofac. Surg. Clin. N. Am.* **2021**, *33*, 197–209. [CrossRef]
20. Storrer, C.L.; Valverde, F.K.; Santos, F.R.; Deliberador, T.M. Treatment of gummy smile: Gingival recontouring with the containment of the elevator muscle of the upper lip and wing of nose. A surgery innovation technique. *J. Indian Soc. Periodontol.* **2014**, *18*, 656–660. [CrossRef]
21. Farista, S.; Yeltiwar, R.; Kalakonda, B.; Thakare, K.S. Laser-assisted lip repositioning surgery: Novel approach to treat gummy smile. *J. Indian Soc. Periodontol.* **2017**, *21*, 164–168. [CrossRef] [PubMed]
22. Farista, S.; Chaudhary, A.; Manohar, B.; Farista, S.; Bhayani, R. Modified laser-assisted lip repositioning surgery to treat gummy smile. *J. Indian Soc. Periodontol.* **2021**, *25*, 355–359. [CrossRef] [PubMed]
23. Aly, L.A.; Hammouda, N.I. Botox as an adjunct to lip repositioning for the management of excessive gingival display in the presence of hypermobility of upper lip and vertical maxillary excess. *Dent. Res. J.* **2016**, *13*, 478–483. [CrossRef] [PubMed]
24. Sánchez, I.M.; Gaud-Quintana, S.; Stern, J.K. Modified Lip Repositioning with Esthetic Crown Lengthening: A Combined Approach to Treating Excessive Gingival Display. *Int. J. Periodontics Restor. Dent.* **2017**, *37*, e130–e134. [CrossRef] [PubMed]
25. Arcuri, T.; da Costa, M.F.P.; Ribeiro, I.M.; Barreto, B.D., Jr.; Lyra e Silva, J.P. Labial repositioning using polymethylmethracylate (PMMA)-based cement for esthetic smile rehabilitation-A case report. *Int. J. Surg. Case Rep.* **2018**, *49*, 194–204. [CrossRef] [PubMed]
26. Foudah, M.A. Lip repositioning: An alternative to invasive surgery a 4 year follow up case report. *Saudi Dent. J.* **2019**, *31*, S78–S84. [CrossRef] [PubMed]
27. Tatakis, D.N.; Silva, C.O. Contemporary treatment techniques for excessive gingival display caused by altered passive eruption or lip hypermobility. *J. Dent.* **2023**, *138*, 104711. [CrossRef] [PubMed]
28. Nourah, D. Digital Smile Makeover: A Multidisciplinary Team Approach. *Eur. J. Dent.* **2023**, *17*, 1349–1355. [CrossRef] [PubMed]
29. Grover, H.S.; Gupta, A.; Luthra, S. Lip repositioning surgery: A pioneering technique for perio-esthetics. *Contemp. Clin. Dent.* **2014**, *5*, 142–145. [CrossRef]
30. Deepthi, K.; Yadalam, U.; Ranjan, R.; Narayan, S.J. Lip repositioning, an alternative treatment of gummy smile—A case report. *J. Oral Biol. Craniofacial Res.* **2018**, *8*, 231–233. [CrossRef]
31. Muthukumar, S.; Natarajan, S.; Madhankumar, S.; Sampathkumar, J. Lip repositioning surgery for correction of excessive gingival display. *J. Pharm. Bioallied Sci.* **2015**, *7* (Suppl. S2), S794–S796. [CrossRef]

32. Abdullah, W.; Khalil, H.; Alhindi, M.; Marzook, H. Modifying gummy smile: A minimally invasive approach. *J. Contemp. Dent. Pract.* **2014**, *15*, 821–826. [CrossRef]
33. Dayakar, M.M.; Gupta, S.; Shivananda, H. Lip repositioning: An alternative cosmetic treatment for gummy smile. *J. Indian Soc. Periodontol.* **2014**, *18*, 520–523. [CrossRef] [PubMed]
34. Rao, A.G.; Koganti, V.P.; Prabhakar, A.K.; Soni, S. Modified lip repositioning: A surgical approach to treat the gummy smile. *J. Indian Soc. Periodontol.* **2015**, *19*, 356–359. [CrossRef] [PubMed]
35. Saleem, R.; Kukreja, B.J.; Goyal, M.; Kumar, M. Treating short upper lip with "Unified lip repositioning" technique: Two case reports. *J. Indian Soc. Periodontol.* **2022**, *26*, 89–93. [CrossRef]
36. Horn, R.O.R.; Elias, C.N.; Joly, J.C. A Lip Repositioning Technique Using Polyester Threads for Gummy Smile Treatment. *Int. J. Dent.* **2022**, 3972150. [CrossRef]
37. Tatakis, D.N. Lip Repositioning Techniques and Modifications. *Dent. Clin. N. Am.* **2022**, *66*, 373–384. [CrossRef]
38. AlJasser, R.N. A Modified Approach in Lip Repositioning Surgery for Excessive Gingival Display to Minimize Post-Surgical Relapse: A Randomized Controlled Clinical Trial. *Diagnostics* **2023**, *13*, 716. [CrossRef] [PubMed]
39. Adel, N. Modified Lip Repositioning Surgery with and without Dual-layered Suturing for Treatment of Gummy Smile Patients. Plastic and reconstructive surgery. *Glob. Open* **2024**, *12*, e5521. [CrossRef]
40. Kazakova, R.T.; Tomov, G.T.; Kissov, C.K.; Vlahova, A.P.; Zlatev, S.C.; Bachurska, S.Y. Histological Gingival Assessment after Conventional and Laser Gingivectomy. *Folia Medica* **2018**, *60*, 610–616. [CrossRef]
41. Lione, R.; Pavoni, C.; Noviello, A.; Clementini, M.; Danesi, C.; Cozza, P. Conventional versus laser gingivectomy in the management of gingival enlargement during orthodontic treatment: A randomized controlled trial. *Eur. J. Orthod.* **2020**, *42*, 78–85. [CrossRef] [PubMed]
42. Ardakani, M.T.; Moscowchi, A.; Valian, N.K.; Zakerzadeh, E. Lip repositioning with or without myotomy: A systematic review. *J. Korean Assoc. Oral Maxillofac. Surg.* **2021**, *47*, 3–14. [CrossRef] [PubMed]
43. Al Jasser, R.N.; AlSarhan, M.A.; Alotaibi, D.H.; Bhola, M. A Modified Approach in Lip Repositioning Surgery: A Prospective Study in a Twin Population with a 3-Year Follow-up. *Int. J. Periodontics Restor. Dent.* **2021**, *41*, e243–e253. [CrossRef] [PubMed]
44. Al Jasser, R. A Comparison of Self-Perceived Oral and Facial Esthetics in Patients After Lip Repositioning Surgery With Modified and Conventional Techniques. *Cureus* **2023**, *15*, e50206. [CrossRef] [PubMed]

applied sciences

MDPI

Article

Toward Quieter Dental Devices: Transient CFD Simulation of Airflow and Noise in Air Turbine Handpieces

Tomomi Yamada [1,*,†], Kazunori Nozaki [2], Makoto Tsubokura [3], Mikako Hayashi [1] and Chung-Gang Li [4,*,†]

[1] Department of Restorative Dentistry and Endodontology, Osaka University Graduate School of Dentistry, Osaka 565-0871, Japan; hayashi.mikako.dent@osaka-u.ac.jp
[2] Division for Oral Dental Informatics, Osaka University Dental Hospital, Osaka 565-0871, Japan; nozaki.kazunori.dent@osaka-u.ac.jp
[3] Graduate School of System Informatics, Kobe University, Kobe 657-8501, Japan; tsubo@tiger.kobe-u.ac.jp
[4] Department of Mechanical Engineering, National Cheng Kung University, Tainan 701, Taiwan
* Correspondence: yamada.tomomi.dent@osaka-u.ac.jp (T.Y.); cgli@gs.ncku.edu.tw (C.-G.L.)
† These authors contributed equally to this work.

Abstract

High-pitched noise generated by dental air turbine handpieces (ATHs) causes discomfort and anxiety, discouraging dental visits. Understanding the time-dependent noise generation mechanism associated with compressed airflow in ATHs is crucial for effective noise reduction. However, the direct investigation of airflow dynamics within ATHs is challenging. The transient-state modeling of computational fluid dynamics (CFD) simulations remains unexplored owing to the complexities of high rotational speeds and air compressibility. This study develops a novel CFD framework for transient (time-dependent) modeling under high-speed rotational conditions. Simulations were performed using a three-dimensional model reconstructed from a commercial ATH. Simulations were conducted at 320,000 rpm using a novel framework that combines the immersed boundary and building cube methods. A fine 0.025 mm mesh spacing near the ATH, combined with supercomputing resources, enabled the simulation of hundreds of millions of cells. The simulation results were validated using experimental noise measurements. The CFD simulation revealed transient airflow and aeroacoustic behavior inside and around the ATH that closely matched the prominent frequency peaks from the experimental data. This study is the first to simulate the transient airflow of ATHs. The proposed CFD model can accurately predict aeroacoustics, contributing to the future development of quieter and more efficient dental devices.

Keywords: dental air turbine handpiece; transient computational fluid dynamics (CFD); aeroacoustics; noise generation; dental fear; high-speed rotation; patient perception

1. Introduction

In dental clinics, the environment is filled with various sounds [1], particularly the high-pitched discomforting noise of dental drills. Studies show that over half the patients feel uneasy due to this noise, which is closely linked to heightened levels of dental anxiety [2,3]. This anxiety can result in patients avoiding dental visits, ultimately compromising their oral health [2,3]. Addressing dental drill noise is therefore crucial for improving patient experience and promoting better oral health outcomes [2,3].

The dental high-speed air turbine handpiece (ATH), a prominent source of high-pitched sound in dental clinics, is defined by ISO standards as a dental drill operating at

160,000 rotations per minute (rpm) or higher, powered by compressed air [4]. Structurally, an ATH consists of a rotor housed in the drill head body, which includes an impeller, bearings, and a spindle [5,6]. When high-pressure compressed air enters the ATH, the impeller rotates rapidly, causing the cutting diamond bar inserted into the spindle to rotate. Given that tooth enamel is the toughest substance in the human body [7], ATHs can sometimes reach speeds of up to 400,000 rpm for effective drilling [6,8,9]. At such high rotational speeds, airflow inside and around the ATH generates complex fluid dynamics, producing noise. The characteristic frequency components of the noise generated by ATHs are primarily determined by the drill's rotational speed [10,11]. The noise generated during ATH idling is different in timbre from the sound of drilling teeth and dental metal, but their frequency components are closely related [10]. Psychoacoustic experiments and acoustic physical measurements have strongly linked both sound pressure levels and high-frequency noise components to patient discomfort caused by ATH noise [10,11]. Therefore, understanding the aeroacoustic mechanisms of ATH noise generation is essential for developing solutions to mitigate these unpleasant sounds from devices and improve patient experiences.

Computational fluid dynamics (CFD) has been widely applied for numerical analysis in various industries, including aerospace, automotive, construction, and chemical engineering. While previous CFD studies on ATHs have focused on torque and rotational speed [12–14], they have been limited to steady-state modeling. Although these studies provide useful insights, steady-state simulations assume fluid properties remain constant over time, which may not capture the transient behaviors critical to aeroacoustic phenomena. Therefore, in systems where transient effects are significant, this approach may lead to incomplete or misleading results. In contrast, transient simulation accurately captures dynamic behavior, transients, and temporal variations, providing a more precise representation of time-sensitive systems and improving the reliability of results. To our knowledge, no previous work has conducted a full transient CFD simulation of ATHs with compressible flow modeling.

Using CFD to assess the transient state for aeroacoustic noise presents unique challenges in simulating airflow in ATHs. The high rotational speed (up to 320,000 rpm), complex small geometry, and significant scale differences in pressure [ranging from 303,975 Pa (3.0 atm) at the inlet of ATHs to 100 Pa for noise fluctuations] demand a compressible flow solver and fine computational resolution. Additionally, transient simulations are essential for accurately predicting decibel levels and evaluating noise impacts on patients, requiring supercomputing resources. These challenges have historically limited research on non-steady airflow and aeroacoustics in ATHs.

To address these challenges, we developed a novel transient CFD framework for ATH noise analysis. By analyzing the flow field of an ATH at high rotational speeds during dental treatment, we aimed to identify the cause of acoustic noise and explore potential improvements. In this study, we simulate transient noise by performing numerical calculations using a novel CFD framework on a supercomputer equipped with a 2.2 GHz, 48-core A64FX multi-core processor. Additionally, comparing the CFD simulation and experimental results, we evaluated the validity of the new transient model in CFD.

2. Materials and Methods

2.1. Physical Model of an ATH for Numerical Calculations

The ATH used in the experiment (TwinPower Turbine, J. MORITA MFG. CORP., Kyoto, Japan) is shown in Figure 1a. To assess the capabilities of the developed framework, we intentionally selected an ATH with a more complex impeller shape among the commercial products, rather than the star-shaped impellers commonly used in numerous dental drill studies [12,13,15]. A three-dimensional (3D) model of the ATH was obtained (Figure 1b) by scanning the realistic geometry of a commercially available ATH. The intricate geometry of the impeller in the rotary is shown in Figure 1b. To obtain geometry data for CFD, we performed the computed tomography (CT) imaging of the body and rotor cartridge separately using a microfocus CT scanner (phoenix v | tome | x m300, Baker Hughes, Houston, TX, USA) [16]. The 3D data were reconstructed by defining a reference plane in the tomographic images. The 3D data of both components were then superimposed and converted into a standard triangulated language (STL) data format. As shown in Figure 1b, the complex 3D shapes of the ATH body and rotor cartridge were accurately reproduced. We adopted the building cube method (BCM) [17–19] to generate the computational grid. The BCM has been proven to be a suitable architecture for running CFD on supercomputers [20]. The concept of BCM is straightforward, as shown in Figure 1c. The computational domain is divided into units called cubes, where each cube is assigned an equal number of cells. By distributing the same number of cubes to each processing rank, high load balancing can be easily achieved. Additionally, the BCM structure offers advantages such as continuous memory access, which enhances the overall computational efficiency.

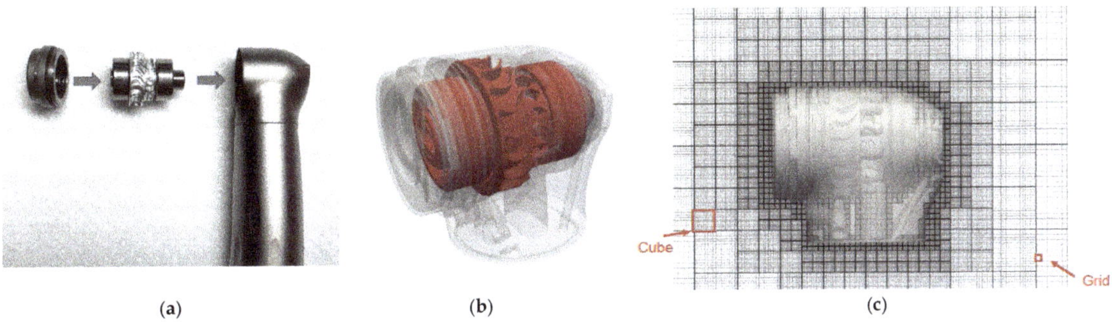

Figure 1. Three-dimensional (3D) geometry of the air turbine handpiece (ATH) and computational mesh generation for fluid dynamics simulations. (**a**) Internal components of the ATH used in this study; (**b**) high-resolution 3D reconstruction of the ATH based on micro-CT imaging. The body (gray) and rotor cartridge (red) are shown separately to highlight the complex internal geometry; (**c**) computational grid generated using the building cube method (BCM), which enables efficient domain decomposition into uniform cubes suitable for high-resolution simulation.

2.2. Numerical Simulation Method

2.2.1. Governing Equation

To capture the aeroacoustic sound, pressure and density fluctuations were calculated using the 3D Navier–Stokes equations while considering compressibility:

$$\frac{\partial U}{\partial t} + \frac{\partial F_1}{\partial x_1} + \frac{\partial F_2}{\partial x_2} + \frac{\partial F_3}{\partial x_3} = 0, \tag{1}$$

where U is the conservative form and F_i is the flux term. Denoting the density of the fluid by ρ, U and F_i are expressed as

$$U = \begin{pmatrix} \rho \\ \rho u_1 \\ \rho u_2 \\ \rho u_3 \\ \rho e \end{pmatrix} \tag{2}$$

and

$$F_i = \begin{pmatrix} \rho u_i \\ \rho u_i u_1 + p\delta_{i1} - \mu A_{i1} \\ \rho u_i u_2 + p\delta_{i2} - \mu A_{i2} \\ \rho u_i u_3 + p\delta_{i3} - \mu A_{i3} \\ (\rho e + p)u_i - \mu A_{ij}u_j - k\partial T/\partial x_i \end{pmatrix}, \forall i = 1,2,3, \quad (3)$$

where $A_{ij} = \partial u_i/\partial x_j + \partial u_j/\partial x_i - 2/3(\nabla \cdot u)\delta_{ij}$. The pressure p is given by the ideal gas equation:

$$p = \rho RT. \quad (4)$$

The dynamic viscosity and thermal conductivity of the fluid at temperature T are based on Sutherland's law:

$$\mu(T) = \mu_0(T/T_0)^{3/2}[(T_0 + 110)/(T + 110)], \quad (5)$$

$$k(T) = \mu(T)\gamma R/[(\gamma - 1)Pr], \quad (6)$$

where $\rho_0 = 1.1842$ kg/m^3, $\mu_0 = 1.85 \times 10^{-5}$ N $\cdot$ s/m^2, $T_0 = 298.06$ K, $\gamma = 1.4$, $R = 287$ J/kg/K, and $Pr = 0.72$.

2.2.2. Numerical Method

To overcome the challenges in simulating ATH aeroacoustics, we developed an innovative numerical framework that combines the immersed boundary method (IBM) with the BCM [20] in a rotational framework. This approach efficiently handles complex geometry and high-speed rotational dynamics by integrating an adaptively switched time stepping (ASTS) scheme [21], thereby enhancing computational stability and precision in capturing transient aeroacoustic phenomena. By addressing the limitations of existing methods, such as grid generation issues and instability at high Courant–Friedrichs–Lewy numbers, our framework provides an unprecedented capability to simulate both internal and external flow fields of ATHs. Table 1 summarizes the numerical scheme adopted; detailed technical implementations and mathematical formulations are provided in the Appendix A.

Table 1. Numerical scheme.

Equation Term	Algorithm	Numerical Method
Time advancement	Implicit	Adaptively switched time stepping
Convective terms	Roe scheme	Low Mach fix Roe [22]
Reconstruction	MUSCL	5th order (without limiter)
Viscous terms	Central difference	2nd order

2.2.3. Computational Setting

To optimize computational efficiency, we conducted simulations using a supercomputer. Our computational domain included both the interior and surrounding environment. The computational parameters are listed in Table 2, and key geometric dimensions of the ATH are shown in Figure 2. The inlet pressure was set to 3.06 atm and the rotational speed was fixed at 320,000 rpm, representing the actual operating conditions observed in the dental clinic. Using the BCM, we generated the computational grid for large-scale simulations within minutes. The simulation conditions were matched to the experimental setup to accurately reflect actual operational conditions, including inlet/outlet pressures and rotational speed. A fine mesh with a spacing of 0.025 mm was applied near the ATH to capture complex flow details. The total mesh cell count reached 100 million, offering precise information on critical regions, such as the gap between the head body and rotor and the region near the airfoil of the impeller (Figure 1c). Although a full grid independence study was not performed due to the high computational cost associated with the mesh size (>100 million cells), the fine spatial and temporal resolutions were validated by the excellent agreement between simulated and experimental results (as discussed in Section 3.3). The time step size was set to 2×10^{-7} s to satisfy the CFL condition for numerical stability near the impeller region, allowing a Nyquist frequency of 2.5 MHz, which is significantly higher than the highest observed acoustic frequency (~21 kHz). This confirms the adequacy of the chosen computational settings for resolving relevant aeroacoustic phenomena.

Table 2. Computation parameter settings.

Category	Parameter	Value
Geometry	Body diameter	9 mm
	Length of the body	13.0 mm
	Impeller diameter	8.1 mm
	Length of the rotor	10.7 mm
	Stage 1 impeller blade count	18
	Stage 1 blade length (axial)	2.0 mm
	Stage 1 blade height (radial)	0.6 mm
	Stage 2 impeller blade count	18
	Stage 2 blade length (axial)	1.2 mm
	Stage 2 blade height (radial)	0.7 mm
Numerical setup	Atmospheric pressure P_0	101,300.0 Pa
	Inlet pressure	3.06 atm
	Outlet pressure	1.15 atm
	Rotational speed	320,000 rpm
	Velocity of the air turbine at impeller tip	135 m/s
	Computational time step (development phase)	4×10^{-6} s flow under development
	Computational time step (after steady state)	2×10^{-7} s after quasi steady state
Mesh	Finest cell size	0.025 mm
	Cell number	104,767,488

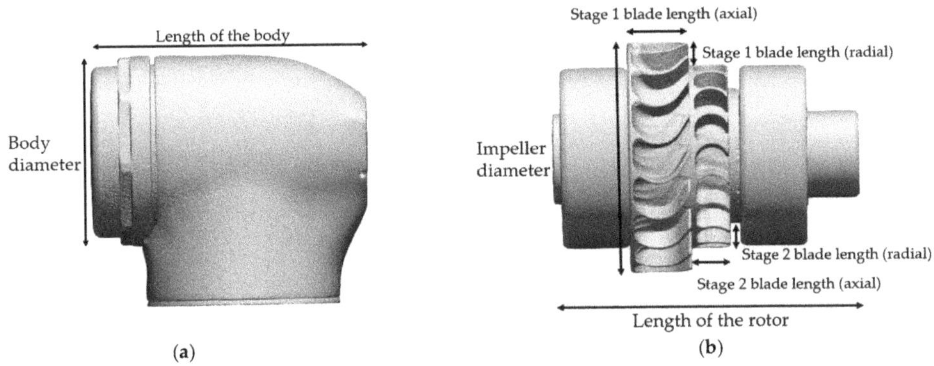

Figure 2. Key geometric dimensions of the air turbine handpiece: (**a**) head body; (**b**) rotor.

To prevent reflections from affecting result accuracy at the boundaries of the computational domain, we adopted an absorbing boundary condition for low-speed flow. Additionally, to accommodate the computational scale of hundreds of millions of cells, we utilized the Supercomputer Fugaku (RIKEN Center for Computational Science, Kobe, Hyogo, Japan). The simulations were performed using the powerful 2.2 GHz, 48-core A64FX processors developed by Fujitsu. Message-passing interface libraries were used to establish communication between neighboring processors. Furthermore, we employed open multi-processing and single-instruction multiple data methods to enhance computational performance.

2.3. Experimental Setting

To validate the CFD simulations, we conducted measurements in a quiet dental clinical room outside of clinic hours at Osaka University Dental Hospital with low noise levels. The background noise level of the clinical room was measured using a sound level meter and was found to be 42 dB. The experimental setup is illustrated in Figure 3. The same ATH model (TwinPower Turbine, J. MORITA MFG. CORP.) and operating conditions were used for both CFD simulations and measurements. Air pressure and rotational speed were regulated using a pressure gauge and a non-contact handheld digital tachometer designed for high-speed measurements (MP-5350 and HR-6800, Ono Sokki, Yokohama, Japan). A 1/4-inch microphone (UC29, Rion, Kokubunji, Japan) with a preamplifier (NH05B, Rion), part of the sound level meter (UN04, Rion), was positioned at a distance of 10 cm in front of the drill head. Data (for rotation speeds up to 320,000 rpm) were collected using a sound and vibration analysis system with a measurement frequency range of up to 40 kHz (O-Solution and DS-5000, Ono Sokki). The recorded data were analyzed using fast Fourier transform (FFT) with dedicated software (Artemis SUITE, Head-acoustics GmbH, Herzogenrath, Germany).

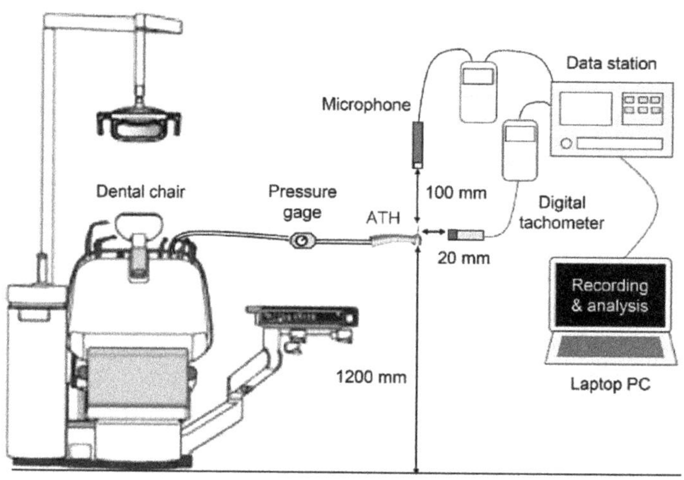

Figure 3. Configuration diagram of the experimental setup for analyzing the noise spectrum.

3. Results

In this section, we present ATH simulations performed using the developed framework. The simulations include both the internal and external flow fields to provide a comprehensive understanding of the acoustic field and noise propagation mechanisms. Our numerical framework proved suitable for running CFD on supercomputers.

3.1. Flow Field

The velocity magnitude (Vmag (m/s)) distribution at different cross-sections inside the ATH is shown in Figure 4, illustrating energy transfer through the turbine before the air exits the system. The ATH comprises two stages of turbine blades (Figure 4a). Figure 4b shows a cross-sectional view at the inlet, where high-velocity airflow enters the first stage of the turbine blades. As high-pressure air enters the ATH through the inlet, it accelerates the turbine blades in the first stage, initiating high-speed rotational motion (Figure 4b). Figure 4c depicts the outlet cross-section, displaying airflow deceleration after interacting with the second stage of turbine blades. The airflow gradually decelerates before the air exits through the outlet. However, not all air exits the ATH through the outlet; a portion flows into the gap between the impeller and capsule, eventually escaping from the front (Figure 4a). This escaping high-pressure air contributes to noise generation, as revealed by the simulation.

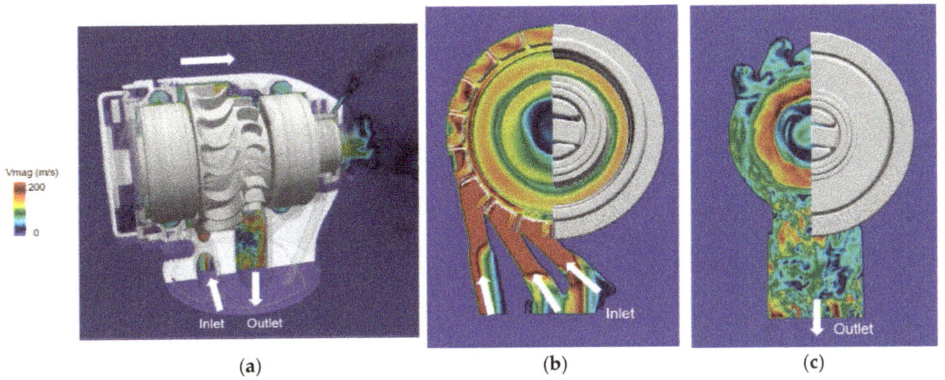

Figure 4. Velocity magnitude distribution inside the air turbine handpiece, showing the airflow behavior across critical regions of the turbine. (**a**) Detailed view of the gap between the impeller and head body; (**b**) cross-sectional view at the inlet plane showing high-velocity airflow entering the first stage of the blades of the impeller; (**c**) cross-sectional view at the outlet plane displaying the deceleration of airflow after interacting with the second stage of the blades.

3.2. Pressure Fluctuation

We achieved a transient simulation that captures the pressure fluctuation in the ATH. Figure 5 presents the instantaneous pressure fluctuation, $P - \overline{P}$, surrounding the ATH head, which represents the acoustic field. It should be noted that the head body of the ATH was fully included in the computational domain, and its shielding effect was accounted for in the simulation. The contours reveal that the primary noise source is located at the front of the ATH, where concentrated pressure fluctuations occur. The pressure fluctuation magnitude is within 100 Pa (ranging from −40 to 40 Pa), approximately 100 times smaller than the dominant pressure generated by the rotational speed at the airfoil tip of the impeller.

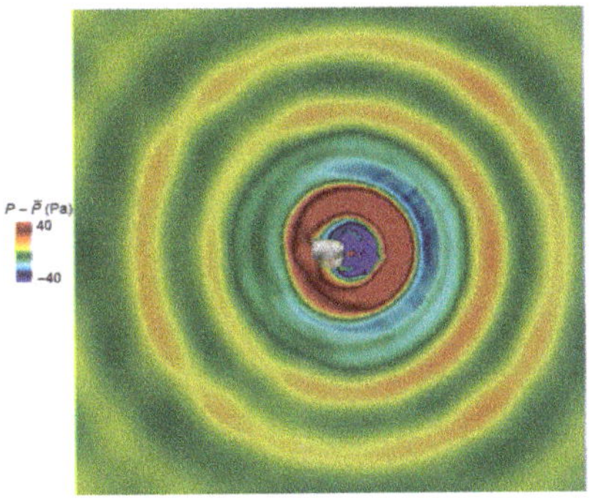

Figure 5. Instantaneous pressure fluctuation contours in the acoustic field around the air turbine handpiece (ATH). The simulation model includes the head body of the ATH.

3.3. CFD Model Validation by Experimental Comparisons and Time Domain Analysis

We validated the simulation results by comparing them with experimental measurements. To investigate the acoustic characteristics, an FFT was applied. Figure 6a presents the FFT analysis of the simulated noise, recorded by a virtual microphone placed 10 cm in front of the ATH head at a rotational speed of 320,000 rpm. Figure 6b illustrates the FFT analysis result (sampling points $n = 2048$, Hanning window) from the actual experiment at 320,000 rpm.

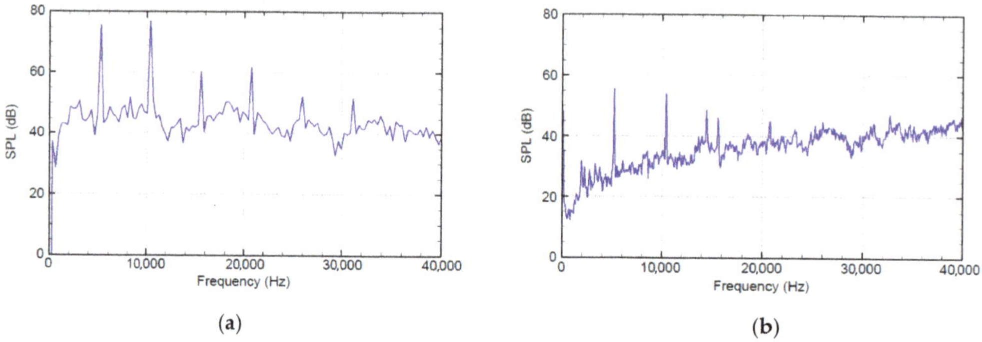

Figure 6. Frequency spectrum analysis of aeroacoustic noise emitted by the air turbine handpiece. SPL = sound pressure level. (**a**) Simulated spectrum at 320,000 rpm; (**b**) experimental spectrum at 320,000 rpm.

Several prominent frequency components appear in both results. The significant peaks in the simulation (5555, 10,555, 16,111, and 21,111 Hz) closely match the experimental results (5200, 10,350, 16,500, and 20,750 Hz). Despite some differences in sound pressure, the predicted characteristic frequencies closely approximate those obtained from actual measurements.

The frequency deviation between the simulated and experimental results was within 7%, with the largest deviation being 6.8% at the first harmonic. These discrepancies are considered reasonable given the high-speed rotational conditions and the complexity of the airflow field. Minor differences may stem from discrepancies between simulation and experimental conditions, such as fluctuations in the experimental rotational speed, as well as geometric simplifications and mesh resolution limitations near the impeller. Despite these factors, the simulation results successfully captured the major spectral features observed in the experiment. Overall, these results indicate that the current framework accurately captures peak frequencies.

In addition to spectral validation, the transient behavior of the pressure field was analyzed to further verify the consistency of the simulated aeroacoustic response. Figure 7 shows the time-resolved contours of the pressure fluctuation field from 5 μs to 60 μs. These snapshots clearly illustrate the outward propagation of concentric acoustic wavefronts originating from the front of the ATH region. The propagation distance of approximately 20 mm over 60 μs corresponds to a frequency of ~17 kHz, which closely matches the third harmonic (16,111 Hz) observed in the simulated FFT spectrum. This time domain validation strongly supports the physical accuracy of the aeroacoustic source modeling and confirms that the dominant noise arises primarily from rotor–stator interaction.

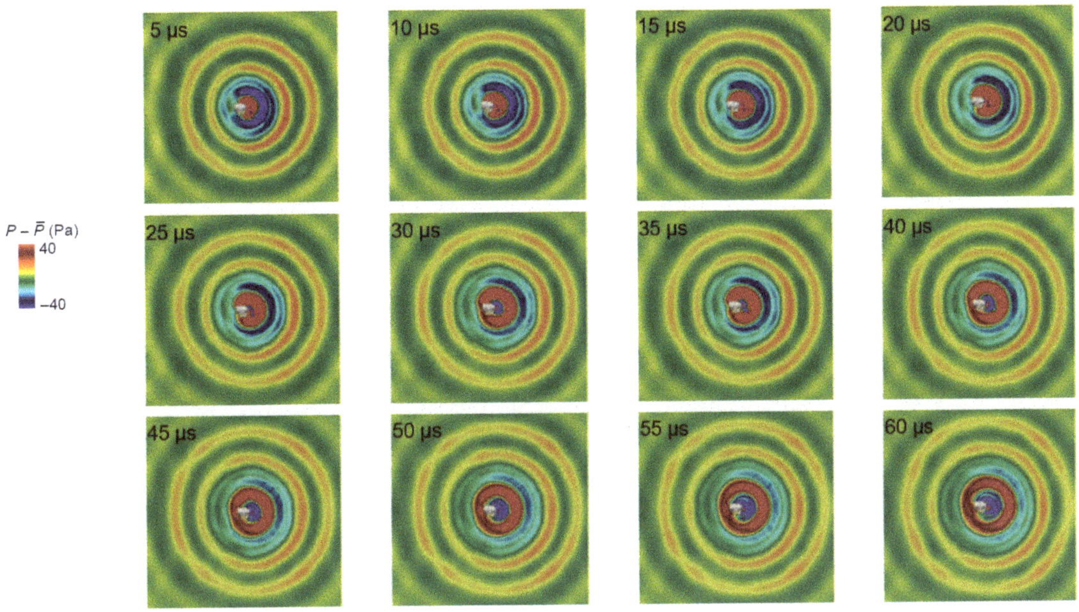

Figure 7. Time-resolved pressure fluctuation contours showing aeroacoustic wave propagation from the air turbine handpiece (ATH). Snapshots are shown from 5 μs to 60 μs at 5 μs intervals. Periodic concentric wavefronts originate in front of the ATH, forming a wave pattern consistent with the third harmonic frequency observed in the simulated spectrum.

4. Discussion

ATHs are indispensable tools in modern dental treatment. While previous studies have focused primarily on enhancing ATH performance metrics such as rotational speed, torque, and power [9,12,15,23,24], this study exclusively investigates the aeroacoustic noise mechanisms that directly impact the patient experience. Although steady-state analyses of ATH aerodynamics have been conducted in prior research [12,13,15], such approaches are fundamentally inadequate for capturing transient pressure fluctuations for noise generation. This study is the first to simulate transient flow to assess aeroacoustic noise.

When detailed analysis of time-dependent effects is required to understand aerodynamic flow and noise during rotation or to optimize control strategies, transient modeling is essential. However, transient calculation introduces complexities such as initial conditions, time step schemes, and convergence, making the setup and analysis more challenging. More computational resources and time are required for managing its multiple time steps and transient data. Our novel CFD framework for transient conditions addresses these challenges. By generating a highly refined mesh near the complex impeller geometry (Figures 1 and 2) and computing over 100 million mesh cells in a few minutes, compared to the several days required by traditional unstructured grid methods, this approach significantly improves computational efficiency. This numerical framework is a suitable architecture for running CFD on supercomputers, enabling simulations at the computational scale of hundreds of millions of cells. The pressure fluctuation magnitude around the ATH was approximately 100 times smaller than the dominant pressure generated by the rotational speed at the airfoil tip of the impeller. The successful capture of these subtle acoustic phenomena demonstrates the high numerical accuracy of our developed framework in resolving acoustic field fluctuations.

Experimental spectral analyses of noise emitted by different ATHs with similar rotation speeds have reported pronounced peaks at approximately 5–6 kHz and their harmonic frequencies [10]. Several studies have explored the relationship between the acoustic properties of sound emitted by ATHs and patient emotions, finding that these prominent frequencies contribute to anxiety and discomfort [10,11]. It has been shown that teenagers are more sensitive to high-frequency components and therefore rate dental drill sounds as more unpleasant than older individuals do [11]. These findings suggest that frequency-specific acoustic design must be adapted to the auditory profiles of different patient groups. Validated against experimental data, our framework accurately captured specific noise frequencies associated with patient anxiety [2,3,11,25,26]. Unlike previous studies [12–14] that focused only on the steady internal flow within the ATH, we employed a comprehensive approach considering both internal flow dynamics and the surrounding acoustic environment. This approach enabled the successful simulation of the complex 3D airflow in an ATH, which is crucial for understanding the mechanisms of sound source generation and accurately predicting noise propagation. Overall, this framework demonstrates a numerical precision that accurately models the sound field.

This study provides valuable insights; however, there are opportunities for further refinement. First, a slightly coarser resolution may have contributed to differences in sound pressure at certain frequencies between the simulation and the experiment. Second, a diamond bar for drilling was not inserted into the ATH, and the water spray used to cool the bar tip was omitted in both the simulation and the actual experimental measurements.

The simulation results also provide a basis for exploring noise reduction strategies, including design modifications to the impeller blades or casing geometry aimed at disrupting coherent tonal sources. By enabling rapid assessment of design modifications, this CFD framework can guide the development of quieter dental tools, fostering a more patient-friendly acoustic environment and improving the overall experience of dental procedures. Future research will focus on using the transient CFD framework to explore the relationship between geometric shapes and noise to further enhance patient comfort.

5. Conclusions

In conclusion, leveraging supercomputing resources, we developed a robust numerical framework capable of simulating the transient flow dynamics and noise generation of ATHs operating at clinical speeds of up to 320,000 rpm. The simulated results closely corresponded with the experimental measurements, effectively representing the frequency components of noise linked to patient discomfort. Our framework provides a foundation for aeroacoustic optimization for ATHs, thereby supporting the development of quieter dental devices that can enhance patient comfort and reduce anxiety in clinical settings.

Author Contributions: Conceptualization, T.Y., K.N., M.H., M.T., and C.-G.L.; methodology, T.Y., K.N., M.T., and C.-G.L.; software, C.-G.L.; validation, T.Y., K.N., and C.-G.L.; formal analysis, T.Y., K.N., and C.-G.L.; investigation, T.Y. and K.N.; resources, T.Y., K.N., and C.-G.L.; writing—original draft preparation, T.Y. and C.-G.L.; writing—review and editing, T.Y., K.N., M.H., M.T., and C.-G.L.; visualization, T.Y., K.N., and C.-G.L.; supervision, T.Y.; funding acquisition, T.Y. and C.-G.L. All authors have read and agreed to the published version of the manuscript.

Funding: This research was funded by the Japan Society for the Promotion of Science, grant numbers 19K10148, 22K09999 and National Science and Technology Council (NSTC) in Taiwan, project No. NSTC 111-2222-E-006-018-MY2.

Institutional Review Board Statement: Not applicable, as this study does not involve human participants.

Informed Consent Statement: Not applicable.

Data Availability Statement: The data presented in this study are available on request from the corresponding author.

Acknowledgments: We thank to National Center for High-performance Computing (NCHC), Taiwan for providing partial computational and storage resources. We also wish to express our appreciation to JMC Corporation, Yokohama, Japan, for their invaluable assistance in acquiring CT imaging.

Conflicts of Interest: The authors have no conflicts of interest relevant to this article.

Appendix A

Appendix A.1. Rotation Framework for the Immersed Boundary

The immersed boundary method (IBM) developed by Li et al. [20] is suitable for treating the moving problem in the current simulation. According to Li et al. [20], because the Courant–Friedrichs–Lewy (CFL) number—expressed as

$$CFL = \frac{u_{conv} \times \Delta t}{\Delta x} \tag{A1}$$

where u_{conv} is the speed of the moving object—cannot be larger than 0.5 in order to avoid the fresh cell problem, the time step is restricted by u_{conv}.

This also implies that if objects have a high rotational speed, resulting in a high angular velocity, the time step must be very small. As a result, a significant consumption of computational resources can be anticipated. To address this issue, the multiple reference frame (MRF) approach is adopted to handle rotating objects. Equation (A2) shows the momentum equation in a rotating frame:

$$\frac{\partial \rho u_1}{\partial t} + \nabla \cdot (\rho V_r u_1) + \rho(\omega \times u_1) = -\nabla p + \nabla \cdot \tau, \tag{A2}$$

where $V_r = u_1 - \omega \times r$ represents the relative velocity, which refers to the velocity observed from the rotating frame, and $\rho(\omega \times u_1)$ represents the term caused by the Coriolis and centripetal acceleration. However, a disadvantage of the MRF method is the challenging treatment of the interface between the stationary and rotating zones. Here, a method combining IBM and MRF is proposed as an alternative approach to handle rotating objects.

Equation (A3) represents the momentum equation with the immersed boundary as a source term ρF_B:

$$\frac{\partial \rho u_1}{\partial t} + \nabla \cdot (\rho u_1 u_1) = -\nabla p + \nabla \cdot \tau + \rho F_B, \tag{A3}$$

where F_B is the body force term, such that the velocity distribution on an arbitrary surface is equal to the desired velocity V_s.

$$u_i^{n+1} = u_i^n + \Delta t(RHS + \rho F_B) = V_s \tag{A4}$$

If the velocity of the next time step u_i^{n+1} is equal to the desired value V_s on the immersed boundary, the source term F_B can be expressed as

$$F_B = \frac{1}{\rho}(\frac{V_s - u^n}{\Delta t} - RHS) \tag{A5}$$

A comparison between Equations (A2) and (A3) reveals that if the relative velocity V_r is zero, which also implies that the angular velocity is a constant, Equation (A6) can be obtained.

$$\rho(\omega \times u_1) = \nabla \cdot (\rho u_1 u_1) - \rho F_B \tag{A6}$$

From an implementation perspective, the impact of rotation on the flow field due to the Coriolis and centripetal acceleration can be directly calculated using Equation (A6). As a result, employing the IBM can address the interface treatment for the rotating zone. However, the application of the MRF method in transient state problems remains controversial owing to the fresh cell problem. Therefore, in the current study, Equation (A6) is utilized solely to expedite the attainment of a quasi-steady state. Once the quasi-steady state is achieved, the time step is gradually reduced to the desired value. The CFL number, which is based on the maximum moving speed of the object, must be kept below 0.5 to avoid the fresh cell problem.

Appendix A.2. Time Stepping Scheme

To alleviate the computational resource requirements imposed by the CFL condition based on the sound speed, the dual time stepping method, which was proposed by Jameson [27], was employed to solve the Navier–Stokes formulation in Equation (1). Thus, the governing equation becomes

$$\frac{\partial U_p}{\partial \tau} + \frac{\partial U}{\partial t} + \frac{\partial F_1}{\partial x_1} + \frac{\partial F_2}{\partial x_2} + \frac{\partial F_3}{\partial x_3} = 0 \tag{A7}$$

where U_p is the primitive form of $[P, u_1, u_2, u_3, T]$; τ and t are the artificial and physical times, respectively; and U is the conservative form of $[\rho, \rho u_1, \rho u_2, \rho u_3, \rho e]$.

$$\begin{aligned} &\frac{U_p^{k+1}-U_p^k}{\Delta\tau} + \frac{3U^{k+1}-4U^n+U^{n-1}}{2\Delta t} + \frac{1}{\Delta x_1}\left(F_1{}_{(i+1/2,j,k)}^{k+1} - F_1{}_{(i-1/2,j,k)}^{k+1}\right) \\ &+\frac{1}{\Delta x_2}\left(F_2{}_{(i,j+1/2,k)}^{k+1} - F_2{}_{(i,j-1/2,k)}^{k+1}\right) + \frac{1}{\Delta x_3}\left(F_3{}_{(i,j,k+1/2)}^{k+1} - F_3{}_{(i,j,k-1/2)}^{k+1}\right) = 0 \end{aligned} \tag{A8}$$

Equation (A6) can be arranged with implicit form as

$$[\frac{I}{\Delta\tau} + M\frac{3}{2\Delta t} + (\delta_{x_1}A_p^k + \delta_{x_3}B_p^k + \delta_{x_3}C_p^k)]\Delta U_p = R^k, \tag{A9}$$

where δ_{x_i} is the central difference operator and $A_p = \partial F_i^k/\partial U_p$ is the flux Jacobian.

With the dual time stepping, only $\Delta\tau$ is restricted by the CFL condition based on the sound speed, and Δt can be free of the CFL condition. However, the inclusion of an artificial time term in the equation leads to Newton linearization error, resulting in reduced accuracy. Therefore, using Equation (A9) is not suitable for aeroacoustic simulations performed in this study as these require high levels of accuracy. The easiest way to solve this problem is to remove the artificial time term. Equation (A9) becomes

$$[M\frac{3}{2\Delta t} + (\delta_{x_1}A_p^k + \delta_{x_3}B_p^k + \delta_{x_3}C_p^k)]\Delta U_p = R^k. \tag{A10}$$

However, a large Δt in Equation (A10) can easily cause divergence because of the lack of the artificial time term.

To address this issue, Lu et al. [21] proposed an adaptively switched time stepping (ASTS) scheme from LUSGS [28]; however, their work focused solely on two-dimensional simulations. In this study, we extend the ASTS scheme to 3D simulations. The concept behind the ASTS scheme is that when the iteration is not yet stable, Equation (A9) should be employed. However, once the iteration reaches a stable stage, Equation (A10) can be used. By automatically switching between the governing equations with and without the artificial time term, we can simultaneously maintain a large time step and high accuracy.

To determine whether the iteration is stable, Equation (A11) suggested by Lian et al. [29] is used as an indicator:

$$\Delta Q_{est} = -\Delta\tau M^{-1}[-(3U^k - 4U^n + U^{n-1})/(2\Delta t) - (\delta_{x_1}\overline{F}_1{}^k + \delta_{x_2}\overline{F}_2{}^k + \delta_{x_3}\overline{F}_3{}^k)]. \quad \text{(A11)}$$

Equation (A12) can be solved only when $|\Delta Q_{est}| < \Delta Q_p^{ref}$, which implies that the iteration is sufficiently stable and that the artificial time term can be eliminated. Conversely, if $|\Delta Q_{est}| > \alpha\Delta Q_p^{ref}$, Equation (A12) is first solved to obtain the allowable CFL number for each grid.

$$CFL_{allowable} = CFL_{specified} \times \alpha\Delta Q_p^{ref} / |\Delta Q_{est}|. \quad \text{(A12)}$$

Then, Equation (A9) is solved to proceed to the next iteration.

ΔQ_p^{ref} for 3D simulations is expressed in Equation (A13):

$$\Delta Q_p^{ref} = \begin{pmatrix} 0.1 \times \max\left[0.5 \times \rho(u_1{}^2 + u_2{}^2 + u_3{}^2), \quad \Delta P_{sur}, \quad P_{global} \times 10^{-9}\right] \\ 2 \times \max[\sqrt{u_1{}^2 + u_2{}^2 + u_3{}^2}, \quad \frac{\Delta P_{sur} \times c}{\gamma P}, \quad V_{global} \times 10^{-9}] \\ 2 \times \max[\ \sqrt{u_1{}^2 + u_2{}^2 + u_3{}^2} \quad \frac{\Delta P_{sur} \times c}{\gamma P}, \quad V_{global} \times 10^{-9}\ ] \\ 2 \times \max[\ \sqrt{u_1{}^2 + u_2{}^2 + u_3{}^2}, \quad \frac{\Delta P_{sur} \times c}{\gamma P}, \quad V_{global} \times 10^{-9}\ ] \\ 0.1 \times T \end{pmatrix} \quad \text{(A13)}$$

where ΔP_{sur} represents the maximum pressure difference between the surrounding points and Pglobal, and Vglobal denotes a global reference value introduced to ensure that all reference values remain positive.

Appendix A.3. Numerical Scheme for the Flux Term

To solve the flux terms in Equation (3), which include the inviscid term F_{inv} in Equation (A14),

$$F_{inv} = \begin{pmatrix} \rho u_i \\ \rho u_i u_1 + p\delta_{i1} \\ \rho u_i u_2 + p\delta_{i2} \\ \rho u_i u_3 + p\delta_{i3} \\ (\rho e + p)u_i \end{pmatrix} \quad \text{(A14)}$$

and the viscous term $F_{visoucs}$ in Equation (A15),

$$F_{viscous} = -\begin{pmatrix} 0 \\ \mu A_{i1} \\ \mu A_{i2} \\ \mu A_{i3} \\ \mu A_{ij}u_j + \lambda\partial T/\partial x_i \end{pmatrix} \quad \text{(A15)}$$

the following numerical methods are utilized.

To solve F_{inv}, we adopted the low-Mach-fix for Roe (LMRoe) [22] method, whereby

$$F_{inviscid,i+1/2} = \frac{1}{2}[F_R(U) + F_L(U)] + F_d, \quad \text{(A16)}$$

where F_d is the Roe upwind dissipation term [30]. To calculate F_R and F_L in Equation (A16), the fifth-order monotone upstream-centered scheme for conservation laws (MUSCL) [31] is adopted. The limiter function in the MUSCL should be removed when the speed is at a low Mach number to reduce dissipation [32]. The fifth-order MUSCL without a limiter function can be written as

$$U_{L,i+1/2} = 1/60 \times (2U_{i-2} - 13U_{i-1} + 47U_i + 27U_{i+1} - 3U_{i+2}), \tag{A17}$$

$$U_{R,i-1/2} = 1/60 \times (-3U_{i-2} + 27U_{i-1} + 47U_i - 13U_{i+1} + 2U_{i+2}). \tag{A18}$$

To solve $F_{viscous}$, the derivatives of A_{ij} in the viscous term of Equation (A15) are computed using the second-order central difference. The numerical scheme adopted in this study is summarized in Table 1.

References

1. Yamada, T.; Nozaki, K.; Hayashi, M.; Kuwano, S. Sound environment during dental treatment in relation to COVID-19 pandemic. *Acoustics* **2023**, *5*, 987–998. [CrossRef]
2. Duker, L.I.S.; Grager, M.; Giffin, W.; Hikita, N.; Polido, J.C. The relationship between dental fear and anxiety, general anxiety/fear, sensory over-responsivity and oral health behaviors and outcomes: A conceptual model. *Int. J. Environ. Res. Public Health* **2022**, *19*, 2380. [CrossRef]
3. Rajeev, A.; Patthi, B.; Janakiram, C.; Singla, A.; Malhi, R.; Kumari, M. Influence of the previous dental visit experience in seeking dental care among young adults. *J. Family Med. Prim. Care* **2020**, *9*, 609–613. [CrossRef] [PubMed]
4. *ISO 14457:2017*; Dentistry—Handpieces and motors. International Organization for Standardization: Geneva, Switzerland, 2017. Available online: https://www.iso.org/standard/66429.html (accessed on 8 July 2025).
5. Dyson, J.E.; Darvell, B.W. Dental air turbine handpiece performance testing. *Aust. Dent. J. Aust. Dent. J.* **1995**, *40*, 330–338. [CrossRef] [PubMed]
6. Dyson, J.E.; Darvell, B.W. The development of the dental high-speed air turbine handpiece. *Part 1 Aust. Dent. J.* **1993**, *38*, 49–58. [CrossRef] [PubMed]
7. Zhang, Y.R.; Du, W.; Zhou, X.D.; Yu, H.Y. Review of research on the mechanical properties of the human tooth. *Int. J. Oral. Sci.* **2014**, *6*, 61–69. [CrossRef] [PubMed]
8. Eshleman, J.R.; Sarrett, D.C. How the development of the high-speed turbine handpiece changed the practice of dentistry. *J. Am. Dent. Assoc.* **2013**, *144*, 474–477. [CrossRef] [PubMed]
9. Brockhurst, P.J.; Shams, R. Dynamic measurement of the torque-speed characteristics of dental high speed air turbine handpieces. *Aust. Dent. J.* **1994**, *39*, 33–38. [CrossRef] [PubMed]
10. Yamada, T.; Kuwano, S.; Ebisu, S.; Hayashi, M. Effect of processing of dental drill noise on subjective impression. *Appl. Acoust.* **2021**, *177*, 107895. [CrossRef]
11. Yamada, T.; Kuwano, S.; Ebisu, S.; Hayashi, M. Effect of age-related extended high frequency hearing loss on the subjective impressions of dental drill noise. *Sci. Rep.* **2024**, *14*, 15655. [CrossRef] [PubMed]
12. Nishi, Y.; Fushimi, H.; Shimomura, K.; Hasegawa, T. Performance and internal flow of a dental air turbine handpiece. *Int. J. Rotating Mach.* **2018**, *2018*, 1826489. [CrossRef]
13. Juraeva, M.; Park, B.H.; Ryu, K.J.; Song, D.J. Designing high-speed dental air-turbine handpiece by using a computational approach. *Int. J. Precis. Eng. Manuf.* **2017**, *18*, 1403–1407. [CrossRef]
14. Beigzadeh, B.; Derakhshan, S.; Shamami, D.Z. A numerical study on performance of dental air turbine handpieces. *Mechanika* **2017**, *23*, 750–755. [CrossRef]
15. Dyson, J.E.; Darvell, B.W. The development of the dental high-speed air turbine handpiece. *Part 2 Aust. Dent. J.* **1993**, *38*, 131–143. [CrossRef] [PubMed]
16. Micro CT Scanner. Phoenix Micro CT Scanner | 3D CT Metrology Scanner. Available online: https://www.bakerhughes.com/waygate-technologies/industrial-radiography-and-ct/phoenix-advanced-industrial-xray-and-ct/phoenix-vtomex-m-high-speed-3d-ct-scanner (accessed on 7 July 2025).
17. Nakahashi, K.; Kim, L.S. Building-cube method for large-scale, high resolution flow computations. In Proceedings of the 42nd AIAA Aerospace Sciences Meeting and Exhibit, Reno, NV, USA, 5–8 January 2004. [CrossRef]
18. Ishida, T.; Takahashi, S.; Nakahashi, K. Efficient and robust Cartesian mesh generation for building-cube method. *J. Comput. Sci. Technol.* **2008**, *2*, 435–446. [CrossRef]
19. Nakahashi, K. Building-cube method for flow problems with broadband characteristic length. In Proceedings of the Computational Fluid Dynamics 2002, Sydney, Australia, 15–19 July 2002. [CrossRef]
20. Li, C.G.; Bale, R.; Wang, W.; Tsubokura, M. A sharp interface immersed boundary method for thin-walled geometries in viscous compressible flows. *Int. J. Mech. Sci.* **2023**, *253*, 108401. [CrossRef]

21. Lu, H.; Li, C.; Tsubokura, M. Adaptively switched time stepping scheme for direct aeroacoustic computations. *AIP Adv.* **2022**, *12*, 035340. [CrossRef]
22. Rieper, F. A low-Mach number fix for Roe's approximate Riemann solver. *J. Comput. Phys.* **2011**, *230*, 5263–5287. [CrossRef]
23. Dyson, J.E.; Darvell, B.W. Torque, power and efficiency characterization of dental air turbine handpieces. *J. Dent.* **1999**, *27*, 573–586. [CrossRef] [PubMed]
24. Dyson, J.E.; Darvell, B.W. Flow and free running speed characterization of dental air turbine handpieces. *J. Dent.* **1999**, *27*, 465–477. [CrossRef] [PubMed]
25. Eitner, S.; Wichmann, M.; Paulsen, A.; Holst, S. Dental anxiety—An epidemiological study on its clinical correlation and effects on oral health. *J. Oral. Rehabil.* **2006**, *33*, 588–593. [CrossRef] [PubMed]
26. McGrath, C.; Bedi, R. The association between dental anxiety and oral health-related quality of life in Britain. *Community Dent. Oral. Epidemiol.* **2004**, *32*, 67–72. [CrossRef] [PubMed]
27. Jameson, A. Time dependent calculations using multigrid, with applications to unsteady flows past airfoils and wings. In Proceedings of the 10th Computational Fluid Dynamics Conference, Honolulu, HI, USA, 24–26 May 1991. [CrossRef]
28. Yoon, S.; Jameson, A. Lower-upper Symmetric-Gauss-Seidel method for the Euler and Navier-Stokes equations. *J. AIAA* **2012**, *26*, 1025–1026. [CrossRef]
29. Lian, C.; Xia, G.; Merkle, C.L. Solution-limited time stepping to enhance reliability in CFD applications. *J. Comput. Phys.* **2009**, *228*, 4836–4857. [CrossRef]
30. Li, X.S.; Gu, C.W. Mechanism of Roe-type schemes for all-speed flows and its application. *Comput. Fluids* **2013**, *86*, 56–70. [CrossRef]
31. Kim, K.H.; Kim, C. Accurate, efficient and monotonic numerical methods for multi-dimensional compressible flows Part II: Multi-dimensional limiting process. *J. Comput. Phys.* **2005**, *208*, 570–615. [CrossRef]
32. Bui, T.T. A parallel, finite-volume algorithm for large-eddy simulation of turbulent flows. *Comput. Fluids* **2000**, *29*, 877–915. [CrossRef]

MDPI AG
Grosspeteranlage 5
4052 Basel
Switzerland
Tel.: +41 61 683 77 34

Applied Sciences Editorial Office
E-mail: applsci@mdpi.com
www.mdpi.com/journal/applsci

www.ingramcontent.com/pod-product-compliance
Lightning Source LLC
Chambersburg PA
CBHW061624210926
51850CB00009B/2424
9783725874361